Disease, Class and Social Change

Disease, Class and Social Change: Tuberculosis in Folkestone and Sandgate, 1880-1930

By

Marc Arnold

CAMBRIDGE
SCHOLARS
PUBLISHING

Disease, Class and Social Change:
Tuberculosis in Folkestone and Sandgate, 1880-1930,
by Marc Arnold

This book first published 2012

Cambridge Scholars Publishing

12 Back Chapman Street, Newcastle upon Tyne, NE6 2XX, UK

British Library Cataloguing in Publication Data
A catalogue record for this book is available from the British Library

ISBN (10): 1-4438-3967-1, ISBN (13): 978-1-4438-3967-9

Dedicated to the memory of Dave Hatton

TABLE OF CONTENTS

LIST OF ILLUSTRATIONS

LIST OF TABLES

PREFACE

The idea underlying this research was to document and analyse accounts and representations of tuberculosis in the late-nineteenth and early twentieth centuries in order to delineate changes in the related spheres of social ideology and medical theory. As tuberculosis was a common chronic condition with a wealth of cultural associations it was felt that references to the social management and experience of the disease - uncovered in medical literature, administrative records, newspapers, health guides, novels, oral histories and any other available public or private sources - could provide what the anthropologist Clifford Geertz referred to as "thick description"; a rich and detailed collection of socially constituted meanings through which the fundamental taxonomic structures and symbolic relationships of a culture are made accessible.[1]

Pulmonary tuberculosis has attracted recent interest amongst historians and literary critics as a disease that derives cultural significance from its complex and contested aetiology.[2] It is associated with various overlapping discourses in late nineteenth and early twentieth century medical and popular culture surrounding infection, degeneration, hygiene, morality and poverty that reveal the diversity of meanings and metaphor that proliferated around it during this period of intense social and cultural

---

[1] C. Geertz, *The Interpretation of Cultures: Selected Essays,* New York: Basic Books, 1973, pp.3-30

[2] K. Byrne, *Tuberculosis and the Victorian Literary Imagination,* CUP, 2011; C. Lawlor & A. Suzuki, The Disease of the Self: Representing Consumption, 1700-1830, *Bulletin of the History of Medicine*, 74, 2000, pp.458-494; C. Lawlor, *Consumption and Literature,* Basingstoke: Palgrave MacMillan, 2006; C. T. Moloney, *George Eliot, Henry James and Consumption: A Shadow on the Lung of the Victorian Psyche*, unpublished PhD thesis, Birbeck College, University of London, 1999; C. T. Moloney, *Inflaming Infirmity: Some Medical-Literary Interfaces of 19th Century Tuberculosis,* (unpublished), 2009; G. S. Rousseau, *Nervous Acts:Essays on Literature, Culture and Sensibility*, Palgrave, MacMillan, 2004; C. Herzlich & J. Pierret, *Malades d'Hier et Malades d'Aujourd'hui: Tuberculeux aux XIXe et XXe Siecles*, Paris: Aubier, 1986; D. Dessertine & O. Faure, *Combattre la Tuberculose, 1900-1940,* Presses Universitaires de Lyon, 1988; S. Sontag, *Illness as Metaphor*, London: Allen Lane, 1979

realignment. Sander Gilman's study of the tubercular Franz Kafka, for example, demonstrates how a variety of explanatory models permitted:

> the coexistence of different views about the meaning of the signs, the significance of the treatment, and the interpretation of the aetiology, both in the lay conception of the illness…as well as in medical discourse.[3]

These coexisting explanations for the causes of tuberculosis provide an opportunity not merely to assess the impact of medical interventions but to examine the socio-political perspectives underlying the various theoretical approaches to the control of the disease.

From the perspective of the second half of the twentieth century, however, and particularly in the post-war climate of confidence in scientific progress, the history of tuberculosis generally came to be regarded as a prime example of the triumph of laboratory medicine and scientific method. By 1970 only 1,465 deaths were attributed to tuberculosis in England and Wales annually[4] compared to between 60,000 to 70,000 at the beginning of the twentieth century.[5]

This triumphalist account of the supplanting of pre-existing explanations of disease causation by a bacteriological model of medicine is misleading and inaccurate. Although it became acknowledged by the early twentieth century that the *tubercle bacillus* was a necessary component cause of tuberculosis, it was also generally understood in the medical world that infection alone was insufficient to cause the active form of the disease.[6] Heredity, lifestyle and the housing conditions and diet of the working classes remained important factors in determining how the disease should be managed.

These precipitating causes of tuberculosis, the factors contributing to the disease by somehow compromising or weakening the immune system, eventually became irrelevant to doctors and public health authorities

---

[3] S. Gilman, *Franz Kafka, The Jewish Patient*, London: Routledge, 1995, p.170

[4] V. H. Springett, Tuberculosis - Epidemiology in England and Wales, *BMJ*, 1, February 12th, 1972, p. 422

[5] *BMJ,* November 22nd, 1902, p.1542

[6] J. A. Mendelsohn, Medicine and the Making of Bodily Inequality in 20th Century Europe, *Heredity and Infection*, eds. J. Gaudillière & I. Löwy, London: Routledge, 2003, p.28

following mass immunisation in the 1950s.[7] Consequently several accounts of the demise of tuberculosis depict the fall in deaths from the disease during the twentieth century as a direct consequence of a revolution in medical theory and practice brought about by advances in bacteriology.[8] These celebrations of biomedical progress issue from a tradition within the history of medicine, mostly contributed to by doctors, focusing on the lives of great men and their contributions to medicine and scientific advancement.

However, as the effectiveness of this bacteriological model of public health was brought into question from the 1960s other commentators have questioned the impact of scientific medicine on the decline of mortality rates in general, and of tuberculosis in particular.[9] Subsequently the historiography of tuberculosis has, particularly in Britain, been overtaken to a large extent by a debate over the reasons for this decline in mortality figures.

This protracted and unresolved argument derives largely from the political standpoints adopted by academics regarding the relative benefits to the health of populations from targeted biomedical intervention and more general improvements in standards of living. Medical historians and sociologists have often been more concerned with understanding the epidemiology of tuberculosis from a contemporary, biomedical perspective than with reconstructing early twentieth century attitudes and approaches to the disease. Consequently the worldviews and cultural values that impelled and informed this expansion of the state into administering and

---

[7] Interestingly, large scale trials in India of BCG, the most commonly used anti-tubercular vaccine, have subsequently reported on the ineffectiveness of the drug, *The Lancet*, editorial, 1980, volume1, pp.73-4, and Holland, the country with the lowest rate of tuberculosis in Europe, has never had a national immunization programme.

[8] S. L. Cummins, *Tuberculosis in History*, London: Bailliere, Tindall, Cox, 1949; R.Y. Keers, *PulmonaryTuberculosis: A Journey Down the Centuries*, London: Baillière-Tindall, 1978; H. Williams, *Requiem for a Great Killer: The Story of Tuberculosis,* London: Health Horizon, 1973; W. Spink, *Infectious Diseases: Prevention and Treatment in the Nineteenth and Twentieth Centuries*, Folkestone: Dawson, 1978; M. Caldwell, *The Last Crusade: The War on Consumption, 1862-1954,* New York: Atheneum, 1988; J. A. Myers, *Captain of All These Men of Death*: *Tuberculosis Historical Highlights,* St. Louis: Warren H. Green, 1977; T. M. Daniel, *Pioneers in Medicine and their Impact on Tuberculosis*, University of Rochester, 2000; F. Ryan, *The Forgotten Plague,* New York: Little, Brown, 1993

[9] T. McKeown, *The Modern Rise of Population*, London: E. Arnold, 1976; *The Role of Medicine: Dream, Mirage, or Nemesis?*, Princeton University Press, 1979; *The Origins of Human Disease*, Oxford: B. Blackwell, 1988

regulating the public health of the nation have been relatively neglected.

This rather narrow focus on the causes of tuberculosis avoids consideration of English *fin de siècle* cultural preoccupations and prejudices, without which historical conceptions of, and responses to, tuberculosis can not be understood. Consequently this study is less concerned with identifying the specific factors that led to the demise of tuberculosis than with understanding the shifting political and ideological currents that continuously shaped and reconfigured medical responses and social attitudes towards tuberculosis between 1880 and 1930.

This analysis of attitudes and reactions to tuberculosis, viewed through the microcosm of a socially polarised health resort, allows us to trace the connections between developments in medical theory, the early twentieth century expansion of public health and changing cultural representations of tuberculosis. It affords a local perspective of conflicting social and political interests operating between borough Councillors and public health officials, religious charities, champions of the poor and rural and urban Boards of Guardians. These conflicts reflect other more centralised struggles for power and control of policy, fought around contested medical and social theory. The concrete effects of these more abstract struggles must be traced in the lives of local doctors, the sick and the destitute in order to approximate any comprehensive historical understanding of the interrelation of ideas and events.

This study of the treatment of tuberculosis, developed initially as a socially exclusive enterprise in Folkestone and later extending to incorporate the poorer classes in Sandgate and, from about 1912, to a state programme intended to eradicate the disease, explores several related areas. It highlights the late Victorian movement towards preventive medicine and the expansion of public health by local, and later, national authorities. It identifies a movement towards arresting the spread of tuberculosis in communities rather than in individuals. It draws attention to broad disparities in health according to social class, and attempts to identify the various scientific and sociological ideas that shaped attitudes to public health and social cohesion. Furthermore it seeks to question how our perceptions and experience of illness are formed and how the medical domain interacts with the cultural.

ACKNOWLEDGEMENTS

Illustration 11.1 is used by permission of Cambridgeshire County Council

Illustration 11.4 is by permission of the Francis Frith Collection. Copyright The Francis Frith Collection R - <http://www.francisfrith.com/

Illustrations 3.1, 4.1, 4.2, 4.3, 11.2 and 12.4 are taken from http://bbhilda.topcities.com/Folkestone/FolkestoneThen_Now.html by permission of Christine Warren

Illustrations 5.1, 5.2, 6.1, 7.1, 9.3 and 9.4 are from http://www.hereshistorykent.org.uk/ by permission of Kent County Council Archives

Other images are in the public domain or the property of the author.

Acknowledgements are made for the quote from *Franz Kafka, The Jewish Patient*, by Sander Gilman, London: Routledge, 1995, p.170, reproduced on p.xii by permission of Routledge.

The quote from David S. Barnes on p.1 is from *The Making of a Social Disease. Tuberculosis in Nineteenth Century France*, Berkeley: University of California, 1995, p.7, and is reproduced by permission of the University of California Press.

ABBREVIATIONS

BMA	British Medical Association
BMJ	British Medical Journal
COS	Charity Organisation Society
EKAC	East Kent Archive Centre
KCC	Kent County Council
LBH	Local Board of Health
LGB	Local Government Board
MoH	Ministry of Health
MOH	Medical Officer of Health
NA	National Archives
NAPC	National Association of Prevention of Consumption, after 1919 referred to as
NAPT	National Association for the Prevention of Tuberculosis
RCPL	Royal Commission on the Poor Law
SER	South Eastern Railway
SMOH	Society of Medical Offers of Health
SUDC	Sandgate Urban District Council

The terms *phthisis, consumption* and *tuberculosis* are used interchangeably throughout the text and refer to pulmonary tuberculosis

poor, on a number of levels.[4]

During the latter half of the nineteenth century tuberculosis came to be equated with urban expansion, industrialisation and immigration as accounts of the squalor of inner city life became known to the public. A social history of tuberculosis, then, allows us to trace the emergence of middle class concerns over the health and control of the urban working classes, and particularly over what was described as the "social residuum", amongst whom the disease was considered most prevalent by the early twentieth century.[5]

Whilst shifting perceptions of tuberculosis can be understood as reflecting particular cultural concerns, tuberculosis can also serve as a focus for seminal changes in the medical understanding of nature and disease. Medical histories celebrating the triumph of germ theory have tended to represent Koch's identification of the *tubercle bacillus* as signalling the birth of scientific medicine and the demise of less objective medical models.[6] Such accounts of the unproblematic acceptance of the contagiousness of tuberculosis are, however, questionable, and a more contextualised approach to medical theory and practice at this time is required in order to better understand the character and motivations of the early public health movement. During the period under study, just as much as today, the infectiousness of tuberculosis was very rarely perceived by the medical establishment as being as virulent as smallpox, measles or scarlet fever, and thus other factors were constantly being sought and

---

[4] G. Sims, *How the Poor Live,* London: Chatto & Windus, 1883; Reverend A. Mearns, *The Bitter Cry of Outcast London: An Inquiry into the Condition of the Abject Poor,* 1883, www.attackingthedevil.co.uk/related/outcast.php; General Booth, *Darkest England and the Way Out*, London, Charles Knight & Co. Ltd, 1890; C. Booth, *The Life and Labour of the People of London,* 9 volumes, London: Macmillan & Co, 1892-97; J. London, *People of the Abyss*, [1903] London: Pluto, 1998

[5] H. de Carle Woodcock, *The Doctor and the People*, London: Methuen, 2nd ed., 1912, p.186

[6] S. L. Cummins, *Tuberculosis in History*, London: Baillière-Tindall, Cox, 1949; R.Y. Keers, *Pulmonary Tuberculosis: A Journey Down the Centuries*, London: Baillière-Tindall, 1978; H. Williams, *Requiem for a Great Killer: The Story of Tuberculosis,* London: Health Horizon, 1973; W. Spink, *Infectious Diseases: Prevention and Treatment in the Nineteenth and Twentieth Centuries*, Folkestone: Dawson, 1978; K. C. Carter, The Development of Pasteur's Concept of Disease Causation and the Emergence of Specific Causes in Nineteenth Century Medicine, *Bulletin of the History of Medicine,* 65, 1991, pp.528-548; F. Ryan, *The Forgotten Plague,* New York: Little, Brown, 1993

identified in order to account for the spread of the disease.[7]

Middle class anxieties regarding the health, habits and living conditions of urban working families at this time were prompted to a great extent by notions of inheritable physical and moral degeneracy. These concerns were further heightened by an awareness of the potential for social unrest and challenges to the *status quo.* Social researches conducted by Seebohm Rowntree, Charles Booth, William Beveridge and Beatrice and Sidney Webb[8] were imbued with a eugenic consciousness and advocated various methods of social engineering.[9] The impact of social Darwinist thought – that is ideas concerned with the biological advancement of the nation – on attitudes to health and illness in Britain has long been underestimated.

Whilst commentators on public health and eugenic thought in England have not previously focused on tuberculosis as a potential object of social engineering there exist many literary, journalistic and medical references to the disease as an inheritable predisposition, even after Koch's isolation of the *bacillus.* Many Fabians and other social reformers were influenced by evolutionary ideas. It was at least the opinion of H.G. Wells, writing at Sandgate in 1900, that the slum, together with the asylum and the prison, would remain a necessary part of society due to their function of reducing the breeding capacity and life expectancy of the "unfit".[10] Whilst these ideas may have rarely been expressed so overtly, it will be demonstrated that they continued to be held by powerful and influential figures and that the influence of social evolutionism in one form or another was pervasive throughout this period.

This study is situated in the period between the discovery of the *tubercle bacillus* in 1882 and the middle of the inter-war years, by which

---

[7] A. Hillier, Tuberculosis and Public Action, *Fortnightly Review*, 71, 424, April, 1902, p.706

[8] C. Booth, *The Life and Labour of the People in London*, 9 volumes, London: Macmillan & Co, 1892-97; B. Seebohm Rowntree, *A Study of Town Life*, London: Macmillan & Co, 1901; W. H. Beveridge, *Unemployment: A Problem of Industry,* London: Longmans, Green & Co, 1909; S. & B. Webb, eds., *The Break-Up of the Poor Law: Being Parts 1 & 2 of the Minority Report of the Poor Law Commission*, London: Longmans, Green & Co, 1909

[9] J. Brown, Charles Booth and Labour Colonies 1889-1905, *Economic History Review,* volume 21, no.2, 1968, pp.349-360; D. Dorling & J. Pritchard, The Geography of Poverty, Inequality and Wealth in the UK and Abroad: Because Enough is Never Enough, *Applied Spatial Analysis and Policy*, 3:81, 106, 2010, pp. 81-105

[10] H.G. Wells, *Anticipations of the Reaction of Mechanical and Scientific Progress upon Human Life and Thought,* London, Chapman & Hall, 1901, pp.80-81

time an elaborate state system for the monitoring, control and treatment of the disease amongst the working classes had become established. This time scale, however, is not rigidly circumscribed, and includes considerations that both precede and follow these date markers in order to look at earlier ways in which the disease was culturally configured, and at the implications of an exclusively biomedical approach to the problem in contemporary society.

In order to examine the widely disparate circumstances of the well-off and the working class consumptive the fashionable late Victorian and Edwardian health resort of Folkestone, together with the adjacent town of Sandgate, have been chosen as the focus of this research. The political wards of Folkestone afford a nice comparison of environmental conditions and cultural backgrounds, as illustrated in chapters six and seven. The congested and impoverished east ward's narrow alleys rising precipitously from the harbour present a stark contrast to the broad, landscaped leas and boulevards of the cliff-top west ward. And, equally, Sandgate's community of residents and visitors from the social elite and officer class are in contrast to the chronically sick and destitute sent there to recuperate by reformist London boroughs.

Folkestone's reputation as a socially exclusive resort for affluent urbanites seeking to escape the unhealthy atmosphere of the city was largely established by the de Bouverie family in the mid-nineteenth century. The natural topography of the town permitted a division between rich and poor that was formalised through strict planning and building regulations. An analysis of the political economy of the town, in chapters six and seven, demonstrates the power of local patronage and provides an opportunity to consider the effectiveness of public health officials and reformist health legislation on this aristocratically managed and conservative coastal town.

In chapter nine the moralising and disciplinarian approach to the sick poor of the predominantly high Anglican Folkestone charitable organisations is contrasted with the work of the evangelical London Samaritan Society and their manager John James Jones and his family, who treated pauper consumptives in the less regulated environment of Sandgate between 1884 and 1915. These exemplify two fundamentally different responses to the problem of tuberculosis. One approach subjected the sick poor to the moral discrimination inherent in the 1834 Poor Law Amendment Act. The other more reformist approach, adopted by some London Boards of Guardians, attempted to provide the destitute with open-air therapy as enjoyed by the leisured classes, rather than merely granting, or refusing, them the means of subsistence. This local study permits an analysis of variations in the experience and treatment of tuberculosis along lines of social class in addition to a consideration of changes in middle class attitudes to poverty and sickness.

The examination of the treatment of destitute consumptives in Sandgate also assesses the extent to which society and the medical profession saw tuberculosis as posing a threat of infection. Parliamentary Select Committee debates initiated by a local Bill that was intended to remedy the purported dangers of infection posed by Jones' enterprise provide a range of contemporary medical opinion concerning the nature of the threat posed to public health by the tubercular. The Parliamentary records of these proceedings, together with reports and analysis of the dispute in contemporary medical journals and records of Local Government Board correspondence, also draw attention to the particularly acute cycle of destitution and tuberculosis existing in urban environments, notably the east end of London, at this time (1904-05).

Research into the public health administration of Folkestone and the provision available for local people suffering from tuberculosis is divided into two sections. Chapter six assesses provision for the tubercular poor prior to the National Insurance Act of 1911. Following the compulsory notification of the tubercular under the Public Health Act of 1912 treatment in a sanatorium was intended to be supplied by the County Council. The operation of this open-air treatment in Kentish sanatoria, discussed in chapter eleven, is contrasted with earlier philanthropic and Poor Law provision for the working classes in order to assess the impact of scientific and medical advances on social health as well as on the increasing medicalisation of working class lives.

Although measures taken to treat or control the disease were, particularly before the provision of sanatorium benefit in 1912, initiated at a local level, other works cited in this study invariably adopt a national overview. No detailed local studies of tuberculosis and its treatment have yet been undertaken.[11]

A significant consequence of the emphasis on national trends and quantitative analysis is the relative absence from the literature of the role of the Poor Law in managing the disease. Although impressions of life in sanatoria have been reconstructed,[12] these institutions probably treated no

---

[11] A. Hardy, *The Epidemic Streets*, 1993, p.212

[12] L. Bryder, *Below the Magic Mountain, A Social History of Tuberculosis in Twentieth Century Britain,* Oxford University Press, 1988; L. Bryder, Papworth Village Settlement: A Unique Experiment in the Treatment and Care of the Tuberculous? *Medical History*, 28, 1984; F. B. Smith, *The Retreat of Tuberculosis 1850-1950,* Beckenham, Kent: Croom Helm, 1988

more than 2% of cases in England until the 1930s,[13] and reference to the extent of treatment in other institutions and in the homes of the tubercular are rare.

The growing middle class demands for state intervention in public health from the end of the nineteenth century, and particularly for the mass treatment and isolation of the tubercular have not yet been fully contextualised by historians. Moreover, these seminal events in the history of medicine and the expansion of the state provide an opportunity to explore the rapidly changing social, scientific and ideological landscape that was unfolding around the birth of the twentieth century.

The overall approach of this research is to examine the ways in which tuberculosis has been understood and treated in order to throw light on the relative influence and interrelation of scientific developments and wider social and ideological forces on attitudes and responses to the disease. Rather than being a purely biological phenomenon, it has long been argued, the continued spread of tuberculosis in developing countries today owes more to the existence of widespread poverty and the political and economic agendas of the affluent and powerful.[14]

Since the Second World War medical theory and practice have been propelled by the myth of a triumphant bacteriological revolution into a vain contest against the natural world. Mutating strains of increasingly deadly bacteria and viruses are becoming multi-drug resistant in the treatment of HIV, tuberculosis, influenza and other diseases.[15] From the mid-1980s there has been a resurgence of tuberculosis in the developed world due to the evolution of strains of bacteria resistant to anti-tubercular drugs, and experts have warned of potential calamity as western overdependence on pharmaceuticals erodes the power of immune systems to resist disease.[16]

In 2002 tuberculosis, described as the most easily preventable infectious cause of death, was declared to be more prevalent than at any time in history due, it was claimed, to increasing social inequalities.[17] In

---

[13] F. B. Smith, *The Retreat of Tuberculosis*, 1988, p.47

[14] P. D. van Helden, The Economic Divide and Tuberculosis, *EMBO Reports*, volume 4 (supplement), June, 2003, S24-28

[15] J. M. Diamond, 'AIDS: Infectious, Genetic, or both?', *Nature*, 328, July 1987, pp.199-200

[16] J. D. Porter & K. P. McAdam (eds) *Tuberculosis: Back to the Future*, Chichester: J. Wiley & Sons Ltd, 1994

[17] M. Gandy & A. Zumla, The Resurgence of Disease: Social and Historical Perspectives on the 'New' Tuberculosis, *Social Science and Medicine*, volume 55, issue 3, August, 2002, p.385

the mid-1990s it was estimated that 3.5 million people a year died of tuberculosis and that one third of the world's population was infected with the *tubercle bacillus.*[18] And yet the question remains; why, when so many are infected, are there not more deaths due to tuberculosis? Perhaps the problem is not how to prevent infection but how to ensure that poverty, conflict and social dislocation do not, yet again, undermine resistance to this chronic infectious disease.

Even during the 1890s tuberculosis was considered by the English medical profession to be a preventable disease. As Albert, Prince of Wales, famously declared at the opening conference of the National Association for the Prevention of Consumption in 1898, "If preventable, why not prevented?"[19] Such persistent high mortality due to tuberculosis, despite over a century of insistence by the medical profession that such deaths were largely avoidable, suggests that a failure to appreciate the social and economic determinants of the disease are as common today as during the period under study, and that purely bacteriological approaches to its control are ultimately ineffective.

The largely uncritical over-reliance on the "magic bullet" of recent decades can be seen as a consequence of the neglect of a tradition of environmental[20] public health in favour of the construction of a chiefly biomedical history of medicine. To better understand the political and cultural determinants that led to this approach to eradicating the disease, an analysis of early twentieth century medical discourse assessing the potential and limitations of laboratory medicine for the treatment of tuberculosis forms part of this study. This analysis questions the still widely accepted understanding of the establishment, at the end of the nineteenth century, of a radically different medical paradigm based on a bacteriological revolution.

Throughout the period 1880-1930 there exists substantial evidence of resistance to a purely bacteriological model of public health, together with

---

[18] P. J. Dolin, M. C. Raviglione & A. Kochi, Global Tuberculosis Incidence and Mortality during 1990-2000, *Bulletin of the World Health Organisation*, 72, 2, 1994, p.217

[19] HRH Albert, Prince of Wales, First NAPT Conference, quoted in Sir Robert Philip, The Outlook on Tuberculosis, *BMJ*, 10th January, 1931, p.43

[20] The term '*environmental*' here, as it was employed in the early twentieth century, refers to diet, exercise and constitution as well as broader public health issues such as sanitation, water, housing and town planning.

the survival of a tradition of holistic, environmentally based therapeutics.[21] This suggests that a focus on the health and natural resistance to disease of the individual was, arguably, as important in English medicine at this time as were approaches aimed at the disinfection and isolation of germs. This reappraisal of the impact of germ theory in England seeks not only to identify the social and scientific forces that impelled state intervention in the treatment of tuberculosis, it also seeks to account for the nearly thirty year delay in England between the discovery of the *tubercle bacillus* and the advent of such intervention.

In summary, the aim of this research is to evaluate how cultural and political factors influenced medical responses to tuberculosis in the late nineteenth and early twentieth centuries, and what effect these innovations in public health had on society. This approach to the understanding of scientific and social change recognises their essential interconnectedness. The past is not viewed as a succession of discrete events – scientific innovations or government legislation – with causal connections occurring on a time-line, but as an ongoing and dynamic process. A constant interaction of actors and ideas – some institutionalised and some challenging the more established offices and axioms – that can best be apprehended in the less abstract and compartmentalised arena of a local study.

---

[21] S. Sturdy, Hippocrates and State Medicine: George Newman Outlines the Founding Policy of the Ministry of Health, *Greater Than the Parts: Holism in Biomedicine 1920-1950*, eds. C. Lawrence & G. Weisz, Oxford University Press, 1998, pp.112-134

PART I:

REPRESENTATIONS OF TUBERCULOSIS

CHAPTER ONE

HEAVEN'S ELECT: THE ROMANTIC IDEALISATION OF TUBERCULOSIS

This section, which investigates shifting social constructions of this devastating disease, points to the way in which particular cultural ideologies have been responsible for framing the epidemiology of tuberculosis – stressing particular symptoms and patterns of causation and neglecting others – and determining its treatment. In England, it will be argued, broad distinctions in the aetiology and treatment of the disease have been established along lines of social class. That is, different aspects and symptoms of the disease have been emphasised in relation to certain social groups. Consequently, tuberculosis signified a different set of meanings for particular classes at different periods in time.

To suggest that a disease is in this way culturally constructed is not to imply that it is in any way unreal. Rather the process of identifying and defining a specific disease is determined according to implicit cultural significations and values that are embedded in linguistic and taxonomical structures that change over time.

During the second half of the eighteenth and the early nineteenth centuries an aestheticised image of the consumptive life and the consumptive death emerged that influenced many sufferers to integrate the disease into their identity as a "disease of the self".[1] From the 1880s into the inter-war period tuberculosis, it will be argued, came to be more commonly viewed as a disease of the "other". The tubercular, together with the inebriate, the "feeble-minded", the indigent, the unemployable and the prostitute came to be perceived as "different manifestations of a degenerate constitution".[2] Consequently, due to its association with what

[1] C. Lawlor & A. Suzuki, The Disease of the Self: Representing Consumption, 1700-1830, *Bulletin of the History of Medicine*, 74:3, 2000, pp. 458-494

[2] N. Rose, Medicine, History and the Present, *Reassessing Foucault: Power, Medicine and the Body*, London: Routledge, eds., C. Jones & R. Porter, 1994, p.57

were perceived as inferior sections of humanity, tuberculosis came to symbolise a threat to the health and moral integrity of the nation.

The Romanticised image of tuberculosis as a disease that particularly affected the creative and overly sensitive, or indeed inspired the imagination, pre-dates the eighteenth century. There is evidence that tuberculosis had been associated with female purity and emotional sensitivity since the Renaissance when the disease had been depicted as a consequence of unrequited love.[3] Popular seventeenth and eighteenth century accounts of the disease as a gentle, almost symptom-free, release from a harsh world, such as Thomas Fuller's seventeenth century aphorism, presented consumption as an ideal death:

> of all the bailiffs sent to arrest us to the debt of nature, none useth his prisoners with more civility and courtesie.[4]

Throughout the eighteenth century and for most of the nineteenth tuberculosis continued to be represented positively in literature[5] and medicine. Reflecting the distinctive sensibilities of the social elite the disease was characterised by a collection of fashionable symptoms - slenderness, pallid skin, intensely bright eyes, flushed cheeks and red lips. This positive symptomatology was identified with the upper and artistic classes into the twentieth century.[6] This representation of the disease, characterised by a growing popular usage of the euphemistic term "decline" from the end of the eighteenth century,[7] disregarded contemporary medical accounts of slow putrefaction and decay.[8]

These positive attributes, which probably benefited both doctor and patient in negotiating the course of the disease, also contributed to what

---

[3] C. Lawlor, *Consumption and Literature,* Basingstoke: Palgrave MacMillan, 2006, p.154

[4] Thomas Fuller, 1656, quoted in C. Lawlor, *Consuming Time*, Narrative and Disease in Tristram Shandy, *Yearbook of English Studies*, volume 30, 2000 p.56

[5] For example Smike's death in Dickens' *Nicholas Nickleby*,[1838-39], Harmondsworth: Penguin, 1994, p.628, and Mordecai in George Eliot's *Daniel Deronda,* [1876], London: Cox & Wyman, 1970

[6] C. Lawlor, *Consumption and Literature,* Basingstoke: Palgrave MacMillan, 2006, p.478

[7] Oxford English Dictionary, second edition, 1989, online version, http://www.oed.com/

[8] R. Porter, The Case of Consumption, J. Bourrau, ed., *Understanding Catastrophe*, Cambridge University Press, 1992, p.195

Roy Porter has referred to as the "commodification" of consumption.[9] From the late eighteenth century aristocratic health resorts became available to the middle classes through the publication of travel guides that included climatological advice for consumptives, and established themselves not only as resorts for the tubercular but also as destinations for the culturally select.[10]

Religious belief also exerted a major influence on the perception and experience of tuberculosis. From the 1830s the rise of a more demonstrative and impassioned evangelical Christianity, which was particularly associated with the urban working classes,[11] contributed to an image of the impoverished consumptive as being somehow *spiritualised,* drawn gradually closer to God. Consumption came to be associated with heightened spirituality and godliness in middle class literary accounts of the urban poor. The disease was often depicted as transformative and redemptive as more emphasis came to be placed on the consolations of the afterlife. Charlotte Bronte's Helen Burns, the consumptive schoolfriend of Jane Eyre, articulated this longing to escape a burdensome life and ascend to a state of purity:

> debasement and sin shall fall from us with this cumbrous frame of flesh and only the spark of the spirit will remain.[12]

Although this *motif* of transformation and redemption, of spiritual advancement and exemplary suffering, was associated with evangelicism, and sometimes parodied by popular writers such as Dickens, the Brontes and Thackeray,[13] it became an increasingly common popular literary theme that pervaded Victorian middle class culture. It gave meaning to chronic disease and signified the sanctity and self-renunciation of the sufferer. This perception of consumption tending to afflict the serious and

---

[9] R. Porter, Consumption: Disease of the Consumer Society? *Consumption and the World of Goods,* London: Routledge, eds., J. Brewer & R. Porter, 1993

[10] T. Smollett, *Travels Through France and Italy,* [1766], Oxford University Press, ed. Frank Felsenstein, 1979; L. Sterne, *Sentimental Journey*[1768] Oxford University Press, 2008*;* J. Clark, *Medical Notes on Climates, Diseases, Hospitals and Medical Schools in France, Italy and Switzerland,* London: T&G Underwood et al., 1820

[11] H. McLeod, *European Religion in the Age of the Great Cities 1830-1930,* London: Routledge, 1995, p.8

[12] C. Bronte, *Jane Eyre*, Harmondsworth: Penguin, 1966, p.91

[13] C. T. Moloney, *George Eliot, Henry James and Consumption: A shadow on the lung of the Victorian Psyche*, unpublished PhD thesis, Birbeck College, University of London, 1999, p.220

spiritually inclined was reinforced by the rise of evangelical religion later in the century, and is illustrated by George Eliot's depiction of the evangelical cleric Edgar Tryon in *Janet's Repentance* and the rabbi Mordecai in *Daniel Deronda*.[14]

However, despite this evangelical reaction from the 1830s against the elitist and narcissistic Romantic image of tuberculosis, the idea of the sensitive and creative consumptive continued in both medicine and literature. The medical acceptance of this association of creativity and tuberculosis also continued to affect the way people experienced the disease. Robert Louis Stevenson, for example, who was diagnosed with tuberculosis in 1880 at the age of twenty nine but who survived an itinerant existence until 1895, adhered to this notion to such an extent that he believed that the quality of his writing declined when his consumption was in remission.[15]

Creativity and emotional intensity were not the only characteristics associated with consumption. More negative personality traits came to be associated with the disease by an expanding and increasingly diverse medical profession. The emergent middle-classes' sense of social distinctiveness led to an affirmation of their identity through attacks on aristocratic values from the 1830s, and on the lower classes during the second half of the nineteenth century.[16]

The emerging values espoused by marginalized middle-class physicians, such as self-reliance, social responsibility and industriousness, served to constitute the medical norm against which pathologies were defined.[17] These socio-medical explanations of the causes of consumption are epitomised by the homoeopath John Epps's observations in 1859. The perceived aristocratic characteristics of lassitude and introspection, often seen as encouraging the habit of self-abuse, were pathologised on the one hand, as were the working-class failings of ill-discipline and immorality

---

[14] G. Eliot, Janet's Repentance, *Scenes of Clerical Life,* [1857], Edinburgh: W. Blackwood, 1878; *Daniel Deronda,* [1876], Edinburgh: W. Blackwood, 1878

[15] H. D. Chalke, The Impact of Tuberculosis on History, Literature and Art, *Medical History*, 6, 1962, p.314. Stevenson is said to have written *Dr Jekyll and Mr Hyde* in three days whilst extremely ill and bedridden at Bournemouth.

[16] E. J. Hobsbawm, *The Age of Revolution,* New York: World Publishing, 1962; K. Figlio, Chlorosis and Chronic Disease in Nineteenth Century Britain: The Social Constitution of Somatic Illness in a Capitalist Society, *Social History*, 3, 1978, pp.176-7

[17] K. Figlio, Chlorosis and Chronic Disease in Nineteenth Century Britain: The Social Constitution of Somatic Illness in a Capitalist Society, *Social History*, 3, 1978, pp.176-7

on the other. However, sexual profligacy or "fast living", in accordance with a "vitalist" model of health and illness, could also be interpreted as a predisposing character trait when applied to consumptive members of more affluent society.[18]

> How often it happens that fast-living men, wrote Epps, die of Phthisis before the age of forty-five. They have lived four years in one year, rather they have exhausted an amount of life-force in one year which ought to have been spread throughout four years. How commonly is Phthisis the result of these sexual excesses.[19]

Potential sufferers were advised to adopt a regimented lifestyle, incorporating regular exercise, more "wholesome" diets and, particularly in the case of aristocratic young women, to pursue practical interests and benevolent "good works". The gentry faced growing criticism in general from the middle-classes regarding their morality and their effectiveness in controlling the poor. Consequently their gradual adoption of middle-class values of piety and social responsibility continued, especially under the influence of Evangelical Christianity, the Oxford Movement, Christian Socialists and other social reformers, throughout the Victorian period.

In the second half of the nineteenth century a perception of tuberculosis emerged, partly informed by a "vitalist" medical model, which viewed the disease amongst the urban poor as being, variously, a consequence of the inadequacies of the parents, constitutional or otherwise, uncleanliness, alcoholic excess or sexual profligacy.[20] The "vitalist" representation of the brief, intense consumptive life, the Romantic ideal of the sensitive and imaginative consumptive, together with the related evangelical themes of transformation and redemption, continued to predominate, however, in literature and art.

As the image of the spiritually transformed female consumptive lingered on, that of the pallid, male Romantic aesthete came to be seen as overly effeminate and self-indulgent towards the end of the century.[21] In a Davos guide book of 1880 an early proponent of open-air therapy, Dr. Johann Weber, typically asserted the necessity of discipline over Romantic values:

---

[18] J. Epps, *Consumption, Its Nature and Treatment*, 1859, p75
[19] Ibid., p.78
[20] H. de Carle Woodcock, *The Doctor and the People*, 1912, p.184
[21] C. Lawlor & A. Suzuki, *The Disease of the Self*, 2000, p.492

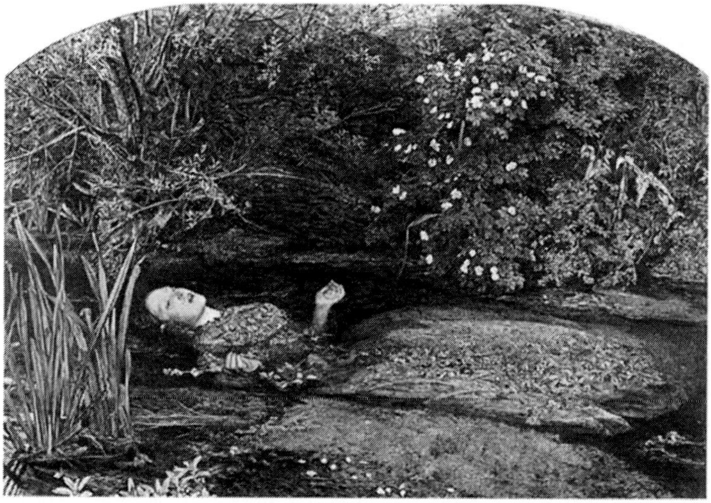

Illustration 1.1: The Romantically influenced Ophelia by John Everett Millais painted in 1852 and modelled by the consumptive Elizabeth Siddal.

> It is a subject for regret that a complaint, the recovery from which depends so much upon the patient's own wisdom and self-denial, should be more or less characteristic of an age when common sense and consistency are still at such a minimum. Thousands die before they are twenty five out of inability to make sacrifices.

And:

> Davos demands qualities the very opposite of resigned sentimentalism in which too frequently the phthisic youth or maiden was encouraged. Here is no place for weak and despairing resignation; here you are not pusillanimously helped to die, but are required to enter into a hard struggle for life.[22]

The stigmatising southern European belief in the infectiousness of tuberculosis also contributed to the decline of Mediterranean health resorts. As middle class values of discipline and duty came increasingly to prominence, so the therapeutic resorts of southern Europe favoured by Keats and Shelley gave way to the harsher physic of the Alps and the English coast. Sanatoria, sea bathing and physical exercise were more

[22] Davos Guide Book, Illustrated Europe Series, London: C. Smith & Son, 1882

readily expressive of manly middle-class virtues than the decadent allure of Menton and Venice. However, as demonstrated above, the ambivalent symbolism of consumption, enshrined in popular religion, literature and science, ensured that notions of redemption through suffering continued to be accommodated within the moral framework of the more socially oriented late Victorian and Edwardian values of civic duty and self-discipline.

The essentially holistic approach of the open-air treatment for consumption continued to emphasise the importance of adapting treatment to the individual constitution. It also facilitated the retention of older Romantic models for the treatment of the disease, predominantly amongst the affluent who were, one imagines, flattered by the positive cultural associations. Therapeutic approaches stressing the importance of the nervous system, and particularly the need to provide the appropriate environment and climate for those of a nervous constitution (often considered as being synonymous with a tubercular *diathesis* or congenital predisposition) were to enjoy a considerable longevity, surviving beyond the middle of the twentieth century.

The delineation of the nervous constitution in the mid-eighteenth century had accommodated more nebulous and subtle gradations of pathology such as hysteria and nervous debility (a condition often employed as a euphemism for consumption), and in the later nineteenth century this medical schema was further elaborated. By the 1880s a new medical taxonomy incorporating what we would today refer to as psychosomatic illnesses – the physiological manifestation of emotional or psychological disorders – had emerged that permitted a broader discrimination of pathologies, predominantly applicable to women, in the form of complaints such as chlorosis, neuralgia and neurasthenia.

These "diseases of refinement",[23] which to some extent can be seen as an obfuscation of complaints that were stigmatised through negative associations with the urban poor, were the preserve of the leisured classes, the intellectual and the artist, and were generally associated with the increasing pressures of modern life.[24] This late nineteenth century elaboration of the medical taxonomy to incorporate these "nervous" diseases sustained and celebrated notions of the delicate and sensitive constitution which had been common earlier in the century. Victorians viewed the nervous system and the "will" as being of prime significance in cases of chronic disease:

---

[23] K. Figlio, Chlorosis and Chronic Disease, 1978, pp.176-177

[24] C. T. Moloney, *George Eliot, Henry James and Consumption,* 1999, pp.287-289

> The immediate cause of chronic disease was their failure in a physical sense, but the predisposing condition was their failure in a mental or moral sense.[25]

Thus diseases of refinement, including tuberculosis, amongst the better off came to be perceived as resulting from a failure of self-control. The power of the will and self-discipline were axiomatic *bourgeois* values reflecting the importance placed on individual endeavour and social aspiration. As middle class doctors reformulated social ideals into a medical, and consequently "objective" domain, the relationship between self control and positive health became naturalised.

A fundamentally holistic construction of the emotional and physical body, predicated on the functioning of the nervous system, persisted into the twentieth century as the foundation of the new discipline of psychiatry.[26] As late as 1926 the psychiatrist D. G. Macleod Munro's observation that "many cases of neurasthenia have proved to be incipient tuberculosis",[27] demonstrates the continuing influence of the "nervous" model on the aetiology of the disease.

In summary, this account of medical and literary representations of consumption during the later eighteenth and early nineteenth centuries suggests that the predominantly exclusive treatment of the social elite led to the construction of a medical model, based on the functioning of the nerves, that tended to emphasise certain positive characteristics of the disease. These Romantic associations of refinement and sensibility, together with a Romantic interpretation of "vitalism" and the holistic conception of constitution were incorporated, by both the medical and literary professions, into the enduring legend of the consumptive genius. This construction of the delicate and refined consumptive can also be seen as contributing to the growth of culturally select European health resorts from the eighteenth century.

The treatment of tuberculosis in the harsher environments of the Alps and the English seaside from the 1850s was due to two main factors. It was both the reaction of an increasingly authoritative medical profession against the Romanticised image of the consumptive, and a manifestation of the more stoical *bourgeois* Victorian values of self-discipline and

---

[25] B. Haley, *The Healthy Body and Victorian Culture,* Harvard University Press, 1978, p.45

[26] G. S. Rousseau, *Nervous Acts:Essays on Literature, Culture and Sensibility*, Basingstoke: Palgrave, MacMillan, 2004

[27] D. G. Macleod Munro, *The Psycho-Pathology of Tuberculosis,* Oxford University Press, 1926, p.7

personal endeavour.

This interaction of medical and popular culture, and the construction of a positive identity for the consumptive, was made possible by the individualised relationships of patient and doctor at the upper end of the medical market. These intimate yet professional connections were structured around a competitive medical system based on patronage. The competition for wealthy patients also encouraged the development of an expanded nervous taxonomy of disease from the later nineteenth century. The emergence of this medicalised language of nerves facilitated the retention of the old Romantic model of tuberculosis in a more scientific form, which served to distinguish the tuberculosis of the elite classes from that afflicting the masses.

Although the disease was more prevalent earlier in the nineteenth century,[28] particularly amongst casual labourers and the unemployed (according to some accounts reaching a peak in the 1840s when 319 deaths per 100,000 of the population were recorded for England and Wales in 1847),[29] tuberculosis was not viewed by the establishment as a "social scourge" until the 1880s. For the working classes there was very little specialised treatment.[30] However, from this time the attention of many in the medical profession, as well as some elements of the political establishment, became increasingly focused on social reform and the health of the working classes. The reasons for this shift of perspective, and of a re-fashioning of tuberculosis as a disease of the "other", of the degenerate, the inebriate and the prostitute, are examined in the following section.

---

[28] Roy Porter claims that by about 1700 one in ten deaths in England and Wales were due to consumption. This rose to one in four by about 1800 and reached a peak of 50,000 deaths per annum in 1875. The Case of Consumption, *Understanding Catastrophe*, Cambridge University Press, ed. J. Bourrau, 1992, p.196

[29] Annual Reports of the Registrar-General of Births, Marriages and Deaths, quoted in A. Salusbury MacNalty, Tuberculosis Work in England, *The Lancet*, 26th January, 1924, p.169

[30] *An Account of the Infirmary for Asthma, Consumption and Other Diseases of the Lungs, Union St., Bishopsgate, established 1814,* Annual Report, 1827, pp.4-5

CHAPTER TWO

PEOPLE OF THE ABYSS: TUBERCULOSIS AND EUGENICS[1]

The previous section has indicated how medical theories in the late eighteenth and early nineteenth centuries interacted with broader ideological trends and economic interests in such a way that tuberculosis came to be Romanticised through being predominantly associated with the social and artistic elite. A contrary and less flattering representation of the tubercular did, however, already exist in the first half of the nineteenth century, although generally applied to those of a different class or race. Consequently, during the nineteenth century, two contrasting characterisations of the consumptive were in evidence. As Sir James Clark, physician to the Royal family, outlined in 1835:

> we have two opposite states of the mental as well as the physical constitution; the one, attended by florid complexion, thin, fair skin, and great sensibility to impressions, along with a corresponding acuteness of mind; the other, characterised by a dark complexion and coarse skin, with a languid, torpid condition of the bodily functions, and a like dulness of the mental faculties.[2]

This more alien image of the dull, brutish and lazy consumptive became far more common from the 1880s when tuberculosis was increasingly perceived as a disease of the urban poor. This shift in perspective reflects a growing tension between social classes and provides an opportunity to consider the influence of science and political ideology

---

[1] The phrase "people of the abyss" was in common usage in the first years of the twentieth century. It was used by Jack London as the title of a novel published in 1903 and by H. G. Wells in *Anticipations,* quoted on page 26, which was written at Sandgate and published in 1902.

[2] J. Clark, Tubercular Phthisis, or Consumption, Phthisis Tuberculosa, Phthisis Pulmonalis, *The Cyclopaedia of Practical Medicine,* volume iv, London: Gilbert & Piper, eds. J. Forbes, A. Tweedie & J. Conolly, 1832-35, p.269

on constructions of the disease during the later nineteenth and early twentieth centuries. In particular the extent to which evolutionist arguments, implicitly or explicitly, influenced responses to tuberculosis as a disease of the working classes.

Many historians have attributed the growing concern with public health from the 1880s as being solely due to the advent of bacteriology, and particularly to Robert Koch's discovery of the *tubercle bacillus* in 1882.[3] However, the impact of germ theory in England during the nineteenth and early twentieth centuries has probably been overstated.[4] In 1897 the physician James Lindsay, reviewing the impact of Koch's discovery in Britain, noted that most of the respondents to an investigation by the BMA did not view tuberculosis as an infectious disease:

> The contagionist view which received a great accession of strength from Koch's discovery is now widely prevalent on the continent, especially in Germany, but never seems to have taken deep root in this country. The results of the inquiry instituted by the Collective Investigation Committee of the British Medical Association were equivocal. A large majority of the medical men who responded had seen nothing to warrant a belief in the contagiousness of the disease…I content myself with giving my opinion that the direct transmission of phthisis from one individual to another is a rare event.[5]

The continued influence of sanitary medicine pioneered by Edwin Chadwick in the 1830s and 1840s and the more recent impact of social Darwinism on middle class attitudes to the poor, and to public health in general, have been underestimated. Conceptions of the emergence of degenerate strains of humanity due to the pathological effects of polluted environments or of immoral behaviour had been advanced by Bénédict Morel in France in the 1850s and 1860s and developed through the statistical eugenics of Francis Galton in the late 1860s. Tuberculosis, syphilis and nervous and mental diseases came to be seen by some as manifestations of a generalised degenerative heredity passed on through

---

[3] For example, S. L. Cummins, *Tuberculosis in History*; R.Y. Keers, *Pulmonary Tuberculosis*; H. Williams, *Requiem for a Great Killer*; W. Spink, *Infectious Diseases*; K. C. Carter, The Development of Pasteur's Concept of Disease Causation and the Emergence of Specific Causes in Nineteenth Century Medicine, *Bulletin of the History of Medicine,* 65, 1991

[4] M. Worboys, Was There a Bacteriological Revolution in Late Nineteenth Century Britain?, *Studies in History, Philosophy, Biology & Biomedical Science*, 38, 2007

[5] J. A. Lindsay, The Problem of the Consumptive Poor, *The Lancet*, 4th December, 1897, p.1437

successive generations, particularly since the hereditary nature of insanity had already been established.[6]

This understanding of biological determinism led to a common perception of paupers and the chronically sick as constituting a "social residuum", a biologically distinct underclass which, it was argued, could not be cured or reformed and which posed a serious threat to the vitality of the national stock.[7] Although Darwin did not himself advocate any form of social engineering in his *Origin of Species* of 1859, subsequent popular interpretations, and works on evolutionary theory by Spencer and Jean-Baptiste Lamarck, lent credibility to the notion of inherited degeneracy.

This biological explanation of chronic sickness served to account for the growing contradiction between national prosperity and empire on the one hand and the persistence of urban poverty and disease on the other.[8] Darwin's apparent scientific endorsement of the hereditary principle appeared to further validate what has been referred to as the "biologisation of poverty".[9] That is to say, a perception of the pauper, who was often chronically infirm, as essentially defective or "feebleminded".

The chronically diseased urban poor were already seen by many as an economic burden to the nation following the publication of Malthus's *Essay on the Principle of Population* of 1798. Malthus's argument was that the future health of society was being threatened by the survival of its weakest members, who were kept alive by charity and thus permitted to reproduce. Such arguments influenced the policy to discourage outdoor relief under the 1834 Poor Law Amendment Act, and contributed to the ongoing reluctance of authorities to provide adequate housing for the poor.[10]

Problems of overcrowding, dampness and inadequate light and ventilation in many working class districts of towns and cities persisted

---

[6] J. Gaudillière & I. Löwy eds. *Heredity and Infection,* London: Routledge, 2001; P. M. H. Mazumdar, The Eugenists and the Residuum: the Problem of the Urban Poor, *Bulletin of the History of Medicine*, volume 54, 1980

[7] A. White, *Efficiency and Empire*, [1901], Brighton: Harvester Press, 1973; F. Galton, *Inquiries into the Human Faculty and its Development*, London: MacMillan, 1883; H. Ellis, Eugenics and St. Valentine, *Nineteenth Century*, 59, 1906; K. Pearson, *The Problem of Practical Eugenics,* London: Dulao & Co., 1909

[8] D. Pick, *Faces of Degeneration, a European Disorder, c.1848-1918,* Cambridge University Press, 1989, p.200

[9] A. Richardson, *Love and Eugenics in the Late Nineteenth Century*, Oxford University Press, 2003

[10] P. M. H. Mazumdar, *Eugenics, Human Genetics and Human Failings: The Eugenic Society, its Sources and its Critics in Britain,* London: Routledge, 1992, p.38

throughout the nineteenth century. Such housing reforms that did occur in the second half of the century were more than offset by rising populations in most towns and cities. Houses for the poor were not built on any scale until government subsidised building programmes were introduced during the 1920s and 1930s.[11]

Although it is difficult to discern how consciously charity workers and Poor Law functionaries withheld assistance from those they considered morally undeserving or constitutionally defective, a pattern of selective neglect often becomes apparent in their treatment of the destitute and the chronically sick. For example, the Charity Organisation Society, originally The Society for the Organisation of Charity and Repressing Mendicity, was guided by social Darwinist principles of limited intervention. Led by Octavia Hill and Helen Bosanquet during the late nineteenth century, the COS foresaw an increase in population amongst the poor and worked to discourage charity for the able bodied.[12]

The COS principles of discouraging charity and refusing assistance to the "undeserving" were also evident in the various small scale housing projects initiated in London during the second half of the nineteenth century. Doctors such as John Simon and Robert Southwood-Smith, and social reformers like Charles Kingsley, Lord Shaftesbury and Octavia Hill were more concerned with the moral and religious reform of the working classes than with effecting improvements to their environment or assisting them financially.[13] Despite a growing awareness of the squalor in which many working class families lived, particularly following sensational reports in the popular press from 1883,[14] the moral and sanitary education of the poor remained the prime objective of reformers in the closing decades of the nineteenth century. Due to the pervasive influence of social Darwinism the regeneration of urban slums was not viewed as a priority for many social reformers and charitable organisations. Indeed for H. G. Wells, writing in 1901 at Sandgate whilst recuperating from tuberculosis, disease ridden slums ensured the weeding out of the unfit:

---

[11] D. Byrne and J. Keithley, Housing and the Health of the Community, *Unhealthy Housing: Research, Remedies and Reform,* London, Routledge, eds. R. Burridge & D. Ormandy, 1993, p.57; N. McFarlane, Hospitals, Housing and Tuberculosis, p.75

[12] P. M. H. Mazumdar, *Eugenics, Human Genetics and Human Failings*, 1992, p.38

[13] A. S. Wohl, *The Eternal Slum: Housing and Social Policy in Victorian London,* New Brunswick:Transaction Publishers, [1977], 2006, p.184

[14] G. Sims, *How the Poor Live,* London: Chatto & Windus, 1883; Reverend A. Mearns, *The Bitter Cry of Outcast London: An Inquiry into the Condition of the Abject Poor,* 1883, www.attackingthedevil.co.uk/related/outcast.php

> Until... it can prevent the birth of just all the inadaptable, useless, or merely unnecessary creatures in each generation, there must needs continue to be, in greater or less amount, this individually futile struggle beneath the feet of the race; somewhere and in some form there must still persist those essentials that now take shape as the slum, the prison, and the asylum.[15]

Only families deemed to be respectable and receptive to the middle class doctrine of cleanliness, sobriety, prayer and industry were selected as tenants.[16] George Sims, one of the first reformers to draw attention to the living conditions of the London poor, expressed the conflated fears of disease and disorder felt by many of the middle and upper classes in 1883 as the disparity in living standards between social classes grew. He warned:

> this mighty mob of famished, diseased and filthy helots is getting dangerous, physically, morally, politically dangerous.[17]

By the 1870s hereditary explanations of disease had gained precedence amongst British doctors over environmental models of health and sickness, largely due to the perceived failure of sanitarian public health initiatives to improve urban environments.[18] And from the 1880s sanitary medicine was increasingly challenged by a social-Darwinist ideology, according to which preventive medicine was seen as contributing to a weakening of the nation by keeping alive "degenerate stock" that would otherwise have naturally died out.

For many, tuberculosis was viewed as a natural purgative of the morally and physically unfit. In 1890, *The Spectator*, a serious news magazine, expressed concern that Koch's discovery of the *tubercle bacillus* would deprive nature of the:

> many bristled besom which sweeps away the feeble......the naturally weak would be preserved to rear up broods of children tainted with their inherent imperfections.[19]

---

[15] H. G. Wells, *Anticipations of the Reaction of Mechanical and Scientific Progress upon Human Life and Thought* , London: Chapman & Hall, 1902, p.79
[16] A. S. Wohl, *The Eternal Slum,* 2006, pp.54-56, p.185
[17] G. Sims, How the Poor Live*,* 1883, p.28
[18] W. F. Bynum, Darwin and the Doctors, 1983, pp.43-53
[19] Doctor Koch's Discovery, *The Spectator*, 65, November 22nd, 1890, pp. 726-727

By the twentieth century calls for preventing the reproduction of the physically and morally degenerate were increasingly in evidence.[20] In 1901 Wells advocated the withdrawal of all state support to the "social residuum" of the unemployable and chronically sick. In his *Anticipations* of 1901 Wells viewed the urban poor as doomed to an early grave and ultimately to extinction:

> either criminal, immoral, parasitic in more or less irregular ways upon the more successful classes, or labouring, at something less than a regular bare subsistence wage, in a finally hopeless competition against machinery that is as yet not so cheap as their toil. It is, to borrow a popular phrase, the "submerged" portion of the social body, a leaderless, aimless multitude, a multitude of people drifting down towards the abyss.... sooner or later, as every East End doctor knows, the ways of the social abyss lead to death, the premature death of the individual, or death through the death or infertility of the individual's stunted offspring, or death through that extinction which moral perversion involves.[21]

Even Sir Arthur Newsholme, the Medical Officer responsible for administering (under the Local Government Board) the National Health Insurance Act of 1911, acknowledged that:

> in regard to the feeble minded, the intermittently insane, and possibly the chronic dependent, it may be hoped that public opinion will ere long demand that these should not be permitted to multiply. It may even be hoped that social pressure will be exercised towards diminishing multiplication in families which are non-supporting.[22]

And, after the passage through Parliament of the Act in 1911, Sir James Barr, President of the BMA, condemned the legislation as likely to:

> increase that spirit of dependency which is ever found in degenerate races, [encouraging the poor and tubercular] to multiply their breed at the expense of the healthy and intellectual members of the community'.[23] [These] moral and physical degenerates [should be] prevented from adding

---

[20] W. H. G. Armytage, The Stock Question, The Social Context of Eugenic Thought, *The Galton Institute Newsletter*, issue no. 15, December, 1994

[21] H. G. Wells, *Anticipations,* 1902, pp. 80-81

[22] A. Newsholme, The Declining Birth-Rate*, New Tracts for the Times,* 3, 1911, quoted in W. H. G. Armytage, The Stock Question, The Social Context of Eugenic Thought, *The Galton Institute Newsletter*, issue no. 15, December, 1994

[23] Sir J. Barr, *BMJ*, 30th December 1911, p. 174.

to the race.[24]

Barr's view was identical to that of Wells. Both men were in favour of allowing nature to "weed out" the weakest and least adaptable members of society. And, for Barr, the *tubercle bacillus* fulfilled that eugenic purpose:

> If we could only abolish the tubercle bacillus in these islands we would get rid of tuberculous disease, but we should at the same time raise up a race peculiarly susceptible to this infection - a race of hothouse plants which would not flourish in any other environment. We would thus increase at an even greater rate than we are doing at present, nervous instability, the numbers of insane and feeble-minded. Nature, on the other hand, weeds out those who have not got the innate power of recovery from disease, and by means of the tubercle bacillus and other pathogenic organisms she frequently does this before the reproductive age, so that a check is put on the multiplication of idiots and the feeble-minded. Nature's methods are thus of advantage to the race rather than to the individual.[25]

These eugenic attitudes also informed medical treatment in the Poor Law system where paupers were, according to one Medical Officer, commonly perceived and treated as being less than human.[26] The view that the chronically sick poor were biologically deficient or bred from degenerate stock was widespread in the later nineteenth and early twentieth centuries.[27] Consumption was the commonest complaint in workhouses, and the Royal Commission on the Poor Law of 1907 reported that in 128 Unions in England and Wales over 21% of indoor cases and nearly 11% of outdoor cases receiving medical relief suffered from pulmonary tuberculosis.[28]

In 1904 William Tyson, senior physician to Folkestone's Victoria Hospital and the Folkestone Charity Organisation Society, asserted that not only hereditary predispositions but also acquired characteristics were visited on one's children [through]:

---

[24] Sir J. Barr, *BMJ,* 27th July 1912, p.158; Sir J. Barr, Doctors' Ultimatum to Ministers, *The Times*, 24th July, 7, 1912

[25] Sir J. Barr, *BMJ,* 27th July, 1912, p.159

[26] M. A. Crowther, Paupers or Patients? Obstacles to Professionalisation in the Poor Law Medical Service Before 1914, *Journal of the History of Medicine and Allied Sciences*, 39:1, January, 1984; J. Rogers, *Reminiscences of a Workhouse Medical Officer,* London: Fisher, 1889

[27] P. M. H. Mazumdar, *Eugenics, Human Genetics and Human Failings*, 1992, p.38

[28] G. Cronje, *Pulmonary Tuberculosis in England and Wales 1851-1910*, University of London PhD thesis, 1989, pp.574-575

> the law of heredity, by which many start in life heavily handicapped, when not only the sins, but the weaknesses, of the parents are visited upon future generations.[29]

Thus, whilst disease was already understood as a consequence of immoral or insanitary behaviour, evolutionism reinforced the view that particular families and racial groups possessed a tendency to disease. Consequently, tuberculosis came to be commonly regarded as an inherent predisposition of individuals or groups who were seen as being somehow morally or racially deficient.

This perspective was supported by Victorian notions of the inter-relatedness of mind and body, which became particularly influential from the 1860s and 1870s, and posited the nervous system, or the "character" or "will" and their inherent moral qualities, as being the fundamental determinants of chronic disease.[30] George Cheyne's model of the centrality of the nervous system, developed in the mid-eighteenth century, readily accommodated conceptions of biological inheritance.[31]

These notions of the predisposition of the individual constitution, or character, to disease were consistent with both the earlier model of Galenic humoural temperaments as well as with an understanding of human "types" informed by evolutionary theory.[32] Consequently, an understanding of tuberculosis as more liable to affect certain families, or individuals possessed of particular characteristics, was well established amongst the medical profession and the public throughout the nineteenth century. This understanding of the hereditary transmission of tuberculosis also associated the disease with the threat of social miscegenation towards the end of the century. One commonly held belief, supported by the arguments of some in the medical profession, was that the Jewish race was particularly predisposed to contracting the disease.[33]

As evolutionary theory contributed to an understanding of how pathologies and aberrations occurred amongst the poorest, it also served to

---

[29] W. J. Tyson, Presidential address to the Preventive Health Section, Reports of Folkestone Health Congress, July, 1904

[30] B. Haley, *The Healthy Body and Victorian Culture*, 1978, p.45

[31] G. S. Rousseau, *Nervous Acts: Essays on Literature, Culture and Sensibility*, Basingstoke: Palgrave MacMillan. 2004

[32] W. F. Bynum, Darwin and the Doctors: Evolution, Diathesis, and Germs in 19th Century Britain, *Gesnerus*, volume 40, pt.1-2, 1983, pp.43-53; F. Galton & F. A. Mahomed, An Inquiry into the Physiognomy of Phthisis by the method of Composite Portraiture, eds. H. G. Howse & F. Taylor, *Guy's Hospital Reports,* 3rd Series, London, J&A Churchill, 1881

[33] S. Gilman, *Franz Kafka, The Jewish Patient*, London: Routledge, 1995

scientifically validate middle class values. The establishment of what Bordieu has termed the "*bourgeois habitus*"[34] can be seen as a post-Darwinian concern with class differentiation. That is to say the control of animal emotion and the "baser passions" which was the prime characteristic of the (male and adult) middle classes, and which distinguished them from the lack of discipline which was seen as a characteristic of the burgeoning mass culture. This concern with emotional control is reflected in many novels of the period, as well as in conduct books and popular health manuals, where the expression of excessive emotion was seen as liable to precipitate illness, particularly in women, and control of the emotions was the distinguishing feature of the English gentleman.[35]

The Victorian maxim *mens sana in corpore sano* epitomised this re-emergent Enlightenment ethos of control. The implicit appeal to right thinking contained in this dictum, urging the adoption of *bourgeois* values and codes, effected a considerable normalising and self-regulatory influence through manipulating the social dread of tuberculosis.[36] Thus the healthy mind, conforming to *bourgeois* notions of moral order and discipline, inhabited a healthy body, whilst the morally or mentally deficient were prone to chronic sickness.

These *fin de siècle* fears of otherness and social contamination, whilst perhaps not being explicit, nevertheless inhabited a part of the middle class psyche, and influenced public health policies directed towards the segregation of paupers, consumptives and others considered to be defective. The activities of organisations such as the Eugenic Education Society also helped foster an awareness of the social applications of evolutionist ideas.[37]

Central to the discourse over the fitness of the nation was the problem of the relationship between disease and poverty. Tuberculosis, the main cause of chronic sickness and death, was seen by some doctors as a consequence of industrialisation and overcrowded cities. Nevertheless the legacy of social Darwinism largely deflected any responsibility for the perpetuation of the disease from the professional classes and captains of industry. The pallid faces and emaciated bodies that were evident on

---

[34] P. Bourdieu, *Outline of a Theory of Practice,* Cambridge University Press, 1977

[35] For example, G. Black, *Family Health Book*, London: Ward, Lock, Bowden & Co., 1892; Anon., *Health for the Household: Based on a knowledge of air, water, food, clothing, drink and the Training of the Mind,* London: Jarrold & Sons, 1858

[36] C. T. Moloney, *Inflaming Infirmity: Some Medical-Literary Interfaces of 19th Century Tuberculosis,*(unpublished), 2009, p.38

[37] G. Stedman-Jones, *Outcast London*, 1971, p.312; G. Himmelfarb, *The Idea of Poverty: England in the Early Industrial Age*, New York: Random House, 1985

London streets around the turn of the century were symbolic, to many, of the physical deterioration, if not degeneration, of the nation. Vice and congenital inferiority, not poverty, were viewed as being responsible for chronic disease.

Here it may be illustrative to note the description of the inhabitants of south and east London in 1886 by Reginald, Lord Brabazon, the twelfth Earl of Meath, imperialist proponent of "national hygiene" and chairman of the Inter-departmental Committee on Physical Deterioration of 1904:

> on all sides pale faces, stunted figures, debilitated forms, narrow chests and all the outward signs of a low vital power.[38]

Revealingly, Brabazon's impression of working class London is characterised by symptoms of consumption. It would appear that images of the gradual physical deterioration of the consumptive had become somehow conflated with conceptions of the hereditary moral and physical degeneration of the urban poor.

Whilst the causes of chronic disease may have been seen as being partially due to the moral and environmental corruption associated with the city, the consequences were also widely understood as being visited on successive generations, so that families were unable to flourish in the city:

> scarcely a man of the highest distinction has been born to parents brought up in the largest towns…London families born and bred do not survive beyond the fifth generation.[39]

These theories of urban degeneration, it has been argued, also served to justify the tendency of employers to favour the more robust, but also the more conformist and docile, rural workers.[40]

The ideology of middle class social reform movements in the 1880s and, in particular, the 1890s, reflected an almost visceral fear and repugnance of the poorest and most desperate urban inhabitants. Widespread support for evolutionism by scientists, intellectuals and politicians ensured the pervasive influence of class consciousness in the future development of public health structures and policies, and a continued focus on the perceived vices and insanitary habits of the poor

---

[38] Lord Brabazon, State Directed Colonisation; Its Necessity, *Nineteenth Century*, volume xxxi, April, 1887

[39] Unidentified author, *The Practitioner*, July, 1901, p.466.

[40] G. Stedman Jones, *Outcast London*, 1971, p.130

throughout the nineteenth and twentieth centuries.[41] In this atmosphere of intense concern over the consequences of rapid industrialisation and urbanisation tuberculosis became a prime source of study for eugenists. Convictions of an inherited predisposition to consumption, if not of its direct inheritance, were particularly common throughout the period under study amongst general practitioners and pathologists.[42]

By the late 1890s conceptions of preventive medicine, inspired by germ theory, began to be employed by some public health officials that emphasised the dangers of infection and which envisaged need rather than worthiness as the principle criterion for delivering therapeutic relief. This increased concern for the health of the poorer classes, however, conflicted with the Poor Law ethos of deterrence and the Charity Organisation Society campaign against outdoor relief.

For the poorest tuberculosis was still not generally acknowledged as a disease requiring medical supervision. As the disease advanced the sufferer had little chance of recovery, particularly if their diet and living conditions were inadequate, and most families were eager to avoid the workhouse. George Lansbury, Labour MP for Lambeth in 1911, acknowledged this widespread unwillingness to resort to the Poor Law in order to claim relief for family members suffering from tuberculosis:

> The other day a mother came to me with three little children, each one of whom, although I am not a medical man, I could see at once was tubercular and ought to have been receiving proper treatment. Not one of these children was going to get proper treatment because the mother, with that spirit of British independence which some people admire so much, would rather see her children suffer than take parish relief to see them dealt with.[43]

Any attempt to treat the disease prior to the development of pronounced symptoms could be interpreted by parish authorities as the unwarranted

---

[41] E. Fee & D. Porter, Public Health, Preventive Medicine & Professionalisation, *Medicine in Society: Historical Essays*, Cambridge University Press, ed. A. Wear, 1992, p.271

[42] J. A. Mendelsohn, Medicine and the making of Bodily Inequality in 20th Century Europe, *Heredity and Infection*, eds. J. Gaudillière & I. Löwy, London: Routledge, 2003, p.6

[43] G. Lansbury, MP for Lambeth, House of Commons debate 11th July, 1911, volume 28 cc325

"pauperisation" of individuals.[44] Poor Law officials were directed to ensure that parish relief remained the last resort of the destitute and chronically sick. Moreover, as will be argued in chapter three, the work of the National Association for the Prevention of Tuberculosis and the Charity Organisation Society tended to reinforce a perception of paupers as a biologically distinct population more in need of containment and moral reform than of therapeutic treatment.

The acceptance of an hereditary predisposition to tuberculosis was still held by many doctors during the early twentieth century. Timbrell Bulstrode's compendious Report on Sanatoria for the Local Government Board, published in 1908, cites the opinion of several experts, including superintendents of sanatoria such as F. W. Burton-Fanning, and Medical Officers of Health such as Arthur Ransome, who asserted that:

> Few medical men who have been long in practice will doubt the existence of family predisposition to tubercular disease.[45]

Bulstrode himself considered that the reproduction of the tubercular constituted a threat to the health of the nation:

> a theory of infection does not count for the facts, and there is an anti-social disregard for national exigencies in the conduct of medical men who can write in the press that the marriage, or even intermarriage, of members of tuberculous stocks is of no social detriment provided they live with a good source of fresh air'.[46]

Similarly, the socialist John Burns, Bulstrode's superior as president of the LGB, expressed the widespread fear of national degeneration when he referred in a House of Commons debate in 1911 to "the accumulated heritage of sickness, invalidity and degeneracy that we have transmitted to us through the centuries", and suggested that the "venue of pauperism" should be transferred from Boards of Guardians to County Councils.[47]

The idea of isolating the unemployed in labour camps first emerged

---

[44] *The Break-Up of the Poor Law: Being Part One of the Minority Report of the Poor Law Commission*, Edited by S. & B. Webb, London: Longmans, Green & Co, 1909, p.243

[45] A. Ransome, 1890, quoted in H. T. Bulstrode, *Report on Sanatoria for Consumption and certain other aspects of the Tuberculosis Question*, Supplement to the 35th Annual Report of the LGB, 1905-6, p.53

[46] H. T. Bulstrode, *Report on Sanatoria for Consumption,* 1905-6, p.55

[47] J. Burns, *Hansard,* Debate on Poor Law Administration, House of Commons, 27th April, 1911, volume 24 cc2029

during the mid-1880s, and the suggestion of institutionalising the "residuum" of the chronically sick and the casual workforce became common in the late 1880s. These ideas were initially inspired by the perceived threat to the middle classes of revolution, but from the 1890s were increasingly motivated by fears of racial degeneration and the spreading moral and physical corruption of the working classes.[48] In 1911 Dr. William Chapple, M.P. for Dumfrieshire, arguing in the House of Commons for the containment of the chronically sick and destitute, urged isolation for paupers as a form of negative eugenics:

> the basic primary cause of destitution is physical, mental and moral defects [which were considered responsible for 90% of cases in Poor Law institutions]...nearly 80% of physical, mental and moral defects are hereditary. We are breeding from defective stock.[49]

A perception of the intrinsically defective character of working class consumptives received further scientific validation in the inter-war years as the emerging discipline of psychiatry contributed to the elaboration of a set of traits associated with the tubercular. In the *Journal of the Royal Sanitary Institute* of 1921 H. Gordon Smith, the Medical Superintendent of Knightwick Sanatorium and Chief Tuberculosis Officer for Worcester County Council, referred to consumptives as being possessed of "an inherent disinclination to work", and recommended the introduction of labour colonies.[50] The tubercular *diathesis* also came to be associated with insanity and neurological disorders such as hysteria and neurasthenia.[51] The disease was characterised not only by physical symptoms but also by behavioural traits, according to a model of nervous pathology:[52]

> There is no disease in which the mental and moral characteristics of the patient are so profoundly modified, and with which psycho-neuroses are so constantly associated, as chronic pulmonary tuberculosis.[53]

---

[48] H. T. Bulstrode, *Report on Sanatoria for Consumption*, 1905-6, p.55; G. Jones, *Social Hygiene in 20th Century Britain*, Beckenham: Croom Helm, 1986

[49] Dr. W. Chapple, *Hansard,* House of Commons debate on Poor Law administration, 27th April, 1911, volume 24, cc2046

[50] H. G. Smith, *Journal of the Royal Sanitary Institute*, volume xli, no 4, March 1921

[51] D. G. Macleod-Munro, *The Psycho-Pathology of Tuberculosis*, Oxford University Press, 1926, p.7

[52] G. S. Rousseau, *Nervous Acts: Essays on Literature, Culture and Sensibility*, Palgrave MacMillan. 2004

[53] D. G. Macleod-Munro, *The Psycho-Pathology of Tuberculosis*, 1926, p.2

The tubercular *diathesis* was acknowledged by physicians up to the middle of the twentieth century, and a family history of tuberculosis would often prevent an individual from being able to purchase a life insurance policy.[54] In 1908 the Birmingham physician Joseph Emmanuel remarked:

> while the medical profession is occupying itself in teaching the public the all importance of the infectious character of tuberculosis, the insurance world still only regards hereditariness of the disease to the total disregard of infectivity.[55]

It would be wrong therefore to assume that with the dawn of the new century tuberculosis had come to be regarded simply as an infectious disease. Karl Pearson's biometric analyses of consumption suggested that cases of tubercular parent and child were more common than both spouses developing the disease.[56] This helped to sustain the belief that tuberculosis was in some way inherited into the inter-war years.

Middle class anxieties over the existence of a biologically distinct "underclass" with a particular predisposition to contracting tuberculosis were further exacerbated by a growing disparity in the birth rate between social classes. By 1914 the national birth rate stood at 24.0 births per 1,000 of the population, representing a continuous decline of more than 33% since a peak of 36.3 in 1876.[57] A trend towards smaller middle and upper class families precipitated fears of class antagonism and social decay.

From about 1910 the idea of tuberculosis colonies and open-air schools for "pre-tubercular" children emerged.[58] The concept of the "pre-tubercular" child implies the acceptance of a recognisable physical "type" who was considered to have inherited a predisposition to contracting the

---

[54] T. Alborn, Insurance against Germ Theory: Commerce and Conservatism in Late-Victorian Medicine, *Bulletin of the History of Medicine*, 2001, 75

[55] J. G. Emmanuel, Tuberculosis and Insurance, *Journal of the Federated Insurance Institute,* 11, 1908, p.1, quoted in T. Alborn, Insurance Against Germ Theory, p.428

[56] K. Pearson, *A Second Study of the Statistics of Pulmonary Tuberculosis: Marital Infection,* London, 1908, p.153, cited in B. R. Mitchell & P. Deane, *Abstract of British Historical Statistics,* Cambridge University Press, 1962, p.29

[57] K. Pearson, *A Second Study of the Statistics of Pulmonary Tuberculosis: Marital Infection,* London, 1908, p.153, cited in B. R. Mitchell & P. Deane, *Abstract of British Historical Statistics,* Cambridge University Press, 1962, p.29

[58] K. Pearson, *A First Study of the Statistics of Pulmonary Tuberculosis*, London, 1907; *Second Study etc*., 1908; L. Bryder, *Under the Magic Mountain*, Oxford University Press, 1988, p.32

disease. The term appears to have been in common use following the introduction of the medical inspection of school children and factory workers in 1907. It has been estimated that in the first two decades of the twentieth century 10% of children were classified as being pre or latent tubercular.[59] And in 1929 Austin Priestman, the Medical Officer of Health for Folkestone, reported in his capacity as School Medical Officer:

> It appears that pulmonary affections indicative of an underlying tuberculosis or tubercular diathesis are much commoner than is generally upheld.[60]

Social evolutionist concepts had inspired considerable research into the individual characteristics of the chronically sick, and particularly the tubercular.[61] Sir Robert Philip had pioneered the "march past" in the 1890s, a procedure designed to ascertain at a glance which family members bore "tuberculous stigmata", and one that was adopted by many Factory Inspectors and School Medical Officers. In 1923 Dr. W. C. Rivers, Tuberculosis Officer for Barnsley, published a paper in *The Lancet* concerned with identifying physical characteristics associated with a tubercular *diathesis*.[62] Quoting from a wealth of European statistical and anthropometric studies on the degenerative traits associated with tuberculosis, various identifying features were found to be more common amongst consumptives than in the general population.

The insane were found to be particularly prone to consumption; whilst the death rate from tuberculosis was recorded as 0.2% of the population of England in 1901 the percentage of deaths from the disease in borough and county asylums was said to be 15.8.[63] In 1911 Arthur Latham claimed that upwards of 24,000 consumptives were "accommodated" in lunatic asylums. The death rates for tuberculosis were high in all such institutions. It seems probable considering the aberrant behaviour associated with the tubercular together with the lack of available accommodation for what was

---

[59] L. Bryder, 'Wonderlands of Buttercup, Clover and Daisies': Tuberculosis and the Open-air School Movement in Britain, 1907-39*, In the name of the child: Health and Welfare 1880-1940,* London, Routledge, ed. R. Cooter, 1992, p.75

[60] A. Priestman, *Report of School Medical Officer,* Folkestone, 1929

[61] The Report of the Inter-departmental Committee on Physical Deterioration of 1904 had recommended the institution of a permanent anthropometric survey of the population.

[62] W. C. Rivers, The Atavistic-Degenerative Diathesis of Tuberculosis, *The Lancet*, 20th January, 1923, pp. 120-123

[63] Ibid., p.120; See also Macleod-Munro, *The Psycho-Pathology of Tuberculosis*, 1926, p.27

coming to be seen by the public as an infectious disease, that some families opted to have troublesome and potentially dangerous consumptive relatives committed to asylums.

Other atavistic or degenerative "stigmata" found to be more common among consumptives included *hypertrichosis* - growth of hair on the back or limbs,[64] a dark complexion in northern Europeans, red hair, squint, *ichthyosis* - the formation of dry scales on the skin, a dislike of fatty food and *lanugo* - fine white hair on the skin. Rivers concluded, citing evidence from Darwin, that miscegenation – the intermixing of races – encourages atavistic traits, a reversion to a more primitive type which, like "primitive" tribal peoples, possess less resistance to tuberculosis.[65] His research proposed some form of eugenic control of working class consumptives and advocated measures to ensure racial purity:

> Practical deductions from all this as regards prophylaxis and diagnosis hardly need mentioning. What does need stress is the eugenic aspect – as regards tuberculous patients bodily degenerate, and without countervailing intellectual superiority.[66]

For many doctors the acceptance of an hereditary factor as a cause of consumption would have tended to bestow a greater recognition of their experience and intuition in the diagnosis and prognosis of a complex condition. If their role were reduced to sending a sputum test to the county analyst and referring the consumptive to a specialist, as seemed possible when the idea of national insurance was first mooted, many clinicians feared a loss of power and prestige.[67] Whilst the recognition of hereditary tendencies might have added another dimension to the work of family physicians, it only served to stigmatise the consumptive in the public mind as a product of "degenerate stock" as well as a possible source of contagion. In the opinion of one influential historian:

> Tuberculosis never fully acquired the status of a medical condition in the British public's mind, but retained strong associations with moral

---

[64] Darwin refers to this as a characteristic of *'delicate children'*, *Descent of Man*, 2nd ed., chapter ii, p.36

[65] W. C. Rivers, The Atavistic-Degenerative Diathesis of Tuberculosis, 1923; Rivers quotes Darwin's *'reconstruction of the primitive jungle guinea fowl by intermixing two modern varieties of poultry'*, p.122

[66] W. C. Rivers, The Atavistic-Degenerative Diathesis of Tuberculosis, 1923, p.123

[67] J. Brand, *Doctors and the State*, Baltimore: Johns Hopkins Press, 1965

inadequacy verging on criminality.[68]

Although a more exclusive focus on the dangers of the *tubercle bacillus* from the late 1890s reflected the inclusion of bacteriology in the training for the Diploma in Public Health,[69] understandings of the causes of tuberculosis became less specific after the First World War as hereditary and environmental factors were reintegrated into the aetiology of tuberculosis.[70]

During the inter-war period the "organic" nature of disease processes was often emphasised in rejection of mechanistic interpretations of the body, which was still generally understood as a dynamic system, constantly adapting to its environment. The fragmentation, reification and standardisation of medical and social science had, to a great degree, been resisted.[71] The causes of disease, and particularly the extent to which they were seen as a consequence of social and economic, hereditary or bacteriological factors, as well as the choice of medical responses, remained contested by the British medical profession throughout the early twentieth century. This interpretation is distinctly at odds with historical accounts of a paradigm shift in medical attitudes following Koch's work on tuberculosis in the 1880s, or a standardisation of medical theory and practice and the sweeping aside of older medical traditions.[72]

Bulstrode's Report on Sanatoria for Consumption of 1905-6 for the Local Government Board, for example, noted that "an increasing number of observers", considered that hereditary factors in the development of tuberculosis had been underestimated since Koch's discovery of the

---

[68] S. Szreter, Healthy Government? Britain c.1850-1950, *Historical Journal*, 34, 2, 1991, p.493

[69] D. Watkins, *The English Revolution in Social Medicine, 1899-1911*, PhD thesis, University of London, 1984, p. 160

[70] M. Pelling, The Meaning of Contagion: Reproduction, Medicine & Metaphor, *Contagion: Historical & Cultural Studies,* London: Routledge, eds. A. Bashford & C. Hooker, 2001, p.33

[71] D. Cantor, The Diseased Body, *Medicine in the Twentieth Century*, London: Harwood Academic Publishers, eds. R. Cooter & J. V. Pickstone, 2000, pp.347-366

[72] K. C. Carter, The Development of Pasteur's Concept of Disease Causation and the Emergence of Specific Causes in Nineteenth Century Medicine, *Bulletin of the History of Medicine,* 65, 1991, p.548

tubercle bacillus,[73] and H. de Carle Woodcock, committee member of the National Association for the Prevention of Tuberculosis, observed in 1912 that:

> since the standard of comfort among the poor has increased ...*phthisis* has declined, and infection as a cause of disease has, at any rate in this country, lost much of its importance.[74]

Contrary to popular conceptions of a linear march of progress in biomedicine inspired by the development of germ theory the impersonal carnage and social dislocation caused by industrial warfare also, perhaps, contributed to a backlash against purely bacteriological accounts of disease causation. As one historian has suggested, without elaborating on this perceived intellectual shift:

> the Great War helped restore the reaction between environment and personal predisposition in etiological explanations and reduce the salience of simple infection. Old romantic notions of *phthisis* returned to fashion.[75]

A reinforcement of holistic and hereditary approaches to medicine and an opposition to reductive, scientised and bureaucratic models on the part of doctors from either side of the political spectrum has also been noted for the inter-war years.[76] It has been suggested that the failure of bacteriological aetiology to predict or respond to the influenza epidemic of 1918-19 also contributed to this ideological shift.[77] George Newman, the Chief Medical Officer of the newly created Ministry of Health, observed in his first publication for that office in 1919 that more attention was being paid to the soil (the environment) than the seed (the germ) than had been the case "in the heyday of germ theory".[78]

---

[73] H. T. Bulstrode, *Report on Sanatoria for Consumption and certain other aspects of the Tuberculosis Question*, Supplement to the 35th Annual Report of the Local Government Board, 1905-6, p.55. Bulstrode was influenced by the eugenicist Karl Pearson, see D. Watkins, *The English Revolution in Scientific Medicine*, 1984, p.223

[74] H. de Carle Woodcock, *The Doctor and the People*, London: Methuen, 1912, p.216

[75] F. B. Smith, *The Retreat of Tuberculosis*, 1988, p.224

[76] P. Weindling, Health and Medicine in Inter-War Europe,2000, pp.39-50

[77] I. Galdston, *Social and Historic Foundations of Modern Medicine*, New York: Brunner/Mazel, 1981, p.80

[78] G. Newman, *An Outline of the Practice of Preventive Medicine; a Memo Addressed to the Minister of Health*, London: HMSO, 1919, p.16

It is significant that this shift of focus from bacteriology to environment and eugenics coincides with middle class concerns over improving the national stock that reached a peak during the inter-war years.[79] Before World War Two the class structure in England was viewed by many as a "natural" order. Those least endowed by nature with health, vitality and intelligence occupied the lowest orders of society and, due to inheriting a feeble or flawed constitution, were more prone to disease. By the 1930s many influenced by eugenics were espousing biological engineering as a means of ensuring the progress of the nation's health.[80] Increasingly it became accepted practice to sterilise consumptive mothers,[81] and there are claims that abortion by mothers with a family history of tuberculosis was encouraged "on a considerable scale".[82]

The Eugenic Society had been supported in its lobbying for sterilisation by the Royal College of Physicians, the Society of Medical Officers of Health, and the Association of County Medical Officers of Health, although not by the BMA. In 1935 Leonard Hill, a physiologist at the National Institute for Medical Research and a member of the Medical Research Council, justified the procedure in terms of the national interest:

> there was one particular disease to which attention should be drawn – namely tuberculosis – which had a strong hereditary background. Consumptives in their own interests but particularly in the interests of the nation, should be sterilised.[83]

An alternative to sterilisation was the tuberculosis colony. Colonists would remain for life, a cure not being considered possible from an hereditary perspective as the disease would remain latent. Despite the Interdepartmental Committee on Tuberculosis of 1919 recommending the expansion of village settlements for working class consumptives only a few colonies were to survive any length of time. Post-World War One financial cut-backs and the disfavour into which social engineering fell after 1945 put an end to this enterprise.[84]

---

[79] G. Jones, *Social Hygiene in 20th Century Britain,* 1986, pp.10-11

[80] A. Richardson, *Love and Eugenics in the Late Nineteenth Century*, Oxford University Press, 2003, pp.184-5

[81] *BMJ*, 5th December, 1931, p.1059; *The Lancet*, 4th November, 1933, p.1056

[82] F. B. Smith, *The Retreat of Tuberculosis*, 1988, p.230

[83] L. Hill, *Manchester Guardian*, 3rd September, 1935, quoted in G. Jones, *Social Hygeine,* 1986, p.22, note 7

[84] Interdepartmental Committee on Tuberculosis, 1919, HMSO, cmd. 317, pp. 139-184

In summary, the normative function of medicine, that is to say its role in defining and monitoring "correct behaviour", can be seen as operating politically as an extension of middle class values. Sanitary, eugenic and infectious medical models were not necessarily mutually exclusive, or in competition, and all were employed in an unprecedented attempt to regulate the behaviour of the lower social orders. These medical approaches served, following the social and demographic upheavals occasioned by the industrial revolution, to deflect attention from the appalling conditions in which men, women and children lived and worked, onto the moral and sanitary failings of the working classes.

The campaign against tuberculosis served to instil middle class mores of cleanliness (or, rather, an antipathy to "dirt"), domestic order, self-discipline, thrift and the benefits of outdoor exercise into a culturally diverse working class population. This created the basis for the first time in England, of a cultural uniformity informed by science, national identity and rationalism. The anti-tuberculosis movement also reflected modernist social aspirations and national values that operated to reinforce and "naturalise" social inequalities.

This eugenic approach to the problem of the unproductive and diseased poor was only ended due to a shortage of funding and, eventually, the ethical backlash following Germany's project to achieve racial purity. As one historian has observed regarding tuberculosis control in the United States, reconfiguring tuberculosis as the first large-scale public health issue provided the structure and impetus to modernise and revitalise working class culture:

> Tuberculosis was in a sense a trope for national degeneration, and as such it became the vehicle for a self-conscious thrust towards national renewal and moral regeneration.[85]

[85] S. Craddock, Engendered/Endangered: Women, Tuberculosis and the Project of Citizenship, *Journal of Historical Geography*, 27, 3, 2001, p.338

CHAPTER THREE

DISEASE, DIRT AND MORALITY: URBAN POLLUTION AND THE OPEN-AIR CURE

The growth of sanatorium treatment from the end of the nineteenth century and the increased supervision of the tubercular in working class districts has generally been assumed to have been the result of a new awareness of the infectiousness of the *tubercle bacillus*. Undoubtedly Koch's identification of the *bacillus* did help to stimulate action to prevent and to treat the disease amongst the working classes. Nevertheless an analysis of approaches to tuberculosis at this time, grounded in their social context, reveals a more complex and dynamic interplay of cultural forces at work.

Representing Tuberculosis in the early Twentieth Century

As argued in the previous chapter a concern with the degenerative effects of urban living was equally, if not more, responsible for stimulating a renewed interest in public health in the late nineteenth century. In addition the sight and smell of overcrowded and insanitary slums resonated with *miasmatic* conceptions of disease propounded by Edwin Chadwick earlier in the nineteenth century.

Notions of corrupt matter and Christian ideas of moral corruption had been inextricably linked in Chadwick's sanitary crusade against "filth", which conjoined the pervasive middle class obsessions of "vice" and "dirt". Victorians were familiar with biblical texts that conflated physical and moral corruption, depicting illness as a divine retribution for sin.[1] The notion of disease and mortal suffering occurring as a consequence of moral transgression was deeply entrenched and persisted beyond the Victorian era.

Moral contagion was also seen as a danger to society during the second

---

[1] K. Thomas, Health & Morality in Early Modern England, Allen M. Brandt & Paul Rozin, *Morality & Health,* London, Routledge, 1997, p.28

half of the nineteenth century. Social commentators such as Arnold White had, in the 1850s, warned that the "social residuum" – the unemployed, itinerant and chronically sick - posed a threat of both moral and physical contamination to the more virtuous and able worker.[2] This *bourgeois* fear and repugnance of moral and material filth is caricatured by Dickens in *Dombey and Son.* In this serial, first published in 1846,

> a dense black cloud... [of] noxious particles... rolling slowly on to corrupt the better portions of town [is linked to] the moral pestilence that rises with them.[3]

And Dickens' almost tubercular depiction of London smog in *Our Mutual Friend* as "a heap of vapour...unfolding a gigantic catarrh",[4] similarly reflects middle class fears of *miasmatic* contagion emanating from the urban poor.

These anxieties were little affected by the advent of germ theory. Until the 1930s the predominant view of the medical profession was that *tubercle bacilli* were spread through the dried sputum of sufferers being attached to dust rather than directly from the breath of the tubercular.[5] Due to this focus on the dangers to health posed by dust, germ theory came to be grafted onto pre-existing *miasmic* conceptions of "filth" as constituting the source of disease.

As it was believed that the *tubercle bacillus* could not survive in the open air,[6] there existed a widespread conviction that tuberculosis was spread in the houses of the poor. Reflecting contemporary social prejudices, the disease came to be associated more with moral irresponsibility and a lack of cleanliness amongst the poorer classes than

---

[2] A. White, *The Nomad Poor of London,* Contemporary Review, May 1855, volume xlvii, pp. 714-727, quoted in G. Stedman-Jones, *Outcast London*, 1971, p.288

[3] C. Dickens, *Dombey and Son,* Harmondsworth, Penguin, 1986, p.738

[4] C. Dickens, *Our Mutual Friend,* London, The New Illustrated Dickens, 1947-58, III, I, p.420, cited in C. T. Moloney, *George Eliot, Henry James and Consumption,* 1999, p.312

[5] J. Tyndall, *New Fragments*, London: Longmans, 1892

[6] According to *The Practitioner,* 1901, fresh air and sunlight killed the bacillus in a fortnight or a month whereas in a dark room it could retain vitality for *'many months'*. In the early twentieth century a popular catch phrase attributed even greater powers to sunlight: "thirty years in the dark but thirty seconds in the sun". Quoted in M. Campbell, What tuberculosis did for Modernism: The influence of a Curative Environment on Modernist Design and Architecture, in *Medical History*, 2005, p.49

with direct contagion.[7] The tubercular poor were, in general, held responsible for their condition, and *bourgeois* conceptions of self-help and self-control, expounded through Chadwick's doctrine of sanitary science, endured into the twentieth century and contributed to a culture that emphasised personal responsibility for health.

Earlier perceptions of tuberculosis as a disease associated with refinement and sensibility were, to a large extent, transformed by social Darwinism and NAPT propaganda into an understanding of tuberculosis as a disease of the poor.[8] Consequently public health initiatives were, from the 1880s, focused exclusively on working class districts.

Many supporters of the NAPT were motivated by fears of the contaminating influence of the diseased working classes, and Sir William Broadbent, their first chairman, advocated the isolation of all working class consumptives for the benefit of the health of the upper classes.[9] For some of the middle classes tuberculosis came to be seen as a symbol of moral and physical degeneration and a threat to civilised society. As one committee member of the NAPT remarked in 1912:

> The beautiful and rich receive it from the unbeautiful poor...Tubercle attacks failures. It attacks the depressed, the alcoholic, the lunatic of all degrees.[10]

Negligence and moral culpability, as well as inheritance, were still seen as factors contributing to the onset of disease in the early twentieth century. In 1904 the Dean of Canterbury, delivering a sermon at Folkestone, warned his congregation that tuberculosis was a consequence of moral as well as hygienic failings:

> if we neglect the discoveries which have been laid before us by physicians and biologists as to the means by which consumption and similar diseases are spread, we must expect to suffer the consequences in the continuance of those diseases, and in the ravages which they commit amongst us…Be assured that in every case it is by the express and deliberate permission of

---

[7] N. Tomes, The Private Side of Public Health: Sanitary Science, Domestic Hygiene and Germ Theory 1870-1900, *Bulletin of the History of Medicine*, volume 64, 1990

[8] A. Hardy, *The Epidemic Streets*, 1993, pp.258-263; Bulstrode, *Report on Sanatoria,* 1905-6, pp.82-86

[9] L. Bryder, Comments on 'The Historical Decline of Tuberculosis' by Leonard Wilson, *Journal of the History of Medicine*, 46:3, 1991, p.361

[10] H. de Carle Woodcock, *The Doctor and the People*, London: Methuen, 2nd ed., 1912 p. 185

God if any disease or harm actually attacks us.[11]

Whilst many social and medical commentators were all too ready to condemn the victims of consumption for their own moral or hygienic failings, alternative epidemiological interpretations, reflecting other political perspectives, were also possible. At the end of the nineteenth century Arthur Ransome, a leading authority on tuberculosis, laid the blame for the prevalence of the disease at the door of the municipal and national authorities:

> It cannot be said that any direct blame attaches to the families of those who have fallen victim to phthisis. The opprobrium rests rather with the supreme health authorities and with the general public for allowing places of public resort to remain in such a condition as to be a serious source of danger to their frequenters. It is a public scandal that places of amusement and our temples of worship should be allowed to remain without adequate ventilation and without frequent and periodic purification.[12]

Some doctors were of the opinion that the prevalence of chronic disease was not an irreversible problem due to inherited degeneracy, but a state of affairs capable of being remedied by reforming the living conditions of the poor. In contrast to a concern with the relationship between heredity, vice and contagion many writers on tuberculosis from the 1890s emphasised the importance of improved sanitation, light and ventilation in housing, public buildings, schools, factories and transport as a means of negating possible sources of infection. Also some doctors acknowledged the benefits of an improved diet in developing resistance to the disease.[13]

Although public health officials like Ransome warned against the dangers posed by infectious buildings, England was not subject to the same degree of *bacillophobia* that affected public health administrations in Europe and the United States. This is demonstrated by the fact that policies of isolation for the tubercular were adopted at least twenty five years later than on the continent.

---

[11] Sermon preached by the Dean of Canterbury before the members of the Folkestone Sanitary Congress, July 1904, at the parish church of St Mary & St Eanswyth, *Journal of State Medicine*, volume xii, January, 1905

[12] A. Ransome, Consumption, A Filth Disease, *The Lancet*, 1st January, 1898, p.17

[13] For example, J. Niven, *Poverty and Disease*, Presidential Address to the Epidemiological Section of the Royal Society of Medicine, 22nd October, 1900, Proceedings of the Royal Society of Medicine, 3, part 2, 1910, pp.1-45; A. Ransome, Consumption, A Filth Disease, *The Lancet*, 1st January, 1898

Ransome was of the opinion that any shift of medical focus towards the continental model of isolation and disinfection would be "folly" considering that "such a magnificent result" had been achieved purely through sanitary reforms and improved ventilation.[14] In 1898 he pointed out that over the previous 60 years deaths from consumption had been reduced to one third of their former incidence. This was generally acknowledged as being due to the sanitary reform of working class housing and improved nutrition:

> Already the simple measures of improved drainage, better house accommodation, better food &c. which have diminished the death-rate from enteric fever have had some effect upon the mortality from phthisis, reducing it by nearly two-thirds.[15]

That English physicians were reluctant to relinquish environmental and holistic approaches to the control of disease in the face of theories emanating from the continent should not be surprising. They were aware that mortality rates for consumption in England had fallen more rapidly than in other nations, and these successes were considered to result largely from the implementation of sanitary legislation from the 1850s.[16] In 1904, for example, Dr. Nathan Raw, physician to the Liverpool Sanatorium for Consumption, presented a paper at the Folkestone Health Congress arguing that the death rate from consumption in Liverpool had fallen from 430 per 100,000 of the population to 234 per 100,000 in the previous 30 years solely in response to general sanitary and hygienic improvements and, as a consequence of such measures, he anticipated that the disease would rarely be encountered in another 30 years.[17]

How pulmonary tuberculosis was understood at this time was central to the debates that informed public health legislation in the first two decades of the twentieth century. Some doctors, like Hubert de Carle Woodcock, one time Poor Law Medical Officer and committee member of the NAPT, saw the disease as particularly affecting the "social residuum". It was a disease of alcoholics, prostitutes, syphilitics, paupers and casual labourers:

---

[14] A. Ransome, Phthisis Rates: Their Significance and their Teaching, *Transactions of the Epidemiological Society*, 1904-5, p. 281

[15] A. Ransome, Consumption, 1898, p.17

[16] A. Ransome, Consumption, 1898, p.17; M. Worboys, *Spreading Germs*, Cambridge University Press, 2000

[17] N. Raw, *Sanatoria for Consumption*, Folkestone Chronicle & Observer and Canterbury Register, July 30th, 1904

> The drunkards who die in common lodging houses, or who die neglected in the common courts, always show *tubercle*, generally active, in some cases so active that you wonder why they dragged along, and also how many they have infected.[18]

Woodcock's alarmist images appear calculated to persuade the middle classes of the threat that the lowest social stratum posed to respectable citizens. He advised that consumptives should be transferred from sanatoria to hygienic labour colonies in order to prevent risking their relapse on returning to society.[19] For many such social reformers intent on reversing the apparent deterioration of the national stock, germ theory appears to have been employed as an additional argument in support of their policy for the institutionalisation of the unfit and unemployed.

Following the humiliating second Boer War of 1899-1902 the health of the working classes became a more urgent concern for the political establishment. Reports of the poor health of military volunteers exacerbated existing anxieties over the "social question" that had been growing since the 1880s. The broader enfranchisement of workers and their increasing political organisation, together with the economic depressions of 1878-79, 1884-87, 1892-95 and 1903-05 helped to focus attention on the appalling conditions of the urban poor. Social surveys of London and York indicated that between 25% and 30% of urban populations were living in poverty.[20] With growing international competition for markets, particularly from Germany and the United States, it was becoming apparent to the establishment that workers represented a valuable and limited resource for industrial production and the defence of empire.[21]

By 1900 the annual deaths from pulmonary tuberculosis in England and Wales had fallen to 140 per 100,000 of the population from 380 per 100,000 in 1838. Nevertheless this still reflected an annual toll of 50,000 deaths.[22] In 1897 the physician James Lindsay conservatively estimated

---

[18] H. de Carle Woodcock, *The Doctor and the People*, 1912, p.186

[19] Ibid., p.221

[20] C. Booth, *The Life and Labour of the People in London*, 1892-97; B. Seebohm Rowntree, *A Study of Town Life*, 1901

[21] G. Stedman Jones, *Outcast London*, 1971, p.313

[22] Figures cited from the NAPT by M. Worboys, The Sanatoria Treatment for Consumption in Britain 1890-1914, *Medical Innovations in Historical Perspective*, London: MacMillan, ed. J.V. Pickstone, 1992; D. Lloyd George, in a speech at Birmingham on June 10th, 1911, claimed that 70-80,000 lives were annually lost to tuberculosis. Cited in E. R. Pike, *Human Documents of the Lloyd George Era*, London: George Allen & Unwin, 1972

the number of people suffering from the disease in Britain to be not less than a quarter of a million, and of these he judged that 200,000 belonged to the working classes.[23] This obviously represented both a great loss of manpower and a financial burden to ratepayers who subsidised the Poor Law.

A concerted national campaign against the spread of tuberculosis was, therefore, increasingly felt to be essential, particularly in view of the fact that both France and Germany had, earlier in the 1890s, created their own national organisations to combat the spread of tuberculosis. Consequently, in 1899 the National Association for the Prevention of Consumption and Other Forms of Tuberculosis was founded.[24]

The first meeting was attended by the Prime Minister, Lord Salisbury, together with the Prince of Wales, the future King Edward VII. This provided both royal and governmental sanction for the movement.[25] The Association was composed largely of tuberculosis specialists and was chaired by the Prince of Wales' personal doctor Sir William Broadbent. The Association's inauguration coincided with the publication by the energetic Malcolm Morris, editor of *The Practitioner* and first Treasurer of the NAPT, of three issues of his journal devoted to the open-air treatment of tuberculosis and its potential benefits for all classes of society. They included contributions from all leading exponents of the therapy.[26] Both Broadbent and Morris were instrumental in organising the London Conference on Tuberculosis of 1901, of which Broadbent was chairman.[27]

Their campaigns proposed sanatorium treatment and, like the COS, aimed at reforming the behaviour of the poor rather than effecting a reduction of poverty or the improvement of living and working conditions. Although some members did cite poor diets and bad housing as major factors contributing to the spread of tuberculosis, lobbying for social reform was not part of their agenda.

The preventive and educational strategies employed by the NAPT and other agencies during this period were mainly directed at the domestic habits of the working classes. Alcoholism and venereal disease were cited by some members as major causes of the spread of tuberculosis through

---

[23] J. A. Lindsay, Inaugural Address on the Problem of the Consumptive Poor to the Ulster Medical Society, 4th November, 1897, *The Lancet*, 4th December, 1897, p.1435

[24] The organisation changed its title in 1919 to the National Association for the Prevention of Tuberculosis

[25] L. Bryder, *Below the Magic Mountain,* 1988, p.15

[26] *The Practitioner,* June, 1898, July, 1899 and July, 1901

[27] *BMJ*, 16th November, 1918, 3020, p.539

compromising the immune system. Drinking and sexual promiscuity were targeted, together with spitting and a lack of cleanliness, in the NAPT's propaganda war against tuberculosis.[28] These campaigns, directed solely at the working classes, attached particular emphasis to the dangers of infection arising from insanitary and immoral habits that were considered particularly prevalent amongst the lower social orders.[29] The NAPT were not simply concerned with propagating domestic hygiene, they were attempting to regulate the behaviour of the working classes in accordance with their own moral codes. It has been argued that, together with related campaigns against physical degeneration and alcoholic mothers, the anti-tuberculosis campaign was "amongst the most powerful assaults on working-class culture mounted in the Edwardian period", and resulted in many sufferers of tuberculosis being treated as social outcasts.[30]

Whilst the catalyst for the founding of the NAPT was the conviction that tuberculosis could be conquered through the isolation of the *tubercle bacillus,* many members were strongly influenced by evolutionist ideas, which held sway into the post-war period. As Malcolm Morris recalled in 1918, an initial focus on the microbe had resulted in hereditary and environmental factors being pushed to the background:

> It may be that even at the present time the predominance given to infection is an obstacle to the full realisation of the importance of the environment...[and] Pre-natal influence has more to do with the spread of consumption than we have of late allowed, and is a more potent factor in the dissemination of effective tuberculosis than is infection.[31]

Paradoxically, as bacteriology redirected the focus of health reformers from the environment to the individual, the eugenic perception of the existence of a fundamental trait that predisposed a certain type of person to contracting the disease was reinforced. Whilst the anti-tuberculosis crusade led to an increasing focus on the dangers posed by the tuberculous individual infection alone did not explain why the majority of individuals who were found to be infected by the *bacillus* failed to develop active tuberculosis. For a majority in the medical profession in the early

---

[28] J. Burns, *Transactions of the NAPT,* Annual Conference, Caxton Hall, Westminster, July 19-21, 1911, Adland & Son, London, p.24

[29] L. Bryder, *Below the Magic Mountain,* 1988, p.19

[30] M. Worboys, Spreading Germs, *Medical Innovations in Historical Perspective*, London: MacMillan, ed. J.V. Pickstone, 1992

[31] M. Morris, The Past and Future of the Crusade Against Tuberculosis, *BMJ*, 16th November, 1918, p.540

twentieth century this anomaly was explained by their inherited predisposition.[32]

Despite periods of quiescence pulmonary tuberculosis was generally a protracted disease, and this chronicity lent the consumptive a particular identity. This construction of a biologically defective "type" who was also considered by many to be a source of contagion further stigmatised sufferers of tuberculosis, causing many to hide their condition. As Folkestone's Tuberculosis Officer observed in 1949 the NAPT's emphasis on infection and predisposition often served to further alienate sufferers:

> the disastrous effect of such prejudice is to drive them to conceal their disease and thus become real or potential dangers to the healthy people among whom they live. Frank acceptance of the active tuberculosis cases among all classes of the community would do much to check the spread of the disease; the fear of isolation and ostracism is one of the primary causes of its spread. The NAPT might not exist for all that has been accomplished towards ameliorating the mental suffering and loneliness of the tuberculous.[33]

In contrast, the dangers posed by financially independent individuals suffering from tuberculosis appeared to warrant little or no regulation. The anti-tuberculosis campaign's focus on the infective potential of dust did, however, have the effect of initiating revolutions in fashion, interior décor, design and architecture, and, arguably, reinforcing anxieties over dirt in general. From the 1890s doctors had warned against the risk of contracting tuberculosis from dust, advising that it be collected on a damp cloth rather than being dispersed with a broom. It was felt that contaminated dust could gather in heavy Victorian fabrics, curtains, tapestries and in ornately carved furniture and thick carpets.[34] Henceforth furnishings inclined towards simplicity; smooth and washable surfaces gradually replaced elaborate and ornamental décor. Linoleum and tiled floors were introduced because they were easy to clean. Washable, rather than flock or embossed wallpapers, came into vogue. Blinds offered an hygienic alternative to heavy drapes and curtains. Clothing became lighter and less layered, and facial hair was considerably reduced by the Edwardian era.[35]

Another consequence of the late-nineteenth century concern with urbanisation, degeneration and tuberculosis - the social effects of industrial

---

[32] J. A. Mendelsohn, Medicine and the making of Bodily Inequality in 20th Century Europe, *Heredity and Infection*, eds. J. Gaudillière & I. Löwy, 2003, p.28

[33] B. G. Edelston, The Ostracism of the Tubercular, *The Lancet*, July 16th, 1949

[34] M. Campbell, What tuberculosis did for Modernism, 2005, pp.466-69

[35] Ibid, pp.477-8

capitalism and urban pollution - was to scientifically validate and reinforce the popularity of climatology and marine health resorts.

The Rise of Seaside Health Resorts

The concept of climatology and the beneficial effects of residence in specific locations can be traced back at least as far as Hippocrates, but it is significant that the Victorians' enthusiasm for health resorts coincided with a growing conviction of the risks to health associated with living in overcrowded industrialised towns and cities. By the middle of the nineteenth century, and for the first time in the history of humanity, more people lived in cities than in the country.[36] Many felt the attraction of a return to a more bucolic existence, and the unsullied climate of the coastal health resort came to be seen as a natural panacea for the corruptions of the city. This quotation adorned the frontispiece of Spencer Thomson's *Health Resorts of Britain*, published in 1860:

> Ye who amid this feverish world would wear
> A body free from pain, of cares a mind,
> Fly the rank city, shun its turbid air;
> Breathe not the chaos of eternal smoke
> And volatile corruption.[37]

The image of the polluted and polluting city permeated nineteenth century religious, literary and medical thought and, as argued above, according to the holistic medical nosology of the time both moral and physical corruption were seen to emanate from the pestilence and excesses of city life.[38] This pathologising of the city as the locus of sin and disease encouraged the nineteenth century growth of marine health resorts. It also shaped the Victorian and Edwardian obsession with the health giving qualities of fresh air, and their perception of the pathological effects of polluted or "rebreathed" air. This preoccupation with respiration reflects a *miasmatically* informed understanding of air as potentially both purifying and contaminating, and illuminates the importance of outdoor activities and natural therapies for the middle classes. As tuberculosis came to be

---

[36] R. Williams, *The Country and the City,* 1975, p.217

[37] J. Armstrong, *The Art of Preserving Health,* quoted in S. Thomson, *Health Resorts of Britain; and how to profit by them*, London: Ward & Lock, 1860

[38] C. T. Moloney, *George Eliot, Henry James and Consumption: A Shadow on the Lung of the Victorian Psyche*', University of London PhD thesis, 1999

seen as a disease of civilisation,[39] of urban pollution and corruption, so its prevention and cure necessitated a return to nature.[40]

Central to this more holistic medical approach was a return to the Hippocratic tradition, fundamental to which was a recognition of the healing powers of nature, and a rejection of the decontextualised and mechanistic basis of the Galenic system.[41] The therapeutic effects of coastal environments came to be recognised in England from about 1800 following the emergence of a general philosophy of Romantic medicine in Germany which emphasised the importance of social and environmental conditions as determinants of health and illness. Both the practice of hydrotherapy and the open-air treatment of pulmonary tuberculosis were established in Silesia before being imported to England.[42]

Although Brighton, Margate and Scarborough were visited for their waters from the late eighteenth century all of these resorts had developed from a tradition of spa towns, originally supplying spring water and, during the early nineteenth century, selling bottled seawater and attracting early adherents of the continental therapy of sea bathing. Only Brighton however, attracted any significant number of visitors before the advent of the railway in the mid-nineteenth century.[43]

In 1840 George Bodington's claims for the efficacy of fresh air, rest and a plentiful diet in treating consumption were critiqued by *The Lancet* as being "very crude ideas and unsupported assertions".[44] At this time, although an elite of the nobility and intelligentsia were embracing the newly discovered tonic properties of the air and sea, much of the population still considered the English coast to be unsuitable for invalids. Humoural models of health and sickness, wherein illness was perceived as the consequence of a systemic imbalance of humours rather than a localised disorder, generally held that a shock to the system, particularly through exposure to sudden changes in temperature, could trigger the

---

[39] A. Latham & C. Garland, *The Conquest of Consumption,* [1910], London, T. Fisher Unwin, 2nd edition, 1911, p.15

[40] L. Bryder, 'Wonderlands of buttercup, clover and daisies', 1992, p.73

[41] H. De Almeida, *Romantic Medicine and John Keats,* Oxford University Press, 1991, p.34

[42] H. Weber, The Croonian Lectures on The Hygienic and Climatic Treatment of Chronic Pulmonary Phthisis, *BMJ*, March 28th, April 4th & 11th, 1885, p.688

[43] J. Hassan, *The Seaside, Health and the Environment in England and Wales since 1800,* Ashgate Publishing Ltd, 2002, pp.15-16

[44] Quoted in R. & J. Dubos [1952], *The White Plague: Tuberculosis, Man and Society,* Rutgers University Press, 1987, p.175. *The Lancet*, however, did acknowledge Bodington's pioneering work on his death in 1882, R. & J. Dubos, *The White Plague,* p.177

onset of disease. Consequently, particularly in the eighteenth and early nineteenth centuries, exposure to the elements was avoided. Patients suffering from tuberculosis, such as John Keats, were nursed in warm rooms with closed windows, fed on a bland and restricted diet and cautioned against the damaging effects of draughts.[45]

René Dubos's seminal work on tuberculosis claimed that until the 1870s the English medical profession "continued to regard abundant food and fresh air as poisons for the tuberculous patient".[46] There is, however, evidence that physicians often recommended the beneficial effects of the English coast decades earlier.[47] Many of the leisured classes had availed themselves of the benefits of English coastal health resorts throughout the nineteenth century, as illustrated in Jane Austen's final, unfinished novel *Sanditon,* written in 1817*,* in which Parker, the promoter of the eponymous health resort, proclaims:

> The sea air and sea bathing together are nearly infallible, one or the other of them being a match for every disorder, of the stomach, the lungs or the blood.[48]

It is also evident from the detailed and sensitive treatise on the treatment of consumption, scrofula and nervous disorders penned in 1853 by George Moseley, surgeon to the Sandgate dispensary, that a number of health resorts on the south coast of England had been established by that time:

> When so many localities have been selected in accordance with tradition, or have been favoured by a species of prescription, along our south coast as resorts for the invalid, it requires some confidence to endeavour to add to the list, and to point to one more spot where nature may be relied on as a kind help-mate to the physician in checking the progress of disease, in recruiting the shattered constitution, and in restoring the shattered energies

[45] R .& J. Dubos, *The White Plague*, 1987, p.12

[46] Ibid., p.175

[47] N. Blundell, *The Great diurnal of Nicholas Blundell of Little Crosby, Lancashire,* Transcribed and annotated by F. Tyrer, ed. J. J. Bagley. 3 volumes Manchester: Record Society of Lancashire & Cheshire, 1968-72 volume I, p.257; B. W. Richardson, *The Hygienic Treatment of Pulmonary Consumption*, London: John Churchill, 1857; J. H. Bennet, *On the Treatment of Pulmonary Consumption by Hygiene, Climate and Medicine*, London: John Churchill, 1866

[48] J. Austen, Sanditon, 1817, *Minor Works,* Vol. VI, ed. R.W. Chapman, Oxford University Press, 1963

of mind and body.[49]

It is undoubtedly the case that the development of the health resort in England achieved wider popularity due to the growing reputation of the practice of open-air therapy in Germany. Hermann Brehmer's sanatorium at Gorbersdorf in the Silesian mountains, which opened in 1854, together with his former patient Peter Dettweiler's sanatorium established at Falkenstein in 1876, have been acknowledged as the progenitors of open-air treatment for consumption, and were responsible for persuading many English doctors of the value of the treatment.[50]

Three distinct periods of health resort development in England have been identified. In the late eighteenth century Brighton, Margate, Hastings and Scarborough were the first resorts to attract the affluent and fashionable. These were superseded by the suburban Regency resorts, such as Hove and St. Leonards, which succeeded them as destinations for the wealthy health seeker following the formers' increased popularity amongst the lower middle classes. The Victorian resorts originated in the mid-nineteenth century,[51] and the rapid development of the majority of these resorts, for example Bournemouth, Blackpool and Eastbourne, from small settlements in the 1850s was due chiefly to the advent of the railway, economic growth, and an increase in the population of the urban middle classes.[52] Although it became easier to visit the coast from the 1850s it was primarily a desire for improved health, together with the medical profession's endorsement of the curative potential of health resorts, that motivated people to visit the seaside at this time.

The rise of the health resort has also been associated with the emergence of that peculiarly nineteenth century phenomenon, the "invalid". Evangelism, self-help ideology, an increase in the status of the medical profession and the development of new diagnostic technologies have all been recognised as facilitating the emergence of the invalid as a specific identity.[53] Certainly the evangelical perception of suffering as denoting a mark of grace and the Victorian obsession with health provided

---

[49] G. Moseley, *Sandgate as a Residence for Invalids*, London: John Churchill, 1853, p.1

[50] R. & J. Dubos, *The White Plague*, 1987, p.176

[51] S. Farrant, London By The Sea: Resort Development on the South Coast of England 1880-1939, *Journal of Contemporary History*, volume 22, no.1, 1987, pp.138-9

[52] J. Hassan, *The Seaside, Health and the Environment*, 2002, p.37

[53] M. H. Frawley, *Invalidism and Identity in Nineteenth Century Britain,* University of Chicago Press, 2004

a strong social sanction for the invalid.[54] Indeed, open air therapy provided a greater opportunity for the social interaction of many wealthy invalids. Whereas, previously, the chronically ill would generally have been confined to bed, from the mid-nineteenth century the more affluent were regularly in evidence on marine terraces and parades in hired bath chairs.

It was not only the confirmed invalid who sought health by the sea. The maintenance of health was equally as important, particularly for those deemed to possess a weak constitution or an hereditary tendency to consumption. Sea bathing and the benefits of sea breezes were seen as fundamental to the practice of preventive medicine during the second half of the nineteenth century, although being generally restricted to a social elite.

The chronic nature of tuberculosis dictated that, until the 1890s, the restorative effects of health resorts were generally only accorded to the financially independent who could afford a lengthy treatment. Many of those afflicted with the disease who were able to take advantage of a good diet, salubrious environment and medical advice, such as John Ruskin, Robert Louis Stevenson and H. G. Wells, were able to extend their lives considerably. In contrast, the fate of even respectable working families was invariably increasing poverty as the disease rendered the victim unable to work, and an early death. Mrs. F. J. Pedlar, biographer of the Peppard sanatorium near Reading, recalled that, until the twentieth century, open-air therapy was generally seen as unsuitable for the working classes. It would have been considered "better for him to be allowed to die quickly, which would be what he would expect".[55]

For most of the nineteenth century the open-air cure and the health resort were predominantly resources available exclusively for the wealthy, whilst the lower classes benefited only through the opportunities this provided for their seasonal employment.

In some resorts, such as Folkestone and Eastbourne, aristocratic landowners were responsible for planning, creating and controlling the environment, and for developing the market.[56] Whilst in other resorts land companies and syndicates were also involved in resort development.[57] The success of the most elite resorts depended on the creation of particularly

---

[54] C. Herzlich and J. Pierret, *Illness and Self in Society*, Johns Hopkins Press, 1987

[55] Mrs. F. J. Pedlar, *The Maitland Story,* Maitland Trust, ca. 1968, p.4

[56] D. Cannadine, *Lords and Landlords: The Aristocracy and the Towns 1774-1967,* Leicester University Press, 1980, pp.412-413

[57] J. K. Walton, *The English Seaside Resort, A Social History, 1750-1914,* D.Phil thesis, University of Kent, 1977, p.105

well controlled and elegantly designed spaces.[58] Often patterns of landholding dictated the character and "social tone" of the town. Single landowners were generally more able to create a style that would attract the elite of society, whilst resorts with multiple landowners, such as Morecombe and Blackpool, were less likely to maintain social exclusivity.[59] Location and topography, as well as the constitution of its local authority, could also contribute to the character of a resort.[60]

The position of Folkestone, possessing a direct travel link to both London and Europe, its titled landowner and the proximity of the Shorncliffe military camp all contributed to its status as a socially exclusive health resort. The social network of the aristocracy was international, and Folkestone provided a convenient and picturesque retreat for both European and British nobility and businessmen. In addition, the topography of the town effectively separated the homes of the working classes from the terraces, parades, apartments and hotels designed for the affluent visitor and resident. Folkestone competed with other resorts with a proximity to London, such as Bexhill and Eastbourne, where the investment of the landowner and the association with an aristocratic name were employed to attract the affluent and fashionable from the snares of the metropolis.[61]

Resorts that depended on maintaining an image of salubrity and social exclusivity would have been characterised by an insistence on social deference and compliance from workers, who competed for limited, seasonal employment.[62] Trade unions were notoriously difficult to organise in such monopolistic economies and potential troublemakers would have been excluded from the workforce.[63]

Most resorts lacked any manufacturing or industrial economy. Corporation jobs would generally have been the most sought after due to their relative security. Public utilities and railways provided some permanent employment, otherwise jobs would mostly have been casual

---

[58] J. K. Walton, *The English Seaside Resort*, 1977, p.103

[59] H. J. Perkin, The '*Social Tone*' of Victorian Seaside Resorts in the North-West, *Northern History* 11, 1976; J. Hassan, *The Seaside, Health and the Environment,* 2002, pp.37-38

[60] J. Hassan, *The Seaside, Health and the Environment,* 2002, p.38

[61] S. Farrant, *London By The Sea*, 1987, p.140

[62] J. K. Walton, *The British Seaside: Holidays and Resorts in the Twentieth Century,* Manchester University Press, 2000, p.6

[63] J. K. Walton, *The British Seaside*, 2000, p.148

and seasonal. Shops and hotels were the worst paid.[64] Construction and related trades were also dependent on the number of visitors the town could attract in the summer. They were also often limited by restrictive building regulations imposed by the ground landlord in order to maintain the town's "social tone".

Resort workers would have been subject to constant insecurity and stress due to the largely casual and unpredictable nature of employment opportunities.[65] In addition the working population was likely to have been fragmented and socially dislocated, with many workers being attracted from poorly paid and arduous agricultural jobs or from industrial centres further afield.[66]

Fishing communities that had generally constituted the heart of the indigenous population were often marginalised and isolated. Possessing their own culture, dialect and knowledge of the local environment, they were regarded by some residents and visitors as lazy, malodorous and morally suspect.[67] Over time fishing communities were forced to adapt to the wider community. There is evidence to suggest that some Kentish locals combined work on the spring sowing with the mackerel fishing between May and July, the summer harvest, and the herring catch in October and November.[68] Fishing was a dangerous and precarious livelihood, being dependent on the weather and fish stocks, and some boat owners would have supplemented their income by providing fishing trips and excursions for visitors.

The economic structure of the health resort was dominated by boarding houses and the letting of apartments and lodgings. Large numbers of, mostly female, workers were employed as servants, cleaners and laundrymaids during the season, assisting the often widowed or spinster landladies who generally ran such establishments.[69] The letting of rooms was so widespread that, quite apart from the hundreds of lodging houses listed in local directories, even working class visitors could be

---

64 R. Tressell, *The Ragged Trousered Philanthropists,* London, Lawrence & Wishart, 1914, quoted in J. K. Walton, *The British Seaside,* p.144; Tressell (Robert Noonan) worked as a signwriter and decorator and died of consumption in Liverpool workhouse in 1911

65 J. K. Walton, *The British Seaside,* 2000, p.144

66 Elham Board of Guardians, April 1904, quoted in *Hythe and Sandgate Standard,* April 9th, 1904

67 J. K. Walton, *The British Seaside,* 2000, p.146

68 T. Richardson, Labour, *The Economy of Kent 1640-1914,* Boydell Press, ed. Alan Armstrong, 1995, p.254

69 J. K. Walton, *The British Seaside,* 2000, p.149

accommodated in out of the way districts of resorts on an informal basis.[70]

Due to the coincidence of the Victorian preoccupation with health, the medical profession's confidence in the beneficial effects of the marine climate on consumption, continued economic growth and the expansion of the middle classes, the population of health resorts expanded rapidly during the second half of the nineteenth century. The sanitary provisions of many towns, such as Bognor Regis and Seaford, were seriously stretched, and local authorities sometimes found themselves unable to manage the increasing demand for water and sanitation.[71] In many instances the short term interests of property owners and investors took precedence over public health, jeopardising the wellbeing of the growing number of workers who were employed to service these health resorts. Local councils were often more likely to invest in schemes designed to attract visitors than in environmental reforms.[72]

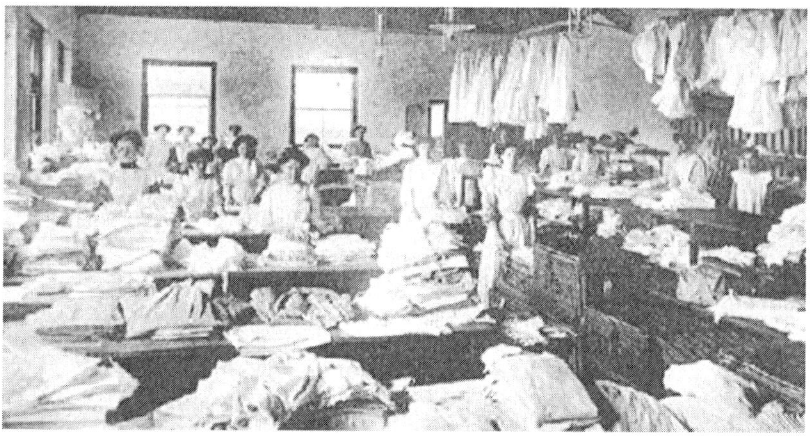

Illustration 3.1: A 1924 photograph of the Sanitary Steam Laundry, one of several laundries in Cheriton, a suburb of Folkestone. Many women moved to Folkestone to find employment there.

In many respects Folkestone and its much smaller neighbour Sandgate, virtually a suburb of the former, are typical of Victorian health resorts. Influential residents and local doctors responded to a demand for

[70] R. Craig & J. Whyman, Kent and the Sea, *The Economy of Kent, 1640-1914*, Boydell Press, ed. Alan Armstrong 1995, p.201
[71] S. Farrant, *London By The Sea*, 1987, p.138
[72] J. Hassan, *The Seaside, Health and the Environment,* 2002, p.44

accommodation by the sea by cultivating an image of refinement and salubrity for the towns. Both resorts successfully developed a reputation for possessing an invigorating climate in a sheltered location where people of a similar social background could meet and interact in an atmosphere of exclusivity.

As argued throughout this section, the causes and symptoms of tuberculosis were interpreted both positively and negatively during the nineteenth and early twentieth centuries. For the fashionable and affluent tuberculosis could be perceived as a gentle, wasting decline. A condition characterised by slenderness, an arresting pallor and flushed cheeks, and an intense, often erratic imagination. This representation became modified later in the century to accord with the emergent middle class values of self-discipline and moral restraint. The coastal and alpine health resort emerged as a popular therapeutic destination for consumptives belonging to the leisured classes, particularly from the 1850s. In contrast tuberculosis amongst the working classes during this period signified economic, moral and physical degradation, the slum, the asylum and the workhouse. Treatment was rarely provided until the sufferer was moribund and incapable of work. The disease was more likely to be associated with degeneration, foul breath, night sweats, spasmodic coughing, spewed blood and putrid clotted sputum.

The following section examines Folkestone's development as a health resort together with the effects of population growth on the health of the town. The topography of the town, a river valley surrounded by steep hills, facilitated the geographical separation of social classes, and it is this feature of the town that provides an opportunity for a comparison of the incidence and experience of ill health, particularly pulmonary tuberculosis and childhood mortality, of different social classes. The time scale of the study permits an appraisal of the impact of bacteriology and notions of infection on the functioning of the health resort as well as on the general public health of the town. The influence of the ground landlord and the Borough Council on the character and economy of the town is assessed, as is the role of successive Medical Officers of Health, their relationship with the Borough Council and their effect on the health of the town.

PART II:

PUBLIC HEALTH AND PRIVATE INTERESTS

Chapter Four

Fashionable Folkestone: The Creation of an Exclusive Health Resort

Folkestone, situated on the south east coast of England overlooking the English channel, was a small fishing town during the eighteenth century until its expansion in 1825. The de Bouverie family, landowners of larger estates in Wiltshire and Berkshire, purchased the 3,266 acre manor of Folkestone and surrounding estates in 1697. William de Bouverie was created Baron of Longford and Viscount Folkestone in 1747. In 1765 his son acceded to the title of Earl of Radnor and Baron Pleydell Bouverie of Coleshill.[1] In 1825 William, the third Earl of Radnor, developed 550 acres of land on the cliffs above the old fishing town.

The town grew rapidly following its connection by railway to London in 1843, the purchase and dredging of its mortgaged and silted harbour by the South Eastern Railway (originally the Harbour Company) in 1848 and the introduction of cross channel packet steamers in the same year. It was, however, predominantly the promotion by the Borough Council and local dignitaries of the beneficial effects to be derived from Folkestone's climate and sheltered seaside location that launched the town's career as a health resort for the affluent and fashionable classes. From this time until the First World War increasing numbers of residents and visitors were attracted to the town.

Sir Astley Cooper, senior physician to Guys Hospital, was the first to recommend the therapeutic qualities of Folkestone to his patients and colleagues. In the 1840s and 1850s he was responsible for filling nearly all available accommodation for visitors in the town.[2] The Souvenir Guide to Folkestone for the Congress of the Royal Sanitary Institute of 1921

---

[1] S. J. Mackie, *A Handbook of Folkestone for* Visitors, London: J. English, Simpkin & Marshall, 1856, p.28

[2] Alderman Sherwood at a meeting of the Association of Public Sanitary Inspectors at Folkestone in 1889, quoted in *Folkestone Express*, September 7th, 1889

recounts that:

> the discovery, by a few London physicians, of the health-giving properties of its atmosphere, led to their sending patients here to recuperate, and also to its rapid expansion.[3]

The de Bouverie family had leased much of the western part of Folkestone to building syndicates and commercial enterprises to develop grand hotels, apartments and restaurants. None of the estate was relinquished freehold until 1910.[4] Consequently, political influence in the town was dominated by a property and business owning elite. The chief concern of Folkestone's landowning and merchant class appears to have been in maintaining the atmosphere of social exclusivity created in the west of the town. In order to deter the lower social classes certain social and economic expedients were employed from the 1870s. Rents in the cliff-top development were kept high in order to restrict residence to the very affluent.[5] The fourth Earl of Radnor (1869-1889) employed a policeman to patrol the Leas and exclude the socially unsuitable. Additionally William Pleydell-Bouverie, the fifth Earl of Radnor (1889-1900), managed to avoid an unwelcome influx of the lower classes by entering into negotiations with the owners of the London, Chatham and Dover and the South Eastern Railways during the 1890s.

Whilst the railway provided a steadily increasing seasonal influx of society health seekers, it also posed a potential threat to the "social tone" of high class resorts during the "railway age" of the later nineteenth century. Radnor, with the support of the Borough Council, ensured that fares for the journey from London to Folkestone remained more expensive than for the roughly equidistant journey between London and Margate.[6] Whereas a fare of £1 was established between London and Margate, a resort increasingly visited by London artisans and shopworkers in the 1890s, a more expensive fare of £1/4 shillings was charged to reach Folkestone. Also no cheap day tickets to Folkestone were available until the end of the century.[7]

---

[3] Souvenir guide to the 1921 Folkestone Health Congress, EKAC Fo-A/Z/7/36

[4] A. Nevill, *The Story of Folkestone*, Eastbourne: A. Rowe, 2009, p.37

[5] G. C. Sharp, *The Aristocracy and the Development of Seaside Resorts*, 1989, p.50

[6] *Folkestone Up to Date,* March 4th, 1893

[7] A. Nevill, *Dickens in Folkestone*, Folkestone and District Local History Society, 2002

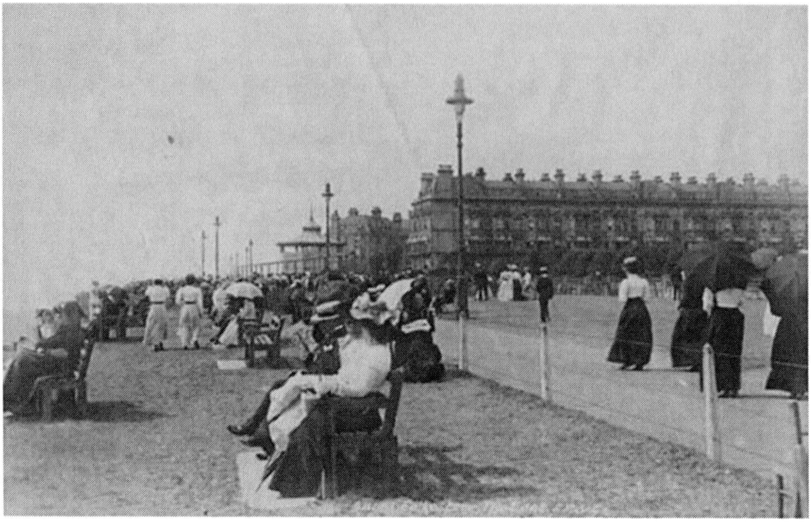

Illustration 4.1: The Leas in 1901

Although the Radnors retained tight control of the planning and development of the town they were often criticised by residents for leaving the running of the estate to their agents. This applied particularly to the fourth Earl who had no residence in the town.[8] As was the case with other aristocratically financed resorts, the local Council did become more involved in the development of Folkestone's reputation from the 1880s.[9] The Borough Council invested in advertising the town's climatological advantages and facilities in London newspapers,[10] and co-operated with Pleydell-Bouverie to oppose the owner of the South Eastern Railway, Sir Edward Watkin, in order to exclude day-trippers.[11]

Thus Folkestone gained its renown in the nineteenth century as a fashionable but quiet health resort catering chiefly for the "upper and travelling classes", and accommodating both long-term and short-term visitors.[12] In 1882 George Hart of Bates' Hotel emphasised the distinctively

---

[8] A. Nevill, *Dickens in Folkestone*, Folkestone and District Local History Society, 2002, p.57

[9] S. Farrant, London By The Sea, 1987, p.138

[10] Folkestone Borough Council minutes, 1899, EKAC-Fo/AMc/5

[11] G. C. Sharp, *The Aristocracy and the Development of Seaside Resorts*, 1989, p.67

[12] J. B. Yeo, *Climate and Health Resorts*, London: Chapman & Hall, 1885

patrician character of the town:

> My houses are patronised almost exclusively by the nobility and aristocracy. The great inducement that they have in coming to Folkestone that it is a quiet and select watering place, unlike Ramsgate and Margate. Any influx of cheap day trippers I should look upon as a disaster.[13]

In support of Folkesatone's reputation for exclusivity research for 1901 shows that Folkestone residents employed a higher percentage of servants than any other town on the south-east coast.[14] The preponderance of private schools established in Folkestone during the late nineteenth century constitutes a further index of the town's reputation as a salubrious and genteel health resort. By 1904 there were 31 private schools for girls and 20 for boys, excluding national schools, private tutors and army "crammers".[15] Mackie's *Guide to Folkestone* of 1883 remarks that no tradesmens' children were accepted at these exclusive educational establishments.[16]

In keeping with Folkestone's image as a prosperous and select health resort the developers of its west ward had taken particular pains to accommodate the bath chair user. The prominent Folkestone physician Charles Egerton Fitzgerald was moved to remark on the "delightfully smooth and level path, far superior to the gravelled parades and flagged pavements of other sea side towns" which the mile and a half long asphalted Leas at Folkestone offered for the bath chair incumbent, augmented after 1885 with hydraulic lifts to transport invalid and conveyance from cliff-top to sea level.[17]

Tuberculosis was the complaint deemed to derive most benefit from a visit to Folkestone or Sandgate, it was certainly the most prevalent chronic disease of the nineteenth century. Promoting Sandgate in 1853 the local dispensary surgeon, George Moseley, claimed:

---

[13] G. Hart, quoted in A. Nevill, *The Story of Folkestone*, Eastbourne: A. Rowe, 2009, p.179

[14] J. K. Walton, *The English Seaside Resort, A Social History, 1750-1914,* D.Phil thesis, University of Kent, 1977

[15] *Folkestone Chronicle and Observer*, 16th January, 1904

[16] S. J. Mackie, *A Descriptive and Historical Account of Folkestone and its Neighbourhood with Gleanings from the Municipal Records*, 2nd edition, Folkestone, J. English, 1883, p.98, cited in Sharp, *The Aristocracy and the Development of Seaside Resorts*, 1989, p.56

[17] C. E. Fitzgerald, *Folkestone as a Health Resort*, p.8, paper delivered at a meeting of the Association of Public Sanitary Inspectors at Folkestone in 1889, Folkestone Library

In cases of scrofula, glandular disease, necrosis and bronchitis, the climate is found assisting the efforts of the physician in a remarkable degree…It is, however, more particularly as a resort of patients threatened with, or actually suffering from consumption, that Sandgate deserves to be noticed.[18]

And in 1895 the promotional brochure for *Beach Rocks* convalescent home declared:

The absence of cold winds and small range of the thermometer render Sandgate particularly favourable for *phthisical* patients…scrofulous patients also derive great benefit.[19]

Writing about Folkestone in 1885 the *London Medical Record* stated:

Folkestone is eminently a place for invalids in the first stage of consumption, as the air is pure and bracing without being too cold.[20]

And in the same year the climatologist and specialist in tubercular complaints, J. Burney Yeo, noted in a guide to health resorts that at Folkestone:

The climate is considered suitable to many forms of chest disease, to cases of early *phthisis*, to cases of chronic *catarrhal* tendencies in the over sensitive and scrofulous.[21]

Likewise, Folkestone physician Arthur E. Larking in his 1889 publication, *Notes on Folkestone,* commends the town as particularly suitable for the treatment of consumption and scrofula, but feels it necessary to add the proviso that the town was not a *lazaret*:

Folkestone does not aspire to attract the common invalid and the consumptive, to the exclusion of all other members of the community. It is not a place where the crowds of pallid and thin faces testify to the sadder side of life, with its illness and suffering.[22]

---

[18] G. Moseley, *Sandgate as a Residence for Invalids*, London: John Churchill, 1853, p.1

[19] *Particulars of Beach Rocks Convalescent Home*, The London Samaritan Society and Homerton Mission, Sandgate, 1895

[20] Quoted in *Folkestone Chronicle*, 27th June, 1885

[21] J. Burney Yeo, *Climate and Health Resorts*, London: Chapman & Hall, 1885

[22] A. E. Larking, *Notes on Folkestone Historical, Climatological and Medical*, London: J&A Churchill, 1889

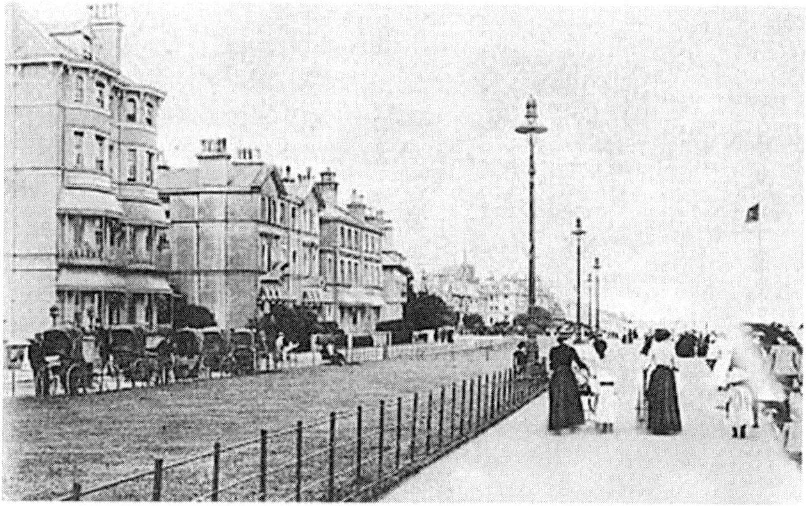

Illustration 4.2: Bath chairs for hire on the Leas. These would have been pulled by hand and fares were regulated by the Council. This photograph probably dates from the late 1890s.

It was well known that health resorts were often used as places of residence by those afflicted with tuberculosis and scrofula.[23] A correspondent to *The Lancet* in 1910 claimed that all seaside resorts attracted tubercular residents:

> it is a matter of common knowledge that in every seaside and health resort in every part of the world consumptives take up their residence with the object of recovery or dragging on an existence, and making a living by letting lodgings

This claim, although difficult to verify due to the reluctance of many victims of tuberculosis to acknowledge their disease, suggests that some sufferers dependent on earning an income may have chosen to invest in a seaside property in the hope of alleviating their condition whilst still making a living. Consequently resorts, or districts of resorts, catering for the lower social classes may have attracted a disproportionately high number of tuberculosis sufferers.

---

[23] Letter to *The Lancet*, 21st May, 1910; also F. P. Weber, *BMJ*, 20th December, 1919

Equally, medical practitioners were to find increasing opportunities to build practices at coastal resorts.[24] In 1875 *The Lancet* noted that:

> The medical profession have regarded [Folkestone] favourably, and a considerable number of persons suffering from chronic affections are annually recommended to reside there.[25]

As metropolitan physicians were often called upon to recommend suitable health resorts where appropriate accommodation, medical supervision and the opportunity for exercise were available, it seems likely that connections soon became established between Folkestone practitioners and their London colleagues.

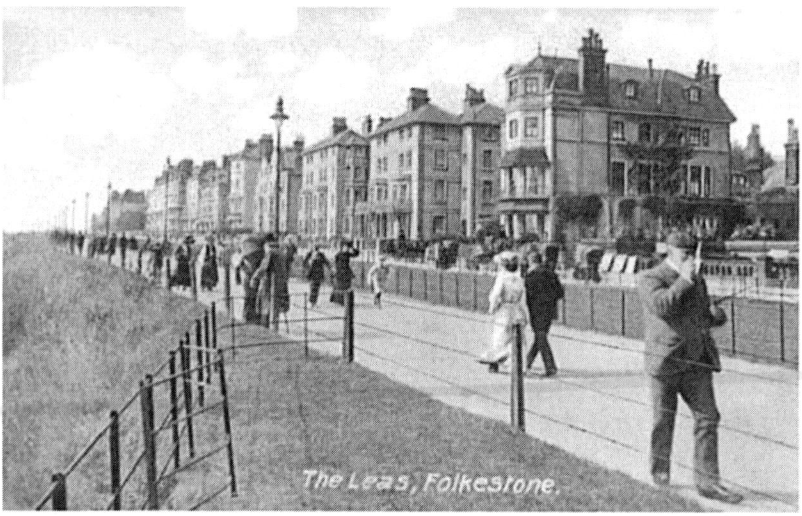

Illustration 4.3: The Leas in 1907

The livelihood of doctors, hotel and property owners and the majority of the town's population depended to a large extent on the publication of favourable health statistics. The regular publication of local mortality data by the General Register Office provided scientific evidence for the sanitary achievements of local administrations that enabled them to

[24] According to the 1899 census there were 22 physicians and 10 surgeons resident in Folkestone.

[25] *The Lancet*, Report on the Sanitary Condition of Folkestone, 17th April, 1875

compete with other towns and cities for commercial expansion.[26] Information regarding the health of towns was particularly sensitive in the case of health resorts, and tended to be used selectively. Comparative medical, climatological and geological data was constantly employed to attract health seekers and to bolster civic pride.[27]

Folkestone's medical practitioners were quick to draw attention to the various natural advantages afforded to the inhabitants and visitors of the town, particularly those which accorded with the latest developments in medical theory. The situation, soil, quality of air, quantity of rainfall, hours of sunshine and range of temperature were all considered propitious for the treatment of tuberculosis at Folkestone and Sandgate. In 1889 Charles Egerton Fitzgerald claimed that:

> for many pulmonary affections where a pure and bracing, but not too keen air is recommended, I know of no place which so effectually combines all these requirements as our own town of Folkestone. It stands to reason that when from any cause, the capacity of the lungs is diminished, the inspired air should make up in quality and in pureness what it lacks in quantity; hence the advantage of high mountain places like Davos Platz, or pure sea air resorts like Folkestone, in the treatment of pulmonary complaints. The day has long passed when warm and enervating places were considered the only suitable winter resorts for invalids.[28]

In addition to the bracing qualities of its air, Folkestone, together with Ventnor, laid claim to being the only town on the south coast situated on greensand, an extremely porous soil permitting easy drainage and discouraging dampness:

> The soil of Folkestone is greensand [which] being a very porous stratum, absorbs the rainfall immediately, so that we have an entire absence of fog, damp and mist, which are inevitable with a heavier soil which allows water to lodge. So porous indeed is the soil that within a short time after heavy rain the roads are dry and clean and ready for walking.[29]

---

[26] S. Szreter, *A Central Role for Local Government? The Example of Late Victorian Britain*, www.historyandpolicy.org, 16.10.08., p.3

[27] S. Szreter, The Importance of Social Intervention in Britain's Mortality Decline c.1850-1914, *Social History of Medicine*, 1, 1988, pp. 21-23

[28] C. E. Fitzgerald, *Folkestone as a Health Resort,* 1889, p.6

[29] Ibid.

A damp climate was seen as notoriously conducive to the development of pulmonary tuberculosis. As William Ewart observed in 1907:

> Great Britain has lost its evil name as the home of *phthisis* mainly thanks to the drainage of its damp soil...The intense sensitiveness of the cutaneous surface of many consumptives to the slightest impressions conducted by damp air, and the excessive response of the mucous mechanisms, are but too genuine.[30]

The situation of the town was also considered particularly favourable for the treatment of invalids. Built upon chalk cliffs overlooking the straits of Dover, Folkestone has a southerly aspect which, asserted one resort guide, afforded it a slightly higher temperature than the east side of Kent, from Herne Bay and Margate to Deal, as well as being sheltered from cold north winds on its landward side by a range of high chalk downs. These topographical features combined, it was claimed, to offer "considerable climatic advantages until December and January",[31] thus permitting hotel and property owners to advertise an extended season in an attempt to optimise their incomes.

The Corporation's attempts to develop a winter season at Folkestone for the wealthy invalid, and also to attract permanent or seasonal residents, involved the employment of highly detailed climatological statistics which would be quoted in guides to health resorts, national newspapers and town guides, as well as in the Medical Officer of Health's annual report. Folkestone was competing with many other coastal towns to be recognised as the driest, sunniest and most salubrious health resort within easy reach of London; the livelihood and prosperity of all social classes and trades depended on successfully promoting the town's natural advantages. The amount of sunshine, recorded on a Jordan photographic recorder, for the years 1894-1898 shows Folkestone to be the sunniest seaside resort for this period, second only to Tunbridge Wells in recorded hours of sunshine.

---

[30] W. Ewart, *Marine Climates in the Treatment of Tuberculosis,* London: Bailliere, Tindall & Cox, 1907

[31] M. Morris, *The Book of Health,* London: Cassell, 1883

Table 4.1: Hours of Sunshine in English Health Resorts 1894-1898[32]

Resort	Hours of sunshine
Tunbridge Wells	1,899
Folkestone	1,871
Torquay	1,817
Brighton	1,814
Eastbourne	1,800
Margate	1,578
Buxton	1,375
London	1,305

The average rainfall between 1888-1898 was recorded as follows, with a rainy day being one in which at least 0.1 inches of rain falls:

Table 4.2: Average Annual Rainfall in English Health Resorts 1888-1898[33]

Resort	Rainy days
Folkestone	126
Bournemouth	164
Eastbourne	165
Torquay	177
London	182
Bath	191
Scarborough	195
Falmouth	204

[32] M. Yunge-Bateman, MOH Report, Folkestone, 1898
[33] M. Yunge-Bateman, MOH Report, Folkestone, 1898

Similarly, tables recording the average mean temperature of health resorts and spas show Folkestone consistently in the top three, whilst the town was also said to experience one of the smallest variations in temperature over twenty four hours, sudden changes of temperature being generally perceived as dangerous to health.[34]

Concerns over the effects of "foul, vitiated or rebreathed" air on the spread of consumption led to more emphasis being placed on the desirability of exposing the tubercular and scrofulous to the "pure and asceptic" air of alpine and maritime resorts, particularly following studies in the early 1880s of "floating matter", or bacteria in the air.[35] Folkestone's reputation for the quality of its air was also enhanced by its renown for possessing a double climate.[36] One at sea level being generally more protected, and that of the Leas on the west cliff where circulating sea breezes were promoted as possessing an added purity through being blown across the English channel:

> after breathing one feels that the heavy poisonous gases of the city have been replaced by a stimulating, tonic and purifying ozone. Not an ozone as at Weston-super-Mare, generated from acres of decayed seaweed, but one that has been wafted by gentle breezes from a region afar, where there is nothing to affect its purity or its strength.[37]

Although the purity of the air was of paramount importance, the quality of the air was much discussed and seen to be of great significance. A "relaxing" climate was believed to induce a feeling of lassitude and loss of appetite, whilst a "bracing" or "tonic" climate could accelerate the metabolism, stimulating renewed vigour and improving the circulation and digestion. George Moseley, for example, took pains to dispel the impression that the climate of Sandgate was relaxing:

> There is, in the health of the inhabitants, not the smallest evidence that the air is relaxing; on the contrary, invalids who have become debilitated in constitution by a residence in warm climates have borne their testimony to the tonic power of the atmosphere.[38]

---

[34] A. E. Larking, *Notes on Folkestone,* 1889, p.76

[35] E.g. G.V. Poore, Climate in its Relation to Health, *Journal of Society of Arts*, 33, 21st November, 1884 – 13th November, 1885

[36] J. Braun, *The Curative Effects of Baths and Waters*, London: Smith, Elder & Co., 1875, p.262

[37] A. E. Larking, *Notes on Folkestone,* 1889, p.65

[38] G. Moseley, *Sandgate as a Residence for Invalids,* 1853, p.50

The invigorating quality of the English climate, even during the winter, was thus emphasised as being more beneficial to consumptives than the torpor-inducing climate of the Mediterranean.

In addition to their exhilarating and remedial effects sea breezes and sunshine were also perceived as effective disinfectants, whether of *miasmatic* effluvia or of bacteria attached to dust. This was, between the late 1890s and the 1930s, generally accepted as the chief means by which the *tubercle bacillus* was spread:[39]

> There are no greater disinfectants than sunshine and breeze. Those who have had to nurse sick friends can always be disinfected gratuitously on the Leas. A brisk walk, making one breathe quicker and deeper, forces out of the recesses of the lungs all the foul residual air accumulated there and replaces it by a fresh pure supply. A stiff breeze forces itself into the meshes of the clothes, removes the dust, and cleans and disinfects the garment.[40]

Augmenting the natural advantages of the town the Folkestone Bathing Company, established in 1869 under the management of Mr. W. D. Fagg, provided salt and freshwater swimming pools at varying temperatures, together with various mineral and vapour baths and massages, under the supervision of MOH William Bateman and local practitioner Robert Bowles.[41] According to one health guide the establishment was "in no sense suggestive of baths, but rather of a first class club".[42] Another amenity operating in the 1880s and 1890s was Mr. H. Court's "Medical Gymnasium" which offered appliances and exercises to remedy all manner of defects and ailments, including those of the lungs, and to which cases were often sent by London physicians.[43] Promenades and sheltered walks were laid out at different levels on the cliffs, and hydraulic lifts and carefully graded walks were provided for invalids.[44]

During the late 1880s at least two convalescent homes were established primarily for the middle classes in straitened circumstances near

---

[39] Report on the Paris Commission on Consumption, *Science,* volume xiv, no.345, September 1899; H. H. Thomson, *Tuberculosis and Public Health*, London: Longmans, 1920, pp. 14-15

[40] A. E. Larking, *Notes on Folkestone,* 1889

[41] Records of Folkestone Bathing Establishment Company Ltd, 1867-1924, EKAC F1954/2

[42] *Views and Reviews* – Special Edition, Brighton: W. T. Pike & Co., 1896

[43] Ibid.

[44] *British Spas & Health Resorts*, Official Publication of British Federation of Spas, Ed. J. Burrow & Co., London, 1920

Folkestone's East Cliff. The St. Gabriel's House of Rest for Gentlewomen in Lennard Road was founded in 1885 with Charles Perry as honorary physician and William Barrett Medical Officer, in 1889 they treated 261 patients. Catering for a "superior class of invalid", and managed by one Sister Miriam with a few lady helpers, their aim was:

> to help the sick and sorrowful and overworked among a rather higher class in society than usually receive it, to replace courage and to fight life's battle.[45]

The wealthier invalid would undoubtedly have rented apartments on the western clifftop near the Leas or taken rooms at a more exclusive hotel, hired a private nurse and been visited by a doctor in their own accommodation. A homoeopathic dispensary was also established on the Parade in 1890, homoeopathy being a system of medicine favoured by the aristocracy at this time.

Folkestone's fashionable western district, then, initiated and regulated by the de Bouverie family as a health resort for the social elite, catered to a large extent for the tubercular and those of a delicate constitution suspected of being predisposed to developing the disease. Although the town's natural advantages were augmented by mechanical bathing machines, a pier and, in 1893, a switchback railway, entertainments and distractions that might have attracted day trippers and holidaymakers were resisted.

If the infectiousness of tuberculosis was accepted by many of the middle classes from the beginning of the twentieth century the financially independent consumptive was still encouraged by the Borough Council to resort to Folkestone for an open-air cure. The spacious gardens, wide boulevards and luxurious hotels and residences of Folkestone's western district would undoubtedly have been considered to provide a healthier environment for affluent sufferers from tuberculosis than did the city. However, the concomitant army of servants, washerwomen, porters, retailers, builders and others on whom they depended were, by the 1880s, living in increasingly crowded and unhealthy conditions. The growing susceptibility of seasonal workers and poor residents to infectious diseases and overcrowded and insanitary housing, particularly during the 1890s, was an unacknowledged consequence of Folkestone's rapid success as a health resort.

---

[45] Letter sent to Archbishop of Canterbury from Sister Miriam, 8th March, 1896, CCA-DCb-F/F/Fo/1

CHAPTER FIVE

SALUBRITY AND SQUALOR: OVERCROWDING AND DISEASE IN EAST FOLKESTONE

Between 1841 and 1861 the population of Folkestone more than doubled from 4,413 to 9,678.[1] Nevertheless this expansion was accompanied by an upgrading of the town's infrastructure. During the 1850s Folkestone's sanitary arrangements were greatly improved due to the Waterworks Act of 1848 and the Local Improvement Act of 1855. This private legislation was encouraged by the state, being relatively cheap and financed by long term government loans. The latter granted Folkestone Borough Council the powers to raise rates for the provision of a sewage system, street paving and other sanitary measures. The former enabled the Folkestone Waterworks Company to levy charges to provide the town with water.

Some contemporary reports indicate, however, that Folkestone's sanitation was so parlous during the early 1850s that intervention by Edwin Chadwick's Board of Health was felt necessary. This evidence indicates that the Board's efforts at improving the sanitary infrastructure of the town resulted in "total failure".[2] This was apparently due, as at neighbouring Sandgate, to a combination of using too narrow earthenware pipes, financial extravagance, underestimating the costs of the operation and the autocratic attitude of the Board's engineers.[3] The sewage system was subsequently engineered by Sir Josiah Bazalgette in 1858, freeing the

---

[1] H. Clunn, *Famous south coast pleasure resorts past and present*, 1929

[2] Anonymous author, (probably T. Hawkesley), *Engineers and Officials; an Historical Sketch of the Progress of 'Health of Towns Works' (between 1838 and 1856) in London and the Provinces,* London: E. Stanford, 1856

[3] Ibid, p.135

Pent stream and the harbour from contaminating effluent.[4]

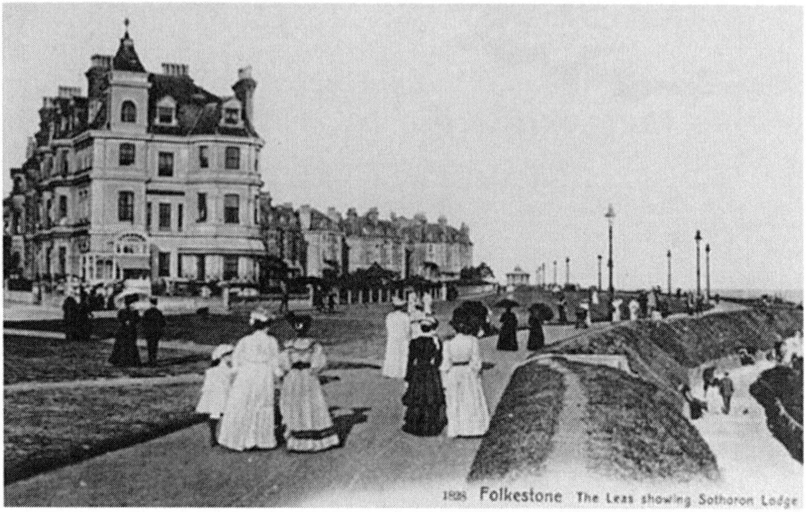

Illustration 5.1: Postcard of The Leas, Folkestone, dated 1828 but probably about 1900.

From the vantage point of 1921 John Pearson, Folkestone's Sanitary Inspector since 1893, recalled the condition of the town prior to this sanitary revolution:

> Up to the year 1850, and even later, the sanitary customs of the town were of the most primitive character, there was no system of drainage, and the stream running through the centre of the town dividing the east from the west portion, and known as the Pent stream, was a kind of elongated cesspool receiving certain drainage and a receptacle of all kinds of solid and liquid filth'.[5]

However, with the spacious planning of broad avenues, crescents and public gardens in the cliff top west ward by Sidney Smirke in the 1850s, Folkestone was, according to Pearson, reinvented as an ideal of salubrity and town planning:

---

[4] J. Pearson, Thirty Years Sanitary Experience in Folkestone with Local Experiences, *Journal of the Royal Sanitary Institute*, volume xlii, no. 1, July 1921, pp.293-297

[5] J. Pearson, Thirty Years Sanitary Experience, 1921, p.294

> whilst dreamers were dreaming of garden cities, Folkestone was being made one, thus anticipating the elysium of the future.[6]

But this vision of *Hygiea* constituted only a partial image of the town. From 1871 to 1891 the town's population virtually doubled again from 12,951 to 24,969. Between 1850 and 1890 about two thirds of this growth was due to an influx of workers migrating to Folkestone in order to service the needs of visitors to the fashionable western part of the town, the majority of these workers being housed in the increasingly overcrowded north and east wards.

Although by 1874 Folkestone could still be depicted as:

> the *ne plus ultra* of health and purity…quite unparalleled in the purity of air, whilst it is free from the pernicious element of town life [associated with Ramsgate and Margate], exquisitely clean, one of the cleanest towns in England. There seems to be no great collection of a very poor dirty class as there is in Boulogne, or most other towns where fishermen and their families abound'.[7]

In the following year the effects of overcrowding were becoming apparent in the east ward as working men and women, particularly from the countryside, were attracted to the town to work in the growing number of hotels, restaurants, dressmakers and laundries. Men were also drawn to Folkestone to seek work as builders or in the brick and cement works.

In 1875 Lord Robert Montagu, the Member of Parliament for Westmeath, in proposing to extend the Artisans' Dwellings Bill to towns with a population of less than 25,000, claimed that in smaller towns there existed "worse evils and more fever dens than were to be found in the large towns" and cited Folkestone as an example. Montagu was a long-term resident of Folkestone. He alluded to a councillor named Robinson, the landlord of properties infested with fever who, Montagu claimed, used the residents' fear of damaging the town's reputation as a health resort to deflect criticism from his overcrowded and insanitary properties.[8]

A report by *The Lancet* of that year found that this part of the town was "disgraceful". However blame for the insanitary condition of the quarter was not directed at the landlord, but apportioned to the residents. Not only were they poor but of another race; "the lowest class of the population, chiefly Irish" who had settled in the town following the construction of the

---

[6] Ibid.

[7] "A medical authority on Folkestone", *Folkestone Chronicle,* 10th October, 1874

[8] *The Times*, Wednesday, 7th April, 1875

railway.[9] Robinson remained in Folkestone as a councillor and landlord until the early 1880s at which time he was apparently forced to leave the town due to local opposition.[10]

Concerns were also raised over the quality and quantity of the town's water supply. Following an unusually high death rate in Folkestone in 1875 *The Lancet* had called for the notoriously intermittent water supply to be remedied immediately. It was suggested that the loose, sandy soil of the town was responsible for its contamination by liquid waste. Folkestone Borough Council, in view of the town's rising population, was advised to properly maintain its drainage system and to take precautions against the possible pollution of its water supplies, both at their source and during storage.[11]

At this time, however, and until his death in 1891, Folkestone's Medical Officer of Health, William Bateman, occupied the position of chairman to the Water Company.[12] His responsibilities for the town's public health may have conflicted with the short term financial interests of this private company, of which both himself and Lord Radnor were major shareholders.[13]

The availability and quality of water was not to improve significantly until the beginning of the twentieth century. In 1893, a particularly dry year, water was available for only two hours in the morning and two hours in the evening.[14] In fact for much of the 1880s and 1890s the supply was limited to about five hours a day; only 600,000 gallons were supplied for a town requiring the consumption of one to one and a half million gallons. As well as the supply being insufficient the reservoirs remained open and unlined and thus subject to contamination; the water was said to have a bitter and mouldy taste that was thought to be caused by rotting vegetation.[15]

---

[9] *The Lancet*, 17th April, 1875, p.566

[10] *Folkestone Up to Date,* 30th March, 1895

[11] Report on the Sanitary Condition of Folkestone, *The Lancet*, 17th April, 1875; *The Times,* 7th & 12th April, 1875

[12] *Folkestone Herald*, 31st October, 1891, p. 114

[13] The Third Earl of Radnor had purchased 300 shares in the company in 1848 at a cost of £5,000. G. C. Sharp, *The Aristocracy and the Development of Seaside Resorts: The Radnor Family and the History of Folkestone 1840-1914*, M.A. Dissertation, University of Kent, 1989, p. 57

[14] *Folkestone Up to Date*, 21st September, 1893, p.3

[15] J. Pearson, Thirty Years Sanitary Progress in Folkestone, *Journal of the Royal Sanitary Institute*, volume xlii, no.5, March 1922

By 1889 local doctor Arthur Larking recognised the threat that the increasing social polarisation and overcrowding posed for the health of the town:

> the low death rate is remarkable when one knows of the very defective condition of many of the old parts of town. Visitors must remember that the modern Folkestone is of recent date, and that long before there were any houses to note on the western side of Bates' Hotel, there existed in Radnor Street, Dover Street, The Narrows, The Bayle, The Stade and High Street numerous old houses crowded together, and thickly populated by the working classes and fishermen of the town.
>
> The Medical Officer of Health has endeavoured to get many parts of these slums condemned as unfit for habitation, but the difficulty always arises as to where these people are to live if turned out of their homes.
>
> It would be a great boon to the lower classes if the authorities would take in hand a scheme for the improvement of these places, and erect decent dwellings on the sites. It would also benefit the town at large, for their existence is a standing eyesore, and a source of danger in the event of any epidemic occurring.
>
> Yet in spite of these crowded and apparently unsanitary spots, Folkestone manages by means of its pure air to maintain its standard among the health resorts of the country.[16]

As in other densely populated and insanitary urban areas in the early 1890s extreme poverty and deprivation were being encountered by religious missionaries and sociological investigators. Civilised society responded in much the same way as discovering an alien and savage race in the outer reaches of the empire. In January 1893 Eric Cady, editor of the *Folkestone Visitors' List,* echoing the national concern generated by recent sociological studies of working class life,[17] published an article revealing the desperate circumstances of many poor people in the town:

> it is not generally known that in Folkestone there exists a class of people among the very poor whose condition is not only utterly deplorable, but a disgrace to nineteenth century civilisation. These people live, herded together in filth and wretchedness, most of them have scarcely any clothing, as the bulk of their poor earnings is swallowed up in payment of

---

[16] A. E. Larking, *Notes on Folkestone Historical, Climatological and Medical,* London: J&A Churchill, 1889

[17] C. Booth, *The Life and Labour of the People in London*, 9 volumes, London: Macmillan & Co, 1892-97; G. Sims, *How the Poor Live,* London: Chatto & Windus, 1883; Reverend Andrew Mearns, *The Bitter Cry of Outcast London: An Inquiry into the Condition of the Abject Poor,* London: J. Clarke & Co., 1883

> their night's lodging and in providing the necessities for keeping body and soul together.[18]

Throughout the 1890s poverty and overcrowding contributed to a rise in infectious diseases in the poorer districts of town, whilst the MOH lacked the authority to demolish slums. High ground rents, local building restrictions and the Radnor family's control of most available land and building materials prevented further house construction for local workers.[19] In March 1893 *Folkestone Up to Date* summarised the situation in an editorial:

> the Corporation cannot prevent overcrowding, because there is not a single cottage in the town to let, and if they close any of the existing insanitary dwellings it increases the overcrowding.[20]

Some Councillors continued, as had Robinson in the 1870s, to benefit from the hardships of the working classes. Aldermen Banks and Sherwood owned many properties in the east of Folkestone and as a consequence were resistant to any proposals to build houses for workers at affordable rents.[21] Investment in cheap tenement properties in the poorer districts of the town was a relatively secure speculation, demand always exceeding supply as immigrants poured into the town in search of work.

Rents ranged from three to ten shillings a week. These high rents, only being affordable by skilled artisans, often led to subletting and crowding. Although apparently partly relieved by house building in the suburb of Cheriton, a *Folkestone Up to Date* editorial of 1895 claimed that these developments were more an attempt by landlords to escape the restrictions of Folkestone's recently introduced sanitary bye-laws.[22]

In 1894 the press disclosed that the MOH's monthly report, revealing that 64 houses had been condemned as unfit for habitation and that there

---

[18] E. Cady, *Folkestone Visitors' List,* 23rd January, 1893

[19] Lord Radnor's estate was said to own, produce and control the supply of building materials in Folkestone, G. Sharp, *The Aristocracy and the Development of Seaside Resorts*, 1989, p.56

[20] *Folkestone Up to Date*, 18th March, 1893; see also *Folkestone Up-to-Date*, 26th October, 1893; LGB Sanitary Papers 1893, Folkestone MOH report, M. Yunge-Bateman, NA MH 12/5045

[21] A. Nevill, *The Story of Folkestone*, 2009, p.104

[22] A. Nevill, *The Story of Folkestone*, 2009, pp.104,155; *Folkestone Up to Date*, 2nd February, 1895, p.3

existed 46 cases of overcrowding, had been repressed by the Council.[23] Councillor George Spurgen, acting as chairman of the Borough Sanitary Committee, appears to have been responsible for the suppression of this report, in addition to stifling a proposed report on overcrowding by councillor John Jones. Spurgen warned Lord Radnor of the consequences to the town in the event of any such report being published:

> I would picture to your Lordship what a serious calamity it would be to the town, and to your Lordship, if any statements should get abroad as to the insanitary condition of the town and the serious overcrowding in our midst.[24]

Some of the more radical London newspapers did, however, expose the consequences of Lord Radnor's management of Folkestone. The ground landlord and local speculators were primarily concerned with attaining maximum profit from Folkestone's reputation as a health resort, claimed *The Star,* whilst disregarding the resulting hardship and suffering caused to the town's poorer residents:[25]

> The cause of this difficulty is that Lord Radnor, who owns most of the land in and about Folkestone, will not have a small house or cottage built on his property. The result is that every small plot of freehold ground that does not belong to him has been inflated to a fictitious value, and secured by syndicates and societies that are wholly indifferent as to the effects of their proceedings on the poor so long as they make a good profit'.[26]

The Council declined to construct any alternative accommodation, and were perhaps unable to do so. In 1894 it was reported that agricultural land offered for sale as a cemetery a few years previously by Lord Radnor for £100 per acre had been valued at £1,000 per acre by his agent when solicited by the Council for artisans' dwellings.

---

[23] *Weekly Dispatch*, 7th October, 1894, quoted in *Folkestone Up To Date*, 11th October, 1894; LGB correspondence, Folkestone Urban October 1894-March 1895, MOH Report 1894

[24] G. Spurgen, Chairman of Folkestone Borough Sanitary Committee, letter to Lord Radnor, General Purposes & Miscellaneous Committees Minute Book, pp.31-32, Fo/AMc5/17

[25] *Weekly Dispatch*, 7th October, 1894, *Reynold's Newspaper*, 7th October, 1894 *The Star*, 6th October, 1894, *Truth*, 11th October, 1894

[26] Folkestone Slums, *The Star*, 6th October, 1894

Aristocratic landlords accumulated significant wealth during the urban expansion of the nineteenth century by keeping undeveloped land off the market and leasing it at extorted prices. It was common for land to be offered on a short leasehold system for consortia to develop, and buildings were, in turn, leased, usually for 99 years, after which they would revert to the ground landlord.[27]

In 1895 one local newspaper reported that the MOH and the Sanitary Inspector had been battling with a prevaricating Borough Council for the past three years in order to enforce the building of houses for the working classes.[28] This ongoing conflict reveals that a growing focus on public health was placing the Borough Sanitary Department at odds with the interests of private property owners and local businessmen:

> This cruel condition of things has enriched the freeholders and the slum owners, but the result to the labouring classes has been overcrowding, ill-health and discomfort. The majority of the Corporation, who seem to be hand in glove with the owners and lessees of the land, cannot avoid ordering the destruction of insanitary property, but at that their reforming intentions end, and they actually suppress the medical officer's report because it suggests that the work of demolition should not be carried out until new houses in Folkestone are provided for the ejected tenants.[29]

Further adverse publicity for the town was generated in 1895 when a handbill was published by an anonymous Folkestone ratepayer describing the town as a "hotbed of diphtheria and scarlet fever".[30]

The Royal Institute of Public Health, which was dominated by MOHs, and its predecessors in the public health campaign,[31] had emphasised that the eradication of slum housing was the key in the struggle against tuberculosis.[32] In 1900 the journal of the SMOH characterised provincial

---

[27] J. Gehrke, Georgist Thought and the Emergence of Municipal Socialism in Britain, 1870-1914, p.5 http://schalkenbach.org/on-line-library/scholars-forum/municipal-socialism-in-britain/

[28] *Folkestone Up-to-Date*, 22nd June, 1895

[29] Ibid.

[30] *Folkestone Herald*, 9th February, 1895

[31] The College of State Medicine (founded 1886) amalgamated with The British Institute for Preventive Medicine in 1893. They changed their name to The Jenner Institute in 1898 and The Lister Institute in 1901. The Royal Institute of Public Health was formed in 1906.

[32] D. Watkins, *The English Revolution in Scientific Medicine*, 1984, p.307; *Journal of the Royal Institute of Public Health*, 1909, volume xvii, pp. 151-157

local government as "oligarchic in the extreme",[33] and local Councillors were often depicted as "jerry builders" and "house farmers" whose interests were opposed to those of the local MOH.[34]

Certainly the majority of Folkestone Councillors were reported to favour the interests of the local monopolies, the South Eastern Railway and the gas and water companies, in which many were shareholders or directors. George Spurgen, for example, manager of the SER's Pavilion Hotel and mayor in the late 1880s, was director of the Folkestone Water Company despite serving on the Council for much of the 1880s and 1890s. Three other Councillors were also directors of the Company during this period when deaths were attributed to contaminated water supplies, and the Council unsuccessfully attempted to take over the Company.[35] In fact many Councillors and Borough officials had stakes in hotels and property to let, and were anxious that Folkestone should attract no adverse publicity in respect of the town's sanitation.

The political and economic structure of Folkestone at this time appears strikingly similar to Robert Tressell's largely autobiographical account of Mugsborough during the first decade of the twentieth century, which was based on the health resort of Hastings situated about thirty miles along the south coast:

> [it] was a favourite resort of the upper classes, but of late years most of these patriots have adopted the practice of going on the Continent to spend the money they obtain from the working people of England. Summer or winter the place was usually fairly full of what were called good-class visitors, either holidaymakers or invalids. [However], the majority of the inhabitants existed in a state of perpetual poverty which in many cases bordered on destitution … a great part of the incomes of the tradespeople and boarding-house-keepers and about a third of the wages of the working classes were paid away as rent and rates … Every public service capable of returning direct profit was in the hands of private companies, and the shares of the private companies were in the hands of the members of the Corporation.[36]

Despite the supposed medical advances achieved through research in bacteriology, the health of Folkestone's working class residents deteriorated

---

[33] Local Misgovernment, *Public Health,* 1899-1900, volume xii, pp. 61-63

[34] D. Watkins, *The English Revolution in Scientific Medicine*, 1984, p.316

[35] Folkestone Sanitary Papers 1899-1900, NA MH 12/5053; *Folkestone Up-to-Date,* 12th October, 1893

[36] R. Tressell, *The Ragged Trousered Philanthropists,* London, Lawrence & Wishart, 1914, appendix, pp.1703-4

during the 1890s. However, due to the topography of the town and the separation of social classes most residents and visitors to the fashionable west of Folkestone would have been largely unaware of the poverty and squalor existing in many parts of the north and east wards. And, judging from the addresses of their practices, the social and professional lives of most doctors would also have been largely restricted to the west ward.[37]

The socially polarised nature of the town, together with the perceived threat posed to the health and lifestyle of the elite by the lower social orders, is exemplified in the recollections of a former pupil of one of Folkestone's many high class schools. As late as the 1930s an invisible cultural barrier still signalled the limits of respectable Folkestone. Further eastwards resided the threat of infection, moral corruption and disease:

> the eastern limits of the town were marked by the William Harvey statue, beyond which there was a risk of being contaminated by the east end of town.[38]

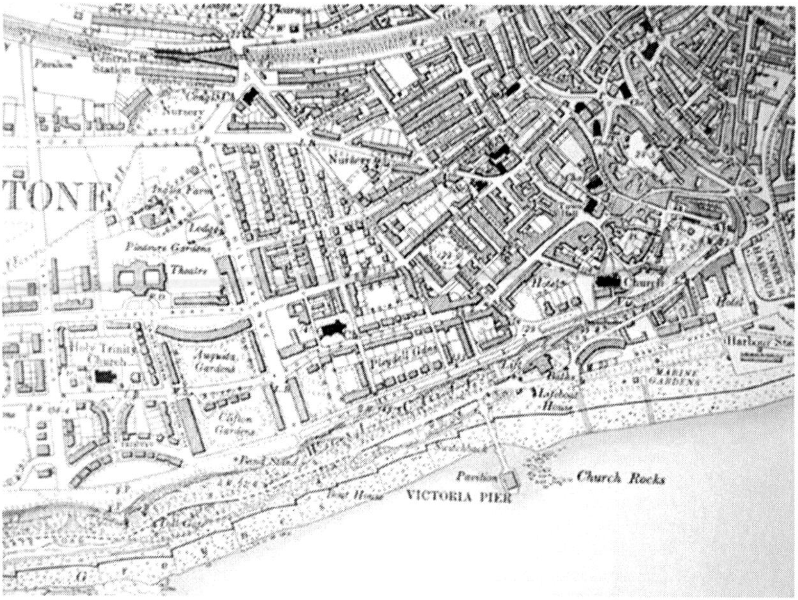

Illustration 5.2: Map of Folkestone in 1881 showing the spacious and well planned west ward in contrast to the crowded eastern ward of the town.

---

[37] Kelly's Directories of Folkestone 1898-9, 1903-4, 1927-30, Folkestone Library,

[38] C. Thomas, 'St.Margaret's, Folkestone', *Bygone Kent* 16/2, February, 1995, p.113.

The poverty, ill health and overcrowding that characterised Folkestone's east ward were largely a consequence of inflated rents and prices charged in the elite west of the town from the mid-nineteenth century, the rigid social planning exercised by the Radnor family and the complete dependency of affluent residents and visitors on a relatively large number of servants, provisioners and tradesmen.

CHAPTER SIX

TUBERCULOSIS AND PUBLIC HEALTH IN FOLKESTONE 1890-1910: CALLS FOR THE SCIENTIFIC MANAGEMENT OF SOCIETY

In the late nineteenth century the social implications of germ theory inspired some doctors to appeal for professional unity and for more powers to be granted to them in the prevention of tuberculosis. This was largely a consequence of social forces operating beyond the sphere of medicine. As demonstrated in Part I, a number of factors combined to make a case for social intervention. Despite the efforts of proponents of environmental reform for the control of tuberculosis, the spur to the eventual provision of a public health policy appears to have derived largely from imperialist and economic motives. During the Boer War of 1899-1902 deaths from sickness had been nearly four times as great as deaths in active service, and the medical examination of recruits had revealed the debilitated condition of British manhood:

> Medical examinations showed that of every nine men of military age in Great Britain, on the average three were perfectly fit and healthy, two were on a definitely infirm plane of health and strength, whether from some disability or some failure in development; three were incapable of undergoing more than a very moderate degree of physical exertion and could almost, in view of their age, be described with justice as physical wrecks, and the remaining man as a chronic invalid with a precarious hold on life.[1]

These concerns for the failing health of the nation, lent additional credibility by social Darwinist theorising and high morbidity and mortality

---

[1] Sir L. Mackenzie, The Production of Fitness, paper delivered at Folkestone Health Congress, 1921, *Royal Society of Health Journal,* volume xlii, no.4, January, 1922, quoting from the National Service Medical Board of 1920.

rates in urban districts, led to urgent demands for government action to improve national fitness and efficiency. They also prompted consideration of the German model of sanatorium treatment. Anxieties focused on the declining fitness of army recruits[2] and the state sponsored public health interventions of European and American trade competitors. The terms of this "social question" encompassed economic, military and political issues.

Calls for reform were made more pressing by the increasingly vocal claims of unskilled workers represented and championed by the Trade Union movement from the 1880s. Social investigators reviewing the conditions of the working classes[3] highlighted the urgency of the problems and potential challenges of the most deprived sections of urban communities. Growing social unrest threatened to engulf the stability of economic life and prosperity of middle class communities.

These anxieties concerning the disintegration of working class health and social order were not experienced in isolation from contemporary scientific understanding. They were articulated through the language of science and expressed in terms of infection. In this way a complex of political radicalism and moral and physical degeneration were conflated. Koch's discovery of the *tubercle bacillus* in 1882 initially had relatively little impact in England. However, from 1898, the year of the founding of the NAPC, germ theory was employed as a means of legitimising a raft of measures and initiatives at a local level such as isolation, disinfection and home inspection by health visitors.

This shift in perception in medical theory is central to an understanding of the formation and development of health policies. These were, it will be argued, informed by social, economic and political responses rather than simply reflecting advances in bacteriology. In Folkestone the action of these various forces can be seen particularly clearly through a focus on the work of successive Medical Officers of Health.

The Medical Officer of Health

As illustrated in chapter five conflicts of interest were likely to be encountered by the MOH in his dealings with Borough Councillors. As the editorial of *The Practitioner* argued in 1904:

---

[2] The health of recruits had not been seen as a problem during the Asante and Zulu wars of the 1870s.

[3] C. Booth, *The Life and Labour of the People in London*, 9 volumes, London: Macmillan & Co, 1892-97; B. Seebohm Rowntree, *A Study of Town Life*, London: Macmillan & Co, 1901

> We cannot but feel that the position occupied in many instances by Medical Officers of Health is unsatisfactory. Their dependence upon local authorities is productive of much mischief. In some instances a Medical Officer of Health may be in active practice himself, and may be called upon in his public capacity to report unfavourably on houses owned by some local magnate who is his best patient. In other cases his tenure of office may depend upon his saying smooth things to the members of the local authority…who may all the time be offenders against the most urgent laws of sanitation.[4]

The Society of Medical Officers of Health felt that part-time MOHs were particularly compromised by having to compete with other private practitioners in order to secure their practice. Unlike metropolitan MOHs, their provincial counterparts were generally employed part-time on low wages and had no security until 1921 when the Public Health (Officers) Act granted them tenure and, in 1929, the Local Government Act abolished part-time appointments.[5] Consequently there often existed little basis for co-operation between the MOH and other local doctors.[6]

William Bateman, employed by Folkestone Borough Council as Medical Officer of Health from 1871 to 1891, was an ex-naval surgeon who, in addition to running a large private practice from 1853, that had been built up by his father, acted as surgeon to local Friendly Societies and the town's voluntary hospital.[7] Bateman had no formal training in public health and it is unlikely that he was in a position to exercise much effect on the sanitary reform of the town. He also occupied the position of Medical Officer to the Elham workhouse and infirmary.

During the nineteenth century there was no separate ward at the Union infirmary for either those suffering from tuberculosis or for children, and the prevention of infection does not appear to have been a major consideration. The Poor Law Medical Service, whose ethos of deterrence was increasingly to come into conflict with the preventive approach to public health espoused by the SMOH from the late 1890s, provided only palliative care of a low standard.[8]

The sanitary condition of Folkestone does, however, appear to have been confronted with less deference to the interests of wealthy property owners and the Borough Council from 1890 when John Pearson, described

---

[4] *The Practitioner*, volume 73, July-December, 1904, p.430

[5] Ibid., p. 165

[6] D. Watkins, *The English Revolution in Scientific Medicine*, 1984, p. 299

[7] *Folkestone Herald*, 31st October, 1891, p. 114

[8] J. Brand, The Parish Doctor: England's Poor Law Medical Officers and Medical Reform, 1870-1900, *Bulletin of the History of Medicine*, 35, 1961, p.106

by one local newspaper as "a Sanitary Inspector who, for his energy, ability and straightforwardness, is unequalled in England",[9] was appointed.

In April 1893, when a prosperous resident appealed to the court against the invasive powers of the local Sanitary Authority, Folkestone Borough magistrates upheld their right to enter and inspect any premises if they suspected sanitary shortcomings. During the case it transpired that Pearson had been obliged to condemn no less than 2,000 water closets in the town out of a total of 5,000 houses during the two years and three months he had held office.[10]

In August, 1893 Pearson summoned future mayor, Councillor Salter, to court under the Public Health Act of 1875 to close two cottages he had leased due to their being unfit for human habitation. In that year 16 houses were found unfit for human habitation, and the MOH noted that the Housing of the Working Classes Act of 1890 could have been better enforced if alternative accommodation had been available for the tenants who were displaced.[11]

In 1892 Marcus Yunge-Bateman, qualified with a Diploma in Public Health, had replaced his late uncle, William Bateman, as MOH for Folkestone at a wage of about six shillings an hour for one hours work every week-day. A *Lancet* editorial bemoaned the Council's parsimony and lack of commitment to securing an experienced practitioner. It described the salary as:

> a remuneration just sufficient to compensate for a perfunctory performance of the ordinary duties of the office, [and continued] The attitude adopted by the majority of the Folkestone Town Council in regard to the appointment of a medical officer of health is not one which is calculated to inspire confidence in the minds of the many visitors who have been in the habit of frequenting that town in quest of health and recreation…More than once the Local Government Board have had to intervene in connexion with preventable disease in and around Folkestone; and it would certainly conduce to the sanitary interests of the place if it were understood that the Town Council desire for the future to place their town above suspicion as regards its sanitary administration.[12]

[9] *Folkestone Up to Date*, 3rd June, 1893, p. 3

[10] Powers of Inspection by Sanitary Authorities (The Folkestone Case), *The Lancet*, 6th May, 1893

[11] LGB Correspondence, Folkestone Sanitary Papers 1893, MOH report, M. Yunge-Bateman, NA MH 12/5045

[12] *The Lancet*, 16th January, 1892, p.156

Whilst the health of Folkestone's working classes may not have been the Council's priority the new MOH and Sanitary Inspector were actively attempting to improve the town's public health from the 1890s. The influence of MOHs on often recalcitrant local authorities at this time have been insufficiently acknowledged. MOHs were responsible for raising the public consciousness with regard to health issues, reporting to the local and regional authorities, as well as to the LGB, on the health of their locality and on measures they deemed necessary for the prevention of disease. In addition, from 1889 they were empowered to notify and isolate suspected cases under the Infectious Diseases Act.

With the reform and standardisation of the Diploma in Public Health in 1889 MOHs and the practice of preventive medicine began to achieve a new legitimacy, despite wider concerns over the infringement of individual liberties. Prospective MOHs were now trained in engineering, geology, climatology, chemistry, practical sanitation, sanitary law, preventive medicine and, from 1896, bacteriology. The health of the community was henceforth the responsibility of a local expert, albeit with only six months training in public health and still poorly remunerated by local Councils.

Yunge-Bateman's recommendations to the Council reveal a reformist approach to the public health of the town. This was undoubtedly inspired by the growing acceptance of germ theory in the 1890s, at least amongst the Society of Medical Officers of Health who, together with the British Medical Association, became increasingly involved in lobbying government for an expansion of public health care during the 1890s in an atmosphere of medical optimism.[13]

There is, however, evidence that this reformist zeal was checked to some degree by vested local interests. Whilst actively proposing action to prevent the spread of infection, MOHs were often constrained to a large degree by the financial and ideological interests of local Councillors and property owners.

The optimism that prevailed in the 1890s was not supported by health statistics. Folkestone's MOH reports reveal a higher death rate for the late 1890s and early 1900s than in the late 1880s. Deaths relative to population were much higher in the east than in the affluent west ward; deaths from tuberculosis being more than twice as high, and infant mortality at least five times higher in the east ward than in the west throughout this period.

---

[13] D. Watkins, *The English Revolution in Scientific Medicine*, 1984, p. 160; C. Bellamy, *Administering Central-Local Relations 1871-1919,* Manchester University Press, 1988; J. Brand, *Doctors and the State,* 1965

Table 6.1: Population Growth in Folkestone 1871-1910

year	North ward	East ward	West ward	Total Population of Folkestone Borough
1871	1,562	4854	6,225	12,641
1881	3,507	6,449	8,846	18,822
1891	5,568	7,720	10,524	23,812
1901	10,460	8,730	11,300	30,490
1910	15,111	9,639	11,880	36,630

Sources: Registrar General census records; H Clunn, Famous south coast pleasure resorts past and present, 1929

Whereas the population of the recently developed, spacious and elite west ward rose by little more than a thousand between 1891 and 1910, the addition of two thousand people in the already congested east ward, and the tripling of population in the working class north ward resulted in increasing inequalities in the burden of sickness and death.

During Folkestone's rapid development as an exclusive resort, building had been restricted by successive Earls of Radnor resulting in inflated rents and prices in the town and overcrowding in the older districts. These areas were populated mainly by dressmakers, laundresses, printers, servants, boarding house proprietors, shopworkers, builders, navvies and fishermen. As income to the town fell in the late nineteenth and early twentieth centuries practically all such local trades, whose incomes were related to the quantity and affluence of visitors in some way, became increasingly subject to underemployment. Consequently the health of the most vulnerable and impoverished, particularly children, in the north and east wards was disproportionately affected by diarrhoea and infectious diseases.

As Dr. G.V. Poore had cautioned in 1885:

> directly a health resort becomes the fashion it is within measurable distance of ruin. Density of population brings with it its attendant evils, difficulties of water supply and drainage, accumulations of filth, and an atmosphere stuffed with microbes.14

[14] G.V. Poore, Climate in its Relation to Health, *Journal of the Society of Arts*, 33, 1885, p.919

Childhood Mortality in Folkestone

Table 6.2 shows that deaths under five years between 1894-1899 accounted for over one third of total deaths in Folkestone. Compared to the national average this was not exceptionally high.

Table 6.2: Childhood Mortality in Folkestone 1894-1899

year	Registered deaths under 5 years	Registered deaths over 5 years	Total deaths
1894	131	232	363
1895	144	258	402
1896	119	219	338
1897	142	281	423
1898	156	284	440
1899	158	288	446

Source: M. Yunge-Bateman, Folkestone MOH reports

Table 6.3 shows that increases in infant mortality (deaths of children under one year old), both in Folkestone and for England and Wales as a whole, occurred in the years 1893, 1895, 1897-1899, 1904, 1906 and 1911. According to Arthur Newsholme in 1899, and Folkestone MOH Yunge-Bateman in 1904, these simultaneous rises in infant deaths throughout urban environments in England and Wales could only have been due to the effects of particularly hot and dry summers on overcrowded and insanitary environments.[15]

In 1897 Yunge-Bateman reported many cases of diarrhoea in the summer, with 29 deaths occurring between July and October, 22 of these being of infants.[16] In 1898 there was "abnormally hot weather" in September and October with 53 deaths from "autumnal diarrhoea", 43 of which were under one year of age and all but one of these occurring in September, mostly in the overcrowded districts of the north and east

[15] A. Newsholme, SMOH Presidential Address, 1899, quoted in Woods et al., The Causes, p.114; M. Yunge-Bateman, MOH report, 1904; R. I. Woods et al, The Causes of Rapid Infant Mortality Decline, Part I, 1988, p.360

[16] M. Yunge-Bateman, MOH report 1897, p.11,

wards.[17]

Table 6.3: Comparison of National and Local Infant Mortality Rates 1892-1913

year	Infant mortality rate England & Wales	Infant mortality Folkestone Borough		year	Infant mortality rate England & Wales	Infant mortality Folkestone Borough	
		rate*	deaths			rate*	deaths
1892	148	127.7	?	1903	132	114.2	84
1893	159	167.2	100	1904	145	143.0	109
1894	137	105.9	66	1905	128	108.3	74
1895	161	150.0	99	1906	132	128.8	87
1896	148	122.0	79	1907	118	97.6	63
1897	156	151.0	101	1908	120	92.7	60
1898	160	178.2	118	1909	109	90.4	57
1899	163	153.2	114	1910	105	60.8	36
1900	154	117.4	82	1911	130	115.3	67
1901	151	160.0	113	1912	95	65.4	39
1902	133	114.1	83	1913	108	65.3	40

*per 1,000 births registered

Source: Registrar General's Annual Reports, LGB records & Folkestone MOH reports

In 1899 55 such deaths were recorded in addition to 16 deaths from typhoid fever.[18] Probably as a consequence, in September 1899 the MOH recommended that all milk entering the Borough be boiled or sterilised. It is debatable whether this suggestion was complied with to any great degree as processed milk was generally considered to be unpalatable and lacking in nutrition at the time.

[17] M. Yunge-Bateman, MOH report 1898, p.8,

[18] Folkestone MOH report, 1898, Wellcome Library, b13562514

Table 6.4: Deaths Due to Diarrhoea in Folkestone Borough 1890-1904

year	Deaths due to diarrhoea	Rainfall 3rd quarter (inches)	year	Deaths due to diarrhoea	Rainfall 3rd quarter (inches)
1890	3	8.02	1898	53	4.05
1891	4	7.02	1899	55	4.54
1892	14	8.90	1900	31	4.14
1893	20	9.15	1901	22	4.00
1894	3	9.78	1902	22	6.25
1895	23	5.68	1903	9	10.75
1896	9	11.44	1904	47	4.14
1897	31	6.62	1905	49	

Source: M. Yunge-Bateman, MOH report 1904, p.24

In 1904 109 infant deaths were recorded in the town, only nine of these occurring in the affluent west ward. The MOH and the Sanitary Inspector were both of the opinion that a major factor contributing to this increase in infantile mortality was the working class practice of bottle feeding babies:

> Can we wonder at the degeneracy of our race, and the appointment of Commissions to enquire into the cause of it, when in the beginning of our life we are denied our natural food, so essential to later development, by our women shirking the highest duty of motherhood, and their infants feed on milk coming from a polluted source, dosed with Boracic Acid, or robbed of its most nutritious parts. Of the 150,000 infants who die annually in this country in the first year of their life, three quarters have been reared on artificial food.[19]

The local health officials acknowledged the role of contaminated milk and water in the typhoid epidemic, although they disagreed as to which constituted the main source of infection. By 1904 about 200 cases of typhoid fever had occurred in Folkestone and Sandgate since 1896, resulting in about 40 deaths. The Sanitary Inspector commented:

---

[19] J. Pearson, *Milk Supplies and their Dangers, with Local Experiences*, Paper at Folkestone Health Congress, 1904, *Journal of State Medicine,* volume xii, no.9, September 1904

> there is no doubt that uncleanly milking, together with a polluted water supply, has been the cause of a continued prevalence of typhoid in Folkestone.[20]

The epidemic was to continue in the town until 1910, contributing to much local unrest and alarm and two Local Government Board enquiries.[21]

Yunge-Bateman included table 6.4 in his 1904 MOH report to illustrate the relationship between dry, hot summers and deaths due to diarrhoea, of which there were 47 that year, 43 occurring in the last quarter of the year and 38 being of children under one year of age.[22] He noted that outbreaks of diarrhoea were generally ended by downpours of autumn rain, as in 1896 and 1903, which served to lay the dust, flush drains and sewers and rid the town of flies which, he observed in 1903, had been very prevalent in previous years.[23] An exceptional number of flies also appears to have contributed to the high infant mortality rate in the hot and dry summer of 1906.[24] He estimated the demographic spread of cases of diarrhoea in 1904 to have consisted of 60 in the north ward, 25 in the east and only four in the affluent west ward.[25] Of these 73 cases occurred among bottle fed infants.

Despite the absence of any major environmental reforms at the end of the nineteenth century a rapid and sustained decrease in infant and childhood mortality occurred from about 1900. This decline of childhood deaths in Folkestone after 1900 does not appear to have been affected by any improvements in housing conditions, overcrowding in the east ward persisting until the 1930s. Nor was the problem of contaminated milk addressed until much later in the century.

Improvements in the water supply may have had an impact on the health of the town at this time. In 1897, the year that 40 cases of typhoid fever had been notified, the water was described as sometimes being "chocolate brown" in colour.[26] Subsequently, in the same year, the

---

[20] J. Pearson, *Milk Supplies and their Dangers, with Local Experiences*, Paper at Folkestone Health Congress, 1904, *Journal of State Medicine,* volume xii, no.9, September 1904

[21] J. Pearson, Thirty Years Sanitary Experience with Local Experiences, *Journal of the Royal Sanitary Institute*, volume xlii, no5, March 1922, p.293; *Folkestone Herald*, 6th September, 1902; P. P. Mortimer, Mr. N. The Milker, and Dr. Koch's Concept of the Healthy Carrier, *The Lancet,* 353, 1999, pp.1354-1356

[22] M. Yunge-Bateman, MOH report, 1904

[23] M. Yunge-Bateman, MOH report 1903, p.14

[24] M. Yunge-Bateman, MOH report 1906, p.12

[25] M. Yunge-Bateman, MOH report 1904

[26] Folkestone MOH report, 1897, p.11, b13562514

reservoirs were lined and covered, the water filtered, and by 1900 additional water supplies were secured for the Folkestone Water Company from the Alkham and Lydden valleys.[27] It would appear, however, that the acquisition of the new water sources was at the expense of its quality. The minutes of the Folkestone Hospitals and Sanitary Committee reveal that due to an increased hardness of the water the health of the town suffered. As a result some residents left and the number of visitors declined, threatening the prosperity of the town.

Following repeated pressure on the private water company by the Folkestone Medical Society, an organisation of local doctors,[28] the supply was improved in 1902. However by this time Folkestone's reputation as a health resort had already suffered. According to the *Folkestone Herald* 1902 had been the poorest ever season for the town, and the value of property was deteriorating.29 Nevertheless, continued pressure from the MOH, influential residents, the LGB and local doctors from 1899 had succeeded in forcing improvements to the sanitary facilities and water supply of the town following growing alarm from local residents due to the typhoid epidemic.[30]

Nationally the rapid decline of infant and childhood mortality rates, after being persistently high during the 1890s, was a major factor in the total decline in mortality in England and Wales from the early years of the twentieth century.[31] Whilst this generally coincides, as at Folkestone, with improvements to the water supply, it was also due to the influence of local health authorities on improved domestic hygiene.

This nationwide campaign to instil hygienic habits into working families, and particularly the promotion of breastfeeding, was a significant factor in improving the nation's overall health. As Folkestone's Sanitary Inspector, John Pearson, had indicated in 1904, three-quarters of deaths occurring during the first year of life were of babies who had been artificially fed.[32] From the late 1890s this was increasingly seen as an

---

[27] J. Pearson, Thirty Years Sanitary Experience, *Journal of the Royal Sanitary Institute*, volume xlii, no.5, 1922

[28] Folkestone MOH Report, 1899-1900, NA MH 12/5053

[29] *Folkestone Herald*, 13th September, 1902

[30] LGB Sanitary Papers, Folkestone Borough 1899-1900, MH 12/5053

[31] R. I. Woods, P. A. Watterson & J. H. Woodward, The Causes of Rapid Infant Mortality Decline in England and Wales, 1861-1921, Part I, *Population Studies*, 42, 1988, p.344

[32] J. Pearson, *Milk Supplies and their Dangers, with Local Experiences*, Paper at Folkestone Health Congress, 1904, *Journal of State Medicine,* volume xii, no.9, September 1904

important factor contributing to infant deaths.[33] Whilst the English medical profession at this time possessed no knowledge of any immunological benefits to be derived from breastfeeding,[34] many doctors were convinced of the harm that could be done to babies and young children by being fed inappropriate foods.[35]

Part of the reason for these fears was the belief that bovine *tubercle* could be communicated to humans, particularly children. At the Folkestone Health Congress of 1904 Councillor Shelmerdine of Liverpool, responding to an interim report of the 1904 Royal Commission on Tuberculosis, suggested that avoiding cows milk could eradicate infant mortality from tuberculosis:

> I should, as a layman, like to have a satisfactory explanation as to why consumption of the Mesenteric glands of the bowels, a common cause of death of infants, is practically unknown amongst breast fed babies but is common in infants fed on cows' milk and is thought to be increasing?'[36]

Consequently, in order to avoid infection from bovine *tubercle*, and to deter mothers from using artificial milk products, breastfeeding was encouraged from the first years of the twentieth century.

This increase in breastfeeding may well have significantly affected the health of the working classes through improving their resistance to disease. The incidence of tuberculosis, as of other infectious diseases, would have been affected not only by external factors such as overcrowding and poor nutrition, but also by improved natural resistance, conferred by healthier nursing mothers, as the more vulnerable and susceptible individuals were "winnowed out" over generations.[37]

Although breastfeeding in England was practised more than in Europe during the later nineteenth century bottle-feeding had been increasingly

---

[33] A. Newsholme, 39th Annual Report of LGB, 1909-10. *Supplement to Report of Board Medical Officer containing a report on Infant and Child Mortality,* (PP 1910/xxix, Cd.5263), p.57; R. I. Woods et al, The Causes of Rapid Infant Mortality Decline, Part II, 1988, p.116

[34] A. Koerber, From Folklore to Fact: The Rhetorical History of Breastfeeding and Immunity, 1950–1997, *Journal of Medical Humanities,* 27, 2006, pp. 151–166

[35] M. Yunge-Bateman, MOH report 1905, p.6

[36] Councillor Shelmerdine, The Distribution and Sale of Humanised and Sterilised Milk, Paper at Folkestone Health Congress, 1904, *Journal of State Medicine,* volume xii, no.9, September 1904

[37] D. Byrne and J. Keithley, Housing and the Health of the Community, *Unhealthy Housing: Research, Remedies and Reform,* eds. R. Burridge & D. Ormandy, London: Routledge, 1993, p. 57

adopted,[38] chiefly due to the emergence of large dairy companies that provided affordable milk. Their advertising campaigns also convinced many of its convenience and safety as an alternative to breast milk.[39] Following the efforts of concerned MOHs to reverse this trend, by 1910 Arthur Newsholme was able to state that 80% of mothers were breastfeeding.[40] This assertive public health campaign, although intended to reduce infection from tuberculous cows, would certainly have improved resistance to diarrhoea and infectious diseases in young children.

MOHs around the country were concerned to improve standards of domestic hygiene and child rearing, particularly following the recommendations of the 1904 Inter-departmental Committee on Physical Deterioration. The Committee's report cited overcrowding, atmospheric pollution and the inadequate nutrition of mothers and children as contributing to the poor health of the working classes. However, its authors chiefly blamed these deficiencies on parental ignorance and neglect rather than poverty. This perception of public health issues resulted in the subsequent emphasis on hygienic education and the relative neglect of environmental reform.

Similarly in Folkestone Yunge-Bateman, in accordance with the views of Arthur Newsholme, James Niven and other MOHs at this time, ignored poverty as a direct cause of poor health amongst the working classes and was more inclined to blame mothers for providing inadequate care for their children. In his 1905 report he indicated that the increase in childhood deaths of the previous year was due to the ignorance and lack of care demonstrated by the poor, who "show a woeful apathy, neglect and want of knowledge in bringing up their offspring". When the mother was working, he claimed, the children were poorly attended and were often fed inappropriate foods such as condensed milk and flour when too young.[41] This condemnation of working mothers for neglecting their children was a typical middle class response at this time, although a mother's income was often the most important factor in keeping her children alive.

Whilst the Committee on Physical Deterioration recognised that social

---

[38] A. Roberts, *Feeding and mortality in the early months of life; changes in medical opinion and popular feeding practice, 1850-1900*, unpublished Ph.D. thesis, University of Hull, 1973

[39] P. J. Atkins, Mothers' Milk and Infant Death in Britain circa 1900-1940, *Anthropology of Food*, 2nd September, 2003, p.10

[40] A. Newsholme, Supplement to Report of Board Medical Officer containing a report on Infant and Child Mortality 1910, p.71; P. J. Atkins, Mothers' Milk, 2003, p.11 claims that evidence from a variety of MOH reports indicates 85%

[41] M. Yunge-Bateman, Folkestone MOH report 1905, p.6

conditions had improved, they concluded that there remained "a considerable class of persons who were physically degenerate".[42] Their report also identified a lack of breastfeeding as being detrimental to the national health and recognised that, together with improvements in domestic hygiene and diet, these were measures that local MOHs and health visitors could implement at little extra cost. It also seems likely that health visitors and charitable agencies would have ensured that new mothers were provided with sufficient nourishment to nurse their children successfully, a problem that had been identified by George Newman in 1906.[43] Furthermore, the Notification of Births Act of 1907 ensured that health visitors knew which families to visit.

In Folkestone Yunge-Bateman initiated the distribution of pamphlets on diet and childrearing from 1899.[44] In 1910 school medical inspections were introduced, and a school nurse was appointed who also visited the homes of sick children.[45] From 1917 a professional health visitor was employed by the Council.[46]

Table 6.5 demonstrates that infant deaths (the usual indicator of the health of a district) were generally falling from 1900 in all wards apart from deaths due to epidemics of diarrhoea in 1904, 1906 and 1911, which occurred almost exclusively in the north and east wards. Infant deaths were, on average, about four times higher per head of population in the poorer north and east wards, far higher than the variation in mortality between wards for the total deaths registered. Births were also falling in all wards suggesting that a reduction in family sizes may have contributed to an overall reduction in infant deaths from the first years of the twentieth century.

Apart from a steep rise in infant deaths during the war, and a smaller increase in deaths from tuberculosis, infant mortality was reduced by about two thirds between 1900-1920 and deaths from pulmonary tuberculosis by about a half. This fall in the death rates for young children and sufferers of pulmonary tuberculosis also reflects national trends at this time.

---

[42] Report of the Inter-departmental Committee on Physical Deterioration, 1904, Cd. 2175 volume 1, part ii

[43] G. Newman, *Infant Mortality. A Social Problem*, London: Methuen, 1906, p.260

[44] Folkestone Borough Sanitary & Hospitals Committee (Amc12/1), Minute Book, January 1898-May 1900

[45] M. Yunge-Bateman, MOH report, 1910

[46] M. Yunge-Bateman, MOH report, 1917

Table 6.5: Distribution of Mortality in Folkestone by Wards 1901-1910

		West ward		
	pop	birth	Total death	Infant death
1901	11,300	122	135	14
1902	11,470	149	112	14
1903	11,560	116	111	14
1904	11,650	117	108	9
1905	11,734	108	101	7
1906	11,641	113	119	12
1907	11,809	106	120	10
1908	11,530	117	103	9
1909	11,636	92	123	8
1910	11,880	98	129	8
1911				3
		North ward		
	pop	birth	Total death	Infant death
1901	10,460	336	179	62
1902	11,030	336	157	41
1903	12,140	375	157	42
1904	12,911	339	169	51
1905	13,780	356	146	38
1906	14,484	339	136	51
1907	14,655	343	124	27
1908	14,691	344	157	39
1909	14,885	316	160	27
1910	15,111	305	126	14
1911				45
		East ward		
	pop	birth	Total death	Infant death
1901	8,730	247	137	37
1902	8,800	242	130	28
1903	8,450	244	124	28
1904	9,139	243	134	49
1905	9,256	218	125	29
1906	9,375	223	122	24
1907	9,566	196	142	26
1908	9,359	186	102	12
1909	9,449	222	111	22
1910	9,639	189	105	14
1911				19

The eradication of tuberculous milk can not be seen as a contributing to this mortality decline. Large financial compensations exacted by agricultural interests considerably delayed the process of animal inspection and testing. Local sanitary authorities had been constrained by a tuberculosis order issued by the Board of Agriculture in 1909 granting compensation to the owners of slaughtered cows for the value of such cows plus 20 shillings per head if the animals were found not to be infected with tuberculosis. As *tuberculin* testing was notoriously unreliable this order probably persuaded local authorities to exercise caution in the slaughter of suspect animals.[47]

As the campaign against tuberculosis became linked to a broader concern for the health of the nation early in the twentieth century, local and national evidence strongly suggests that a consequent focus on the welfare and conduct of mothers and children, including an increase in breastfeeding amongst the working classes, contributed significantly to an overall reduction of mortality rates.

Tuberculosis in Folkestone

In 1899, coinciding with independent action taken by Arthur Newsholme in Brighton, and the campaigning work of the NAPT, Yunge-Bateman proposed various measures designed to prevent the spread of pulmonary tuberculosis. These proposals were confounded by a Council reluctant to raise rates for social reform as well as by local agricultural interests. His detailed report on tuberculosis emphasised the infectious nature of the disease and urged the Council to take immediate action:

> Consumption, in one form or another, is the cause of forty eight deaths on an average per annum in this Borough; and until recent years has been considered to be an hereditary disease, this opinion still holding good among the general public. Research, during the last few years, has proved it to be an infectious disease, and one which is easily preventable. With this knowledge before you, and in view of the measures now being commenced throughout the country for its prevention, it becomes your duty to consider what steps should be taken.[48]

A common, if conservative, estimate of the number of active cases of pulmonary tuberculosis in a community was arrived at by multiplying the

---

[47] M. Yunge-Bateman, Sanitary & Hospitals Committee Minute Book, 1907-1910

[48] Folkestone MOH Report on Consumption, Folkestone Sanitary & Hospitals Committee Minute Book, 1899, Fo-Amc12/1

number of deaths from the disease by 10. Thus, in 1899, it can be judged that there existed about 480 consumptives requiring medical supervision, and the number giving a positive reaction to a tuberculin test would have been "vastly greater".[49]

Yunge-Bateman's faith in the practical application of germ theory is evident in his communications with the Council at this time. He was convinced that the discovery of the *bacillus* heralded the imminent eradication of tuberculosis. He recommended a variety of preventive measures, the most significant of which, such as the reduction of overcrowding in tenements, the provision of public slaughterhouses, and obtaining powers from Parliament to inspect all cows from which milk supplied to the district originated, were not adopted by the Council.

In October 1901 Yunge-Bateman, recognising the inadequacy of voluntary notification for locating cases of consumption, recommended the adoption of compulsory notification for all cases:

> At present the only means of cases being brought to my knowledge is by returns of deaths and the return of new cases taken from the District Medical Officer's relief book, which are furnished me weekly. This is only a small percentage of the cases that really exist.[50]

If notification were enforced, Yunge-Bateman advised the Council, the homes of all consumptives could be inspected and thoroughly disinfected, and the occupants educated as to the infectious nature of tuberculosis and instructed in measures to control the spread of the disease. Despite growing alarm, in part due to the influx of consumptives sent chiefly by the Poor Law Guardians of London boroughs to nearby Sandgate, the Council deferred their decision.

The desirability of compulsory notification was, however, recognised by some local practitioners, despite its threat to the confidential relationship between doctor and patient and to the short term prosperity of the town. W. J. Tyson, senior physician to Folkestone's Victoria Hospital, felt compelled to urge the adoption of notification at the Folkestone Health Congress of 1904:

> Such a state of things as is at present carried on at Sandgate should be impossible, for there, in a town of 2,000 people, in its most crowded streets

---

[49] R. W. Philip, Progressive Medicine and the Outlook on Tuberculosis, *The Lancet*, 31st July, 1909, p. 284

[50] Report of MOH, October, 1901, Folkestone Council Sanitary & Hospitals Committee Minute Book, 1900-1901, Fo-A/M/c/12/4

> are placed at times some 300 or 400 persons suffering from pulmonary tuberculosis. Many of the medical profession have never been very strongly in favour of the compulsory notification of *phthisis*, and, I think, for some good reasons; but when such a condition of things exists as in Sandgate, a change of opinion will rapidly come about...'[51]

Nevertheless, in March 1906 the Borough Council's Sanitary and Hospitals Committee felt this measure could threaten the town's reputation for health and voted against applying to the Local Government Board to make consumption a notifiable disease.[52]

In 1908 Yunge-Bateman advised the Committee to adopt a comprehensive system of isolation, education and health visiting of infected houses. "The idea to be aimed at" he emphasised "is that wherever [the consumptive] is, his powers of infectivity shall be reduced to a minimum". As consumption was a disease of protracted duration Yunge-Bateman viewed long term isolation as impracticable. He suggested that the working life of a patient could be extended by occasional visits to a sanatorium of about a month which, he advised, could be provided by the Council under section 131 of the Public Health Act of 1875. These visits would, he claimed, improve the patient's condition, inculcate "desirable habits", reduce infection, and permit the early diagnosis of other infected members of the household. Home treatment, he warned, often failed to prevent infection, besides failing to cure the patient.[53]

The Council continued to oppose any overt public health interventions. They rejected the MOH's proposals for the public treatment of consumptives at a dispensary, the employment of a tuberculosis nurse to visit patients at home and the provision of sanatorium treatment and isolation.[54] In addition to baulking at the cost of such a scheme, Councillors were apprehensive of drawing attention to the existence of infectious disease and damaging Folkestone's popularity as a health resort. As it had only recently been claimed that tuberculosis posed a problem of infection Folkestone Borough Council apparently felt that the workhouse infirmary, conveniently situated outside the Borough, could continue to accommodate destitute consumptives. And those suffering from the disease

---

[51] W. J. Tyson, Presidential Address to the Preventive Medicine Section, Folkestone Health Congress, *Journal of State Medicine*, volume xii, no.9, September 1904

[52] Report of MOH, October, 1901, Fo/A/M/c/12/4

[53] Sanitary & Hospitals Committee Minute Book, 1907-1910, Fo/A/M/c/12/6

[54] Report of sub-committee on tuberculosis, September, 1912, Sanitary & Hospitals Committee Minute Book, Fo/A/Mc/12/7

with families to support them would invariably be housed out of sight of visitors to the town's elegant west ward.

This policy of inaction and concealment was further consolidated in September 1910. Following a communication from Margate Town Council suggesting that the records of infectious disease in health resorts be kept confidential, Folkestone Council voted to approve such a course of action.[55] Undoubtedly, continuing to attract the more affluent health seeker afflicted with tuberculosis, who may have been deterred by the introduction of public health regulations, was also a consideration for the Council.

During the first two decades of the twentieth century a singular emphasis on the role of the *bacillus* in causing active tuberculosis tended to sidetrack environmental reforms. The medical profession's focus on infection, although it threatened to publicise the incidence of disease in towns, also served to accommodate local interests by deflecting attention away from the need for radical housing and environmental reforms and towards the dangers posed by the infectious individual.

Even Folkestone's Sanitary Inspector and MOH, recently trained in the new germ theory of disease, were still inclined to blame the insanitary habits of the poor whilst ignoring the effects of poverty and a lack of planning in the poorer districts of the town. Moreover, they were unable to persuade the local Council to effect a reduction of overcrowding or to adopt any course of action that might be detrimental to the town's reputation as a health resort.

The intransigence of Folkestone's Council to adopting preventive measures designed to avoid the spread of tuberculosis was not an isolated instance. Local government structures had traditionally served land and property interests, and in many Boroughs these interests prevailed against public health interventions recommended by their MOHs. There was at this time, it has been argued, considerable resistance throughout the country to raising rates for housing reform, the municipal ownership of water companies, and the control of milk supplies and slaughterhouses.[56]

Although some Boards of Guardians and Friendly Societies had, since the early 1880s, sent consumptive patients to convalescent homes and hospitals for tuberculosis, it was not until 1898, even in the more socially progressive London Boroughs, that local government authorities took any action against the spread of the disease. Even then the majority of

---

[55] Folkestone Borough, Sanitary & Hospitals Committee Minute Book, March-October, 1910, Fo-A/M/c12/6

[56] C. Bellamy, *Administering Central-Local Relations*, 1988, p. 66; D. Watkins, *The English Revolution in Scientific Medicine*, 1984, p. 46

Councils restricted their interventions to offering to disinfect the rooms, clothes and bedding of consumptives, a service that was, as in Folkestone, rarely accepted due to the complex and stigmatising image of the disease.[57] Furthermore the disinfection of houses occupied by the tubercular remained unenforceable until the implementation in 1912 of the National Insurance Act as tuberculosis had not been classified as infectious under the Infectious Diseases Act of 1898.

Tuberculosis and Milk

Little concerted action was taken in England before the late 1920s to control the production and sale of milk. But during the 1890s a nascent interest in bacteriology did stimulate some interest in the relationship between tuberculosis in man and animals. Three Royal Commissions were established to consider the question in 1890, 1901 and 1911 but little consensus was established, partly due to Koch's refutation of the notion of any cross-infection at the London Tuberculosis Conference of 1901, and partly owing to the powerful economic interests vested in the meat trade, the Board of Agriculture and the farming community in general. Consequently there was little action taken to eradicate the disease from the national herd at this time.[58]

Although it was eventually to prove the source of a considerable amount of death and disease in the town, the production and consumption of milk in the Folkestone area was subject to no official regulation or inspection until part of Yunge-Bateman's recommendations to combat tuberculosis were adopted in March, 1899. The MOH recognised that debilitated children were particularly at risk of contracting scrofula, tuberculosis of the bones and joints, and other diseases:

> Cows are known to suffer from a tubercular disease of the udders, and milk procured from such a cow is the chief cause of infection in children of tender years, especially those who have been weakened or rendered susceptible by diarrhoea or catarrhal conditions of the intestines. Statistics prove that quite 30% of the cows in England are suffering from

[57] A. Hardy, *The Epidemic Streets*, Oxford University Press, 1993, pp.260-261; Report of MOH, Folkestone Borough, Sanitary & Hospitals Committee Minute Book, 1900-1902, Fo/A/M/c/12/3

[58] K. Waddington, The Science of Cows: Tuberculosis, Research and the State in the U.K., 1890-1914, *History of Science*, xxxix, 2001

tuberculosis.[59]

He advised that a qualified man should be appointed as milk inspector, that educational pamphlets on the hygienic production of milk be sent to all suppliers, that regulations be instituted for the operation of dairies and cowsheds and that contracts for tuberculosis free milk be recommended for all hospitals, convalescent homes, workhouses and institutions receiving children in the district. These measures were, however, unable to prevent infected milk being consumed in the town. The Council voted against obtaining powers to inspect milk imported from outside the district, and in 1896 it was estimated that nine tenths of milk came from outside the Borough directly to the consumer.[60]

The MOH suspected that the chief danger of disease being spread by milk was as a consequence of it being polluted in the homes of the working classes, particularly in hot weather.[61] Nevertheless he continued to press for the inspection of imported milk. In 1899 he had additionally recommended that the Council seek authority under a local act of parliament to examine all milk, cows and dairies involved in supplying the town, whether from inside or outside the district. This advice was, however, not acted upon. As late as 1921 the mayor of Folkestone, R.G. Wood, was left to decry a situation whereby the benefits granted to some towns who had obtained such private acts twenty years previously had not been accorded to the rest of the nation:

> why should Manchester, which has powers to inspect Dairy herds and cowsheds outside its area, be more favoured than other parts of the country in view of the advantages which have accrued by the reduction of tubercular infected milk supplies, one of the chief causes, I am informed, of tuberculosis.[62]

In May 1899 Mr. H. Hogben was employed by Folkestone Council, at 25 guineas a year, to inspect milk and examine cows as required by the MOH. By the end of the year Hogben reported that the periodical analysis of milk supplies was an insufficient safeguard, there being about 500

---

[59] M. Yunge-Bateman, Report on Prevention of Consumption to Folkestone Sanitary and Hospitals Committee, March 1899, Fo/A/M/c/12/1

[60] Ibid; MOH Report, 1911, Wellcome Library, b13562514; Folkestone MOH report, 1896, NA MH 12/5049, p.20

[61] Folkestone MOH report, 1906, Fo-A/M/c/12/3, p.12

[62] R.G. Wood, Presidential Address to Folkestone Health Congress, 1921, *Journal of the Royal Sanitary Institute*, volume xlii, no. 4, January 1922

different suppliers, and that the inspection of cows was essential.[63] Given the lack of powers afforded sanitary authorities to prohibit the sale of suspect milk imported from outside the district, and the time involved in obtaining the results of bacteriological analysis, milk would have remained a considerable source of disease. The Sanitary Inspector, John Pearson, observed that:

> often polluted milk which is known to be creating disease cannot be prohibited under 14 days, thus adding considerably to the number of cases, and the length of the epidemic.[64]

Infection and Control

These conflicts in Folkestone in the late nineteenth and early twentieth centuries between the MOH and the Borough Council illustrate the clash of values associated with a shift from a culture emphasising the freedom of the individual, favouring a *laissez faire* style of government, to a more integrated conception of society based around notions of civic duty and responsibility.

This ideological opposition was paralleled by totally incompatible approaches to public health. On one hand a positivist model centred on the prevention of infection demanded social co-operation and the constant surveillance and early treatment or institutionalisation of individuals identified as potentially pathological – paupers, the indigent, alcoholics, the sexually delinquent and the feeble-minded. On the other hand the Poor Law and Charity Organisation Society ethic of deterrence and self-responsibility encouraged the chronically sick and destitute to be independent of the state until they were *in extremis* and their relatives and neighbours were no longer able to support them.

This demand for a more centralised control of society emerging in the late 1890s, characterised by direct intervention in the lives of the working classes, is exemplified by Charles Egerton Fitzgerald, President of the Folkestone Medical Society. In 1898 Fitzgerald published a paper in *The Lancet* applauding the action of the New York City Board of Health in notifying and isolating consumptives and calling for notification to be

[63] Folkestone Borough Council, Sanitary & Hospitals Committee minute book, 1898-1900, Fo-A/M/c/12/1

[64] J. Pearson, *Milk Supplies and their Dangers, with Local Experiences*, Paper at Folkestone Health Congress, 1904, *Journal of State Medicine,* volume xii, no.9, September 1904; M. Yunge-Bateman, 1896 MOH report, p.9, b13562514

"rigidly enforced in all cases of tuberculosis".[65] Fitzgerald felt that it was the duty of the medical profession to place the health of the community above the rights of the individual:

> The liberty of the subject has to be curtailed in the case of individuals who are imperilling the safety or lives of the community; why, then, should there not be restrictions on those who, by their carelessness, ignorance, or wilfulness, entail sickness, suffering, and death on millions of their innocent fellow-creatures, aye, and on millions yet unborn?[66]

Fitzgerald's concern to curtail the liberty of the tubercular from spreading disease appears to have conflicted with the promotion of Folkestone as a health resort. The social tensions surrounding this stigmatising disease and the partial and class based nature of measures enacted for its prevention are illustrated by the case of Radclyffe Radclyffe-Hall, a middle class victim of tuberculosis who succumbed to the disease in a local hotel.

Shortly after the publication of his article Fitzgerald had been called to the Leas Hotel to treat Mr. Radclyffe-Hall who had recently arrived from Cannes. On the following day Radclyffe-Hall expired in his room. Fitzgerald gave the cause of death as pulmonary tuberculosis and informed the manager of the hotel that the disease was infectious, despite it not being included in the list of notifiable diseases at that time, and advised that the furniture and bedding should be destroyed, the wallpaper removed, the woodwork repainted and the room disinfected.

Subsequently a claim for the costs of these procedures was made on behalf of the hotel against the executors of Mr. Radclyffe-Hall's estate. The defendants, understandably reluctant to admit to a history of tuberculosis in the family, claimed that several eminent physicians had attended the deceased and that he had never been diagnosed with chest disease. The judge, whilst commenting that in his experience the case had no precedent, accepted Fitzgerald's diagnosis, as well as the evidence of MOH Yunge-Bateman, that the medical profession now regarded tuberculosis as infectious. He found for the plaintiffs, and awarded the hotel costs. The defendants asked for leave to appeal, contending that the case raised issues of serious import for hotel patrons, but appeal was denied.

This decision to legally impose restrictions and costs on the tubercular

---

[65] C. E. Fitzgerald, The Prevention of Tuberculosis, *The Lancet,* 8th October, 1898, pp.932-933

[66] Ibid, p.933

for the danger they posed to public health was unprecedented in Britain, and appears to have been the exception that proved the rule. Although regulations excluding the tubercular had long been enforced in many hotels in southern Europe where the infectiousness of consumption had traditionally been acknowledged, this judgement seems to have had no effect on the subsequent reception of the tubercular at English seaside hotels.[67]

This example strongly suggests that although many doctors were, following the initial crusading enthusiasm of the campaign against tuberculosis in 1898, convinced of the risks of infection, regulations to limit its spread were not uniformly accepted or applied. The crusade against tuberculosis was essentially a mission directed exclusively at working class behaviour.

Whilst similar social interventions in public health to those recommended by Fitzgerald had been under way for most of the decade in Germany and France it would be another fifteen years before similar regulations would be adopted in England. Fitzgerald recognised the cultural difficulties that such action would have entailed:

> The government of the United States is democratic, but the sanitary measures adopted are sometimes autocratic and the functions performed by the sanitary authorities paternal in character. I freely admit that in this country public opinion is not yet ripe for radical measures.[68]

Even the NAPT, many of whose members advocated the segregation of working class consumptives, had rejected the adoption of coercive practices. As the Prince of Wales had observed at their first conference in 1900, the Association had chosen the path of instructing public opinion and stimulating interest rather than advocating measures involving compulsion.[69] There existed a strong tradition of resistance to interventionist social policy in Britain; the Contagious Diseases Act of 1869 had been repealed and the 1873 Vaccination Act nullified. Nevertheless Fitzgerald envisioned a future when the medical profession were:

> not simply medical advisors but a species of "beneficient autocrats" with the power of enforcing our salutary policy in spite of the prejudice, timidity, and sentimental conventionality which step in and ofttimes

[67] The Infectiousness of Phthisis, *The Lancet*, 18th March, 1899, p. 782
[68] C. E. Fitzgerald, The Prevention of Tuberculosis, 1898, p.933
[69] HRH Prince of Wales, First NAPT Conference, quoted in Sir Robert Philip, The Outlook on Tuberculosis, *BMJ*, 10th January, 1931, p.43

> prevent us from carrying our scientific convictions to a philosophical conclusion.[70]

Fitzgerald, although a supporter of the Conservative Party, was in favour of social intervention and believed that sentiment should not be allowed to interfere with a scientifically validated programme directed at confining the tubercular in institutions. The implementation of these measures would not, however, be permitted to interfere with the operation of Folkestone's function as an elite health resort. Despite Fitzgerald's notification to the local MOH of Radcliffe-Hall's death from pulmonary tuberculosis, and the subsequent court case and attendant publicity, it is evident that resort hotels and apartments remained unregulated and available to middle and upper class sufferers of the disease.

Certainly Folkestone continued to be promoted as an all year round resort for consumptives. Unsupervised cures were advertised into the inter-war years, apparently facilitated by the latest technology. A health resort guide of 1919 stated:

> Tubercular cases do extremely well, especially cases of *phthisis* without much bronchial catarrh. There are many houses facing south, on the front and elsewhere, in which a fresh air cure can be carried out with ease all through the winter; a number of them are fitted with verandahs. One of the largest hotels has "loggias", which are veritable sun traps, with arrangements for keeping them ventilated with fresh air while warding off the wind if excessive.[71]

Owners of hotels and apartments were also able to offer the tubercular an alternative to the strict regimes which operated even at sanatoria for the middle classes, such as the King Edward VII at Midhurst in Sussex:

> catarrhal lung cases of tuberculous origin do well, and an open air cure can easily be carried out without call for sanatorium, owing to the common provision of balconies and spacious verandahs in the roomy houses facing the front.[72]

---

[70] C. E. Fitzgerald, The Prevention of Tuberculosis, 1898, p.933

[71] N. Wood, *Health Resorts of the British Isles,* University of London Press, 1919

[72] T. D. Luke, *Spas and Health Resorts of the British Isles*, London: A.&C. Black, 1919.

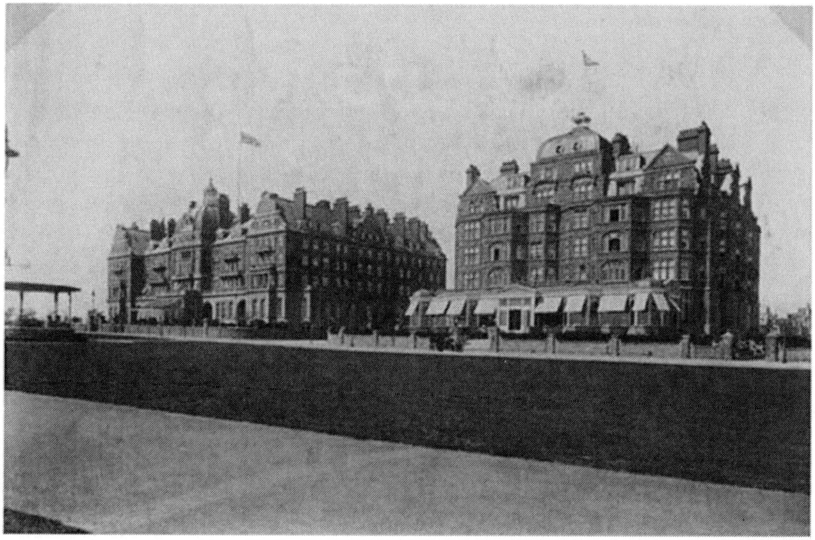

Illustration 6.1: Folkestone 1905 - The Grand Hotel on the right and the Metropole.

For the more privileged the doctor/patient relationship remained a governing factor that was not essentially compromised by scientific developments, and the older medical models of constitution and heredity were retained. Pursuing an individually prescribed regimen under their personal physician may well have been more attractive to those who disliked the atmosphere of an institution. The middle classes were accustomed to personalised medical care being provided in their own rooms and, particularly in the case of such a protean disease as pulmonary tuberculosis, any course of treatment, it was felt, needed to be especially suited to the constitution and character of each particular case. Hermann Weber had emphasised the necessity of accounting for individual manifestations of the disease in 1885:

> The difference between different cases of *phthisis* is so great, that it is impossible to lay down fixed rules for climatic treatment. In deciding between different climates and localities, the circumstances connected with the aetiology, the stage of the disease, the amount of destruction, the complications with diseases of other organs, are very important; but still more so, the distinction between a weak and a strong constitution, an excitable or a torpid nature, between progressive or retrogressive, active or stationary cases. Mental peculiarities too, ought not to be overlooked – the

habits of the invalid, the circumstances in which he has lived.[73]

Even after the compulsory notification of the disease the more affluent and independent consumptives continued to follow a peripatetic existence, often moving from one resort to another in order to benefit from the appropriate climate at any season of the year. A speaker at the NAPT annual conference of 1927 acknowledged that health regulations were not enforced in hotels, and that the tubercular posed a danger to the health of seaside towns. In particular he drew attention to:

> the dangers of migratory cases of tuberculosis. Patients came to health resorts from London or from various sanatoriums; they did not call in a doctor; they came in the busy season and the rooms were not disinfected after them.[74]

The epidemiology of tuberculosis remained difficult to determine. Resort doctors whose practices depended on affluent consumptives maintained that the risk of infection was minimal. This conviction was evident at a meeting of the new British Health Resorts Association at Hastings in 1932, where notable doctors claimed:

> The fear of infection…was practically baseless, and the public must learn that there was no danger in using a health resort both for the sick and healthy.[75]

Financially independent consumptive visitors to health resorts such as Folkestone were rarely subject to any public health controls. The early twentieth century crusade against tuberculosis was exclusively focused on the hygienic and social control of the working classes and their domestic habits. But despite the urgings of Medical Officers of Health little action was taken by local or national authorities to alleviate overcrowding, improve housing conditions or to rid cattle of tuberculosis for a further quarter of a century.

---

[73] H. Weber, The Croonian Lectures on The Hygienic and Climatic Treatment of Chronic Pulmonary Phthisis, *BMJ*, 28th March, 4th & 11th April, 1885, p.688

[74] Anonymous speaker, NAPT 13th Annual Conference, *The Lancet*, 9th July, 1927, p.69

[75] Dr. R. A. Young, physician to Middlesex Hospital, and Dr. L. Findlay, physician to the East London Hospital for Children, The Coastal Health Resort, *The Lancet*, 12th March, 1932, p.583

Tuberculosis and Inheritance

By 1900 there were, as noted in chapter two, increasing demands from social commentators and the public for the isolation of destitute consumptives. There were also concerns that the Poor Law system was unsuited to cope with them and unable to prevent their reproduction. In 1908 the *British Journal of Tuberculosis* referred to a:

> great army of tuberculous derelicts [whom it considered responsible for] dragging into destitution and disease their families and friends, and only too frequently multiplying the evil by the propagation of delicate and tuberculously disposed children.

The editorial noted the common dread of the workhouse infirmary and the refusal of the vast majority of consumptives to apply for relief under the Poor Law, but insisted that isolation was the only solution:

> No satisfactory advance towards the elimination of the Great White Plague can be effected until rational means are found for the effective segregation and proper care of these infectious consumptive cases for whom no other aid is possible than that which should, and must, be provided by the State.[76]

As this article indicates, it was not only the fear of infection posed by this "army of tuberculous derelicts" that concerned the middle classes, but also their continued propagation. The influence of evolutionism was, however, not restricted to the middle classes. In Folkestone not only establishment figures, such as Dr. William Tyson (quoted in chapter 2), held that pauperism and sickness were largely due to the operation of "laws of heredity". Samuel Pilcher, one of the first working class Folkestone Councillors and resident of the east ward for which he continually urged social reform during the late nineteenth and early twentieth centuries, similarly viewed disease and moral weakness as being passed from generation to generation.

Despite being a rare champion of the working classes in Folkestone, Pilcher considered that England had become a drunken nation, lacking in self-control, and that there was an increase of paupers, lunatics, criminals

---

[76] Editorial, Tuberculosis and the Poor Law, *British Journal of Tuberculosis*, 1908, pp. 155-8

and debtors.[77] Pilcher felt, in common with many others at the turn of the century, that the nation was in decline and argued that people should consider the health of their antecedents before marriage:

> the present generation are suffering with certain maladies inherited from parents of previous times indulging in certain excesses...in one form or another there may be consumption, insanity, hereditary sin, drunkeness, morbid appetites, laziness, selfishness or another of the hereditary diseases innumerable either of mind or body...the taint of blood is bound to show itself in either a new or remote generation.

Pilcher believed that social reform was possible, overcrowding was the main problem confronting the health of the poor, and that with the "proper physical and moral training" these undesirable qualities could be checked.[78]

This view of the potential dangers posed to the fitness of the nation from the biological inheritance of a sickly and degenerate urban working class, together with an advocacy of both environmental and moral reform, reflects a view of social evolution which, it has been argued, was largely embraced by the Liberal party in the early twentieth century. A more collective society was now envisioned where economic, social and physiological progress was guided by the state rather than being left to market forces. Whilst "new" Liberal thought accommodated eugenic assumptions, some individuals, such as the influential Arthur Newsholme, believed that the negative effects of biological inheritance could be offset by a form of moral evolution of the working classes initiated by the state.[79]

The Liberal party had formulated no specific policy to address the problems of poverty and the apparent deteriorating health of the poor. Proposed responses included isolation of the chronically sick and destitute, the moral reform of the working classes and environmental improvements. They reflected a diversity of medical approaches towards public health at a time when medical experts exerted increasing influence over social policy. Inspired by evolutionary theory and an almost evangelical compulsion for the moral reform of the working classes as much as by bacteriology, these planned interventions were not mutually exclusive, or even necessarily in

---

[77] *Folkestone Herald*, 7th October, 1899; Manuscripts of Samuel Pilcher 1839-c.1912, F/1987/8 EKAC
[78] *Folkestone Herald*, 7th October, 1899
[79] J. M. Eyler, Poverty, Disease, Responsibility: Arthur Newsholme and the Public Health Dilemmas of British Liberalism, *The Millbank Quarterly*, volume 67, supplement 1, 1989, pp.117-123

competition.[80]

It can be argued, for example, that a concern to promote "national efficiency" prior to the First World War manifested itself in the anti-tuberculosis campaign through withholding relief to the poor consumptive who drank or was considered sexually profligate, as much as through the indoctrination of domestic hygiene by health visitors. All these approaches to improving the health of the nation, which increasingly required some form of centralised co-ordination, served to placate complex *bourgeois* anxieties relating to health and social order and promised to reinvigorate the national economy.

[80] The potential cultural reversal of negative traits was accommodated in Lamarck's notion of the inheritance of "acquired characteristics".

CHAPTER SEVEN

TREATING THE TUBERCULAR POOR IN FOLKESTONE, 1880-1912

This chapter identifies the provision, either medical or financial, that would have been available to the working man or woman who contracted tuberculosis in Folkestone prior to the National Insurance Act of 1911. The work of Friendly Societies, voluntary hospitals, charities and the Poor Law is assessed together with the motives of lay and medical contributors, the type and quality of care offered and the responses of those in receipt of assistance.

Self Help and Mutual Aid Societies

The medical care of the working classes during this period can be divided between that supplied through institutions created and administered by members of the middle classes, such as charities, the Poor Law and the dispensary or voluntary hospital, and organisations established by and for the working classes, such as Friendly and Co-operative Societies and Trades Unions operating on principles of mutual aid. The increasing impact of charitable, state and municipal medical agencies and institutions on the lives of the working classes from the late nineteenth century has been attributed to a variety of factors including local civic pride, humanitarian and religious impulses, fears of disease and a desire for more efficient control of the labour force.[1] However, throughout the nineteenth century and into the twentieth, it has been argued, medical treatment for the working classes was predominantly self prescribed and administered.

If medical advice was sought it was far more likely to be from a

---

[1] H. Marland, *Medicine and Society in Wakefield and Huddersfield, 1780-1870,* Cambridge University Press, 1987, p.2

chemist than a doctor.[2] Whilst some patent medicines appealed to all social classes, chemists were mostly patronised by the lower middle and working classes[3] where traditional medical recipes, often handed down through families, could be made up.[4]

Various patent medicines were advertised from the late nineteenth century as remedies for pulmonary tuberculosis. These included *Congreve's Elixir for Consumption, Dr. William's Pink Pills for Pale People, Hardy's Brompton Cough Specific, Angier's Emulsion,* and J. Collis Browne's[5] *Chlorodyne*. They were generally opium based specifics, indeed opiate addiction was not uncommon amongst consumptives,[6] and possibly this added to the perception of the consumptive as being emotionally temperamental. In Folkestone the number of chemists, predominantly located in working class districts, rose from three in 1847 to seventeen in 1909. Allowing for the increase in population this represents a constant of one chemist for about every 1,700 inhabitants.[7]

Cures were also advertised in the local and national press and were available by post. As about 20% of active cases were thought to recover spontaneously,[8] and as there existed no established remedy, tuberculosis provided a ready market for both quacks and herbalists. One of the more notorious and enduring cures was Stevens' *Umckaloabo,* a herbal remedy from South Africa.

The ethos of self-help and a determination to avoid charity is also evident in the history of British Friendly Societies. Prior to the National Insurance Act of 1911 membership of Friendly Societies and sick clubs provided the only affordable means available to the working man of securing himself and his family against destitution and the workhouse in the event of chronic sickness.

---

[2] V. Berridge, Health and Medicine, *The Cambridge Social History of Britain: Social Agencies and Institutions,* ed. F. M. L. Thompson, Cambridge University Press, 1993 p.186; H. Marland, *Medicine and Society in Wakefield and Huddersfield*, p.378

[3] V. Berridge, Health and Medicine, 1993, p.181

[4] Ibid, p.190

[5] Collis Browne was born in Maidstone in 1819, and later lived in Ramsgate where he died in 1884.

[6] V. Berridge, *Opium and the People: Opiate Use and Policy in 19th Century and Early 20th Century Britain*, London: Free Association Books, 1999, p.187

[7] *Chemist & Druggist*, 31st July, 1909, p.164. The population of Folkestone was about 5,000 in 1847 rising to about 33,000 in 1908

[8] Dr. A. Latham, in evidence for the BMA at the Select Committee on Patent Medicines of 1912, quoted in S. W. B. Newsom, Stevens' Cure: A Secret Remedy, *Journal of the Royal Society of Medicine*, volume 95, 2002, p.464

Tuberculosis, apart from being the most deadly disease at the turn of the century was also, according to the Report of the Royal Commission on the Poor Law of 1909, the most likely disease to lead to destitution.[9] The chronic nature of the disease generally led to financial ruin for the working man, leaving himself and his family to be relieved under the Poor Law, despite a widespread reluctance to apply for medical relief.[10]

Although there is some evidence to suggest that Friendly Society physicians may have prescribed rest at an earlier stage of the disease towards the end of the nineteenth century,[11] there would have been enormous social pressure on both working men and women to provide for their families while they were able, and the disease was, therefore, generally well advanced before it prevented work. In 1915, even after the provision of a limited period of state sickness benefit in 1912, Godfrey Dixon, Birmingham's Chief Tuberculosis Officer, advised that consumptives should work as long as possible:

> Acting upon the medical advice given to him, and following his own instincts in too many instances, he discontinues his work unnecessarily, and the resulting state of semi-starvation aggravates his disease.[12]

Whilst Friendly Societies and sick clubs did provide some security it was generally less than adequate and mediated through over-committed doctors. Sickness benefits were no more than three or four shillings a week, Friendly Societies did not usually treat wives or children [13] and, according to Beatrice Webb's evidence to the Poor Law Commission, neither medical clubs nor Friendly Societies would accept people with "incipient disease or constitutional defects".[14] Consequently, any form of insurance for workers known to come from a family with a history of consumption would probably have been difficult to obtain.

Nevertheless, whether due to the cursory nature of initial examinations of potential members or to members succumbing to the disease after joining a society, one seventh of all Friendly Society deaths were

---

[9] Royal Commission on the Poor Law, volume xxxvii, p.51

[10] RCPL, appendix, volume iv, 1905-9, notes that neighbours tended to rally round and support the sick and their dependants

[11] J. C. Riley, Ill Health During the Mortality Decline: The Friendly Societies' Experience, *Bulletin of the History of Medicine*, 1987, p.583

[12] G. B. Dixon, The Domiciliary Treatment of Tuberculous Patients, *British Journal of Tuberculosis*, volume 9, p.21

[13] D. G. Green, *Working Class Patients*, 1985, p.180 states that there was an increase in provision for women and children from the early twentieth century.

[14] B. & S. Webb, *The State and the Doctor*, London: Longmans, 1910, p.138

reportedly due to consumption.[15] In 1910 it was reported that, due to the chronic nature of the disease, Friendly Societies in England were paying out three times as much in sick pay to consumptives as the average sick pay to members dying from other causes.[16]

It seems probable that the thoroughness of medical examinations performed before candidates could be admitted to membership varied considerably. One researcher comments that admission to a society was easier than joining the army, whilst other sources suggest that it was in the interest of doctors to provide a strict initial examination in order to preclude candidates with potentially serious conditions.[17] In a survey conducted by the BMA in 1905 a doctor in Kent claimed that whilst he was content with club practice he knew of others who faced heavy workloads due to conducting lax examinations.[18]

Societies were also sometimes founded under local patronage,[19] although this may have compromised members' independence. In Folkestone the Baptist minister the Reverend Jeffrey, also a member of the Board of Guardians, founded the teetotal True Blue Friendly Society during the 1890s.[20] This form of sponsorship exemplifies the socially conservative position of many working men at this time; an organisation founded on the principle of mutual aid was often more likely to be motivated by notions of Christian fellowship than by socialist idealism in southern provincial towns at the turn of the century.

The COS considered that families who failed to make provision for times of sickness and unemployment were undeserving of relief.[21] Many of Folkestone's local oligarchy, the aristocrats, property owners, businessmen, military officers, churchmen and professionals, from whom the memberships of the local COS, as well as the Borough Council, were comprised, were also vociferous in their condemnation of families who, they felt, relied on the rates or charity to support them.

---

[15] *Daily Telegraph*, 3rd June, 1909, p.11

[16] From the South London District of the Ancient Order of Foresters, quoted in *The Englishman*, 12th January, 1910

[17] J. C. Riley, Ill Health During the Mortality Decline: The Friendly Societies' Experience, *Bulletin of the History of Medicine*, 1987, p.569; D. G. Green, *Working Class Patients*, 1985, p.103

[18] BMA Medico-Political Committee, An Investigation into the Economic Conditions of Contract Medical Practice in the United Kingdom, *BMJ* Supplement, 22nd July, 1905, p.44

[19] D. Weinbren, Mutually Beneficial, *Ancestors*, June, 2004, p.61

[20] http://www.leshaigh.co.uk/folkestone/folkestone page/cook family

[21] B. Abel-Smith, *Hospitals 1800-1948*, London: Heinemann, 1964, p. 101

They considered that the poorer elements of the town were behaving irresponsibly by not joining a club, particularly due to the seasonal nature of most employment in the town. Captain A.H. Bradshaw condemned this lack of foresight and social responsibility at a Folkestone COS meeting in 1904:

> How many there were in all our cities who were simply in the summer never thinking of what was to occur in the winter, and then when the winter came, hurling themselves headlong upon the various charity societies… Another thing was that Folkestone, like a good many other towns, was a season town. Any wage that had to be earned must be earned in eight months. For the greater part of the population there was absolutely nothing to be got in the other four.[22]

However, whilst the Friendly Society sickness benefits paid to subscribers may have kept them from the workhouse, there is evidence that examination, diagnosis and treatment were often perfunctory, institutional treatment was rare and waiting lists for admission were long.[23]

The "club doctor"[24] was the lowest paid in his profession. He often struggled to maintain a respectable living, and was charged not only with care of the sick but also with preventing misuse of society funds and detecting malingerers.[25] It has been claimed that doctors would only work in club practice out of financial necessity [26] but, equally, it has been argued that club practice was profitable and socially rewarding for some doctors. It certainly provided a regular income rather than *per capita* fees, which were often left unpaid by the poorer patients of general practitioners.[27] A large percentage of private doctors' accounts could be written off as "bad debts", although these would be less in an established practice.[28]

Although the mortality rate for consumption had fallen by 25%

---

[22] Charity Organisation Society Annual General Meeting, July 10th, 1904, Folkestone COS Journals for Weekly Relief; EKAC Fo-Z/1/F/1

[23] T. Alborn, Insurance Against Germ Theory: Commerce and Conservatism in Late Victorian Medicine, *Bulletin of the History of Medicine*, 75, 2001

[24] Exemplified by Blenkinsop, the down-at-heel, but committed and hard working consumptive doctor in George Bernard Shaw's 1906 play *The Doctor's Dilemma,* London: Penguin, 2004

[25] J. Harris, *Private Lives & Public Spirit: Britain 1870-1914*, London: Penguin, 1993, p.58

[26] B. and S. Webb, *The State and the Doctor*, London: Longmans, 1910, p. 141

[27] D. G. Green, *Working Class Patients*, 1985, pp.51-53

[28] Ibid, p.59

between 1871 and 1899,[29] there was a significant increase in the duration of episodes of ill health for this period recorded in the archives of the Independent Order of Odd Fellows. As consumption was the major killer throughout these decades,[30] the evidence suggests that, towards the end of the century, more consumptives were surviving, but in poor health.[31] Nineteenth century estimates of the average duration of pulmonary consumption increased on average from around eighteen months in the 1850s to three, four or even five years in the 1890s and 1900s.[32]

The rudimentary nature of "club" treatment dictated by the size of such practices is suggested from an account of the work of Dr. J. W. T. Gilbert, the "working man's doctor of Folkestone". In December 1895 he undertook one of the largest practices in the town, the Medical Friendly Society. During the first month of his appointment he treated over 1,000 patients and, on becoming doctor to the Prussian Hermits' Lodge in July 1896, saw 14,198 members in one year and paid 4,000 visits to patients' houses.[33] In order to undertake this Herculean schedule consultations could have lasted little longer than two or three minutes.

Club practice, intended to provide financial security to artisans and their families in times of sickness was, by the late 1890s, increasingly viewed by the medical profession as adversely affecting their earnings and status. More affluent members of the community were enrolling as members of societies for the subscription of a few pence a week, drugs included, and the undercutting of fees by doctors was "all too common".[34]

Eventually, in a few towns, the profession rebelled supported by the General Medical Council and the British Medical Association. Particularly in small towns, established doctors were able to socially and professionally ostracise incomers attempting to undercut their fees.[35] In December 1895 doctors at Folkestone formed "a sort of trades union" to boycott the Provident Societies Medical Association by refusing to work

---

[29] Sir H. Beevor, *An Oration on the Declension of Phthisis*, London: n.p., 1899

[30] In 1890 Arthur Ransome stated that '*phthisis at ages between fifteen and forty-five...kills more than a third of people who die and nearly half between fifteen and thirty*-five', quoted in J. A. Lindsay, The Problem of the Consumptive Poor*, The Lancet*, 4th December, 1897

[31] J. C. Riley, Ill Health, 1987, p.564

[32] *The Lancet*, 22nd November 1851, p.480, 2nd July, 1892, p.3, 4th December, 1897, p.1435, 28th December, 1901, p.1781, 8th August, 1903, p.363, 30th January, 1904, p.282

[33] *Folkestone Up-to-Date*, December 1895, 2nd May, 1896

[34] D. G. Green, *Working Class Patients*, 1985, p.114

[35] Ibid, p.118

for it. They also opposed the practice of canvassing for members by medical associations, which they considered medically unethical.[36] In February 1896 Folkestone practitioners formed their own Provident Medical Association that limited treatment to families earning less than 35 shillings a week.[37]

In some areas the control of medical societies was being, in effect, wrested from co-operative groups of working men through a consolidation of the medical profession. The BMA encouraged the founding of medical clubs run by doctors rather than lay associations.[38] It has been suggested that the growing financial power and popularity of Friendly Societies prompted a campaign by the BMA, from about 1909, to discredit them for improper use of funds and the exploitation of doctors.[39] Lobbying by the medical profession prior to the National Insurance Act resulted in Lloyd George being persuaded by their calls for a free choice of doctor under the new insurance scheme. This ended the power of Friendly Societies to appoint and dismiss doctors and to set their own rates of contribution and doctors' fees.[40]

Apparently unwittingly, Lloyd George had been responsible for a shift in power from the consumer to the registered medical profession.[41] Between 1910 and 1912 the incomes of doctors nearly doubled.[42] Evidence suggests that this advancement of the medical profession, largely as agents of the state, did not signal any improvement in the quality of medical care, any reduction in the caseload of doctors under the new insurance scheme, or any further provision for the treatment of women.[43]

Furthermore, it can be argued that at least nine million of the twelve million covered under the National Insurance scheme already possessed medical cover with Friendly Societies.[44] The provision of institutional

---

[36] *The Lancet*, 22nd December, 1894, p.1498; 29th December, 1894, p.1574, 18th March, 1905, p. 378; *Folkestone Up-to-Date,* 14th December, 1895, p.6

[37] *The Lancet*, 1st February, 1896, p. 327

[38] D. G. Green, *Working Class Patients*, 1985, p.55

[39] Ibid, p.57

[40] J. Lewis, Providers, 'Consumers', the State and Health-care Services in Britain, *Medicine In Society,*ed. A. Wear, Cambridge University Press, 1992, p.327; D. G. Green, *Working Class Patients*, 1985, p.126

[41] J. Lewis, Providers, 'Consumers', the State and Health-care, 1992, p.327

[42] D. G. Green, *Working Class Patients,* 1985, p.114

[43] S. Yeo, Working Class Associations, Private Capital and the State in the late Nineteenth Century and Early Twentieth Centuries,*Social Work, Welfare and the State,* eds. N. Parry, M. Rustin and C. Satyamati, London: E. Arnold, 1979, pp.48-71; D. G. Green, *Working Class Patients*, 1985, p.150

[44] D. G. Green, *Working Class Patients,* 1985, p.95

treatment for tuberculosis, including sanatoria,[45] by Friendly Societies and Trade Unions was growing in the early twentieth century. Their treatment and insurance of women and children was also increasing.[46] Nevertheless the enactment of compulsory national insurance undermined membership of these societies and strengthened the financial independence of doctors.

From this perspective the 1911 National Insurance Act can be seen as legislation designed to wrest control of working class health care from mutual aid societies and put it in the hands of medical professionals who were directly responsible to the state and operating in accordance with government legislation.[47]

The Voluntary Hospital

Throughout the nineteenth century working men from local firms regularly contributed a penny or twopence from their wages every Saturday towards the maintenance of their local hospital or dispensary. In return subscribers' letters were sent from the hospital to employers, who could endorse a letter in the name of a particular employee if he was in need of a consultation at the outpatients department or had to be admitted for treatment.[48] Robert Tressell describes how, although workers felt obliged to contribute to the fund, they resented having to request a letter testifying to their being of suitable character to receive the "charity", and were generally fearful of being experimented on as "free" patients if admitted.[49]

The protagonist of Tressell's novel, Owen, a signwriter and decorator suffering from consumption in the first decade of the twentieth century, as was the author,[50] remarks on his "horror" of visiting the hospital. He concludes that, taking into account his loss of earnings after hours of waiting and the ineffective medicine he had to buy, he would have been

---

[45] The Benenden sanatorium in Kent, established by the National Association for the Establishment and Maintenance of Sanatoria for Workers Suffering from Tuberculosis, was intended as the first of a chain of workers' sanatoria founded on Friendly Society principles.

[46] D. G. Green, *Working Class Patients*, 1985, p.180

[47] Ibid, p.149

[48] B. Abel-Smith, *Hospitals 1800-1948*, London: Heinemann, 1964, p.338-9

[49] R. Tressell, *The Ragged Trousered Philanthropists,* [1914], http://www.unionhistory.info/ragged/php, p.1672

[50] D. Harker, *Tressell: The Real Story of the Ragged Trousered Philanthropists,* Zed Books, 2003

better off visiting a doctor.[51] Certainly, there is evidence that outpatients could wait up to six hours for a consultation of about three minutes,[52] and some patients may have preferred to pay for the services of a doctor. Due to the competitive nature of the medical profession, some doctors charged variable fees in the early twentieth century, sometimes reducing them to one shilling for artisans.[53] However, for lower paid workers, earning about £1 a week around the turn of the century, the hospital or the Poor Law may have been their only realistic options in a crisis if they were not a member of a sick club or Friendly Society.[54]

In Folkestone there existed little provision for the sick poor until a dispensary was established in July, 1846 in Rendezvous Street by Dr. William Donnelly, a retired naval surgeon who also founded dispensaries at neighbouring Hythe and Sandgate at about the same time. The dispensary was open two days a week and those too sick to visit were treated at home. In 1863 the dispensary moved to Glennie House in Dover Road and acquired a small inpatient ward. In 1868 an infirmary was built at Elham workhouse, about six miles distant from Folkestone, containing 50 beds, at a cost of £2,300. However, provision for the sick poor of the town continued to be inadequate for the burgeoning population, and in 1889-90 Victoria Hospital was built in Radnor Park at a cost of £7,300, including operating and consulting rooms as well as a dispensary.[55]

Contributions towards the maintenance of the hospital came not only from local dignitaries, physicians and the aristocracy, but also, in some measure, from local Friendly Societies and groups of employees. In 1893 the Friendly Societies' and Trades Unions' Carnival Fête Committee collected £60-15-3, and seven other Friendly Societies made small contributions. And in 1894 contributions were made by builder William Dunk's workmen, the Gas Company and Corporation workers.[56]

Although the hospital depended on legacies, donations and subscriptions to survive, the proportion of contributions by local Friendly Societies grew and, by February 1905, the United Friendly Societies of Folkestone had two representatives on the Victoria Hospital management committee in return for contributing their Saturday and Sunday Fund

---

[51] R. Tressell, *The Ragged Trousered Philanthropists*, p.1673

[52] A. Digby, *The Evolution of British General Practice, 1850-1948*, Oxford University Press, 1999, p.284

[53] D. G. Green, *Working Class Patients*, 1985, p.179

[54] J. Lewis, Providers, 'Consumers', the State and Health-care, 1992, p.325

[55] Royal Victoria Hospital Committee Minutes, April 1897-October 1909, MH/SEK6/1/1/4

[56] Royal Victoria Hospital Annual Report, 1893-1904, EKAC MH/SEK6/1

donations. Some paying patients were also admitted, their ability to pay being assessed by an almoner.[57]

A sanatorium for the isolation of infectious diseases had also been built in 1879 on the East Cliff. In 1889 the Council adopted the Infectious Diseases Notification Act, which provided for the notification and isolation of cases of diphtheria, scarlet fever, whooping cough and typhoid, and in 1898, when the Infectious Diseases Act was instituted nationally, the sanatorium was enlarged to house four wards.

The number of outpatients to Victoria hospital fell after 1895 when consumptives appear to have been refused treatment, although tuberculosis of the bones, joints and skin was still treated. According to the records of the COS consumptives were treated as outpatients from at least 1905.[58]

By the mid 1890s general hospitals were not normally considered suitable for cases of pulmonary tuberculosis, more due, it would appear, to the poor responses of tubercular patients than for any concern over infection:

> It is certainly bad for the *phthisical* patients, probably bad for the other patients. It was strongly condemned by the International Congress on Tuberculosis a few years ago and it is quite time for all hospital physicians and those interested in hospital administration to make a resolute stand against it. No *phthisical* patient ever recovers in a general hospital and his treatment there – with the exception of the relief of urgent symptoms – is little better than a farce.[59]

Until 1895 consumption was recorded as the most common cause of death for inpatients as well as outpatients of the Victoria hospital. From that year consumptives were no longer accepted, and 25 patients were discharged as incurable or unsuitable. No domestic servants were treated except by the recommendation of the Medical Officer, and both inpatients and outpatients required a letter of recommendation, generally from the COS. Otherwise cases were only admitted in the event of a serious accident.

Outpatients suffering from consumption would probably have received cod liver oil, a renowned specific for tuberculosis, and perhaps laudanum and chalk for pain relief and to counter diarrhoea. Beatrice Webb, together

---

[57] Royal Victoria Hospital Minute Book, April 1897-October 1909, EKAC MH/SEK6/1/1

[58] Royal Victoria Hospital Annual Reports, 1893-1904, EKAC MH/SEK6/1

[59] J. A. Lindsay, The Problem of the Consumptive Poor, *The Lancet*, 4th December, 1897, p.1438

with the COS, condemned outpatient dispensaries at voluntary hospitals as ineffective and likely to spread disease.[60] It should also be noted that the voluntary hospital was part of a paternalistic system that prioritised the male breadwinner, and for most working class women and children there existed no access to health care apart from the chemist.

Folkestone Charity Organisation Society

Although tuberculosis was understood by charities and social reformers as a disease that could lead to poverty if the sufferer was irresponsible enough not to have provided for such an eventuality,[61] it was not generally seen by the middle classes as a disease that was caused by poverty. Despite continued warnings by doctors that a damp environment, lack of light and ventilation and an inadequate diet could engender or exacerbate the disease, most charities restricted their activities to a limited and selective award of vouchers for coal and groceries to families they deemed to be deserving.

In addition lady visitors, who have been characterised as "almost entirely ladies from at least moderately well-to-do homes with little experience of working class life",[62] called to investigate the domestic circumstances and habits of the potential "case", and to encourage thrift, hygiene, morality and pious stoicism.

Although charitable organisations could temporarily relieve the plight of an impoverished consumptive the circumstances that bred and sustained the disease were in no way alleviated or even addressed. The reputation of donors was of course enhanced by having their names published in society newsletters. The impracticality of this approach to the disease, stemming from an entrenched middle class belief in individualism, self-help, and an aversion to state interference was, however, clear to elements of the working class. Robert Noonan, writing in the early years of the twentieth century at the nearby south-east coast health resort of Hastings, understood that tuberculosis was a disease caused by poverty:

> The majority of those who profess to be desirous of preventing and curing the disease called consumption must be either hypocrites or fools, for they ridicule the suggestion that it is necessary first to cure and prevent the poverty that compels badly clothed and half-starved human beings to sleep

---

[60] B. & S. Webb, *The State and the Doctor,* London: Longmans, 1910, pp.131-2; B. Abel-Smith, *Hospitals*, 1964, p.101

[61] Report of the Royal Commission of the Poor Law, volume xxxvii, 1909, p.51

[62] G. Slater, *Poverty and the State,* London: Constable & Co., 1930, p.25

in such dens as this.[63]

The conviction that poverty could be overcome through hard work was commonly held by those involved with charities well into the twentieth century, and was epitomised by the Charity Organisation Society. This was particularly the case in the south of England which lacked the community self-help networks that came to prominence in industrial northern towns with the emergence of the Guilds of Help in the early years of the twentieth century.[64]

The value placed on self-sufficiency is well illustrated by the fact that, after the Education (Provision of Meals) Act in 1906, permitting free school meals to be provided for malnourished children, by 1912 only one third of local authorities had made use of the provision.[65] Kent was particularly resistant to the Act.[66] This is perhaps also indicative of the moral stigma that was attached to the receipt of charity.

As described in chapters five and six, Folkestone's rapid growth during the later nineteenth century, together with strict building regulations imposed by the lord of the manor resulted in inflated rents that adversely affected the poorer classes in the town during the 1890s and the first decade of the twentieth century. In addition high levels of unemployment and a slump in the building trade added to these hard times for many in this unpredictable seasonal economy.

In February 1903 W. Linton, the chairman of the Folkestone branch of the Charity Organisation Society, remarked in a letter to the chairman of the London branch that "the unemployed are much in evidence".[67] Winter poverty was endemic in even the most elite seaside resorts in the nineteenth century[68] and, according to one Folkestone newspaper in December 1903, there existed "a great deal of poverty in this town",[69] and financial prosperity had "decreased to a considerable extent" in the

---

[63] R. Tressell, *The Ragged Trousered Philanthropists*, 1914, p.834

[64] K. Laybourn, The Guild of Help and the Changing Face of Edwardian Philanthropy, *Urban History*, 20, 43-60, 1993

[65] D. Dwork, *War is Good for Babies and Other Young Children: A History of the Infant and Child Welfare Movement in England 1898-1918,* London: Routledge, 1987, pp.167-184

[66] P. Hastings & N. Yates, Health and Social Welfare, *Kent in the Twentieth Century,* ed. N. Yates, Woodbridge: Boydell & Brewer, 2001, pp.230-231

[67] Correspondence of W. Linton to Major General Sandham, 15th February, 1903, Folkestone COS Minute Book

[68] J. K. Walton, *The English Seaside Resort, A Social History, 1750-1914*, Leicester University Press, 1983

[69] *Folkestone Up-to-Date*, 7th December, 1903

previous 25 years following the construction boom of the 1860s and 1870s.[70]

In this atmosphere of growing hardship for the most vulnerable the Folkestone Charity Organisation Society had been founded in 1885 under the chairmanship of Lord Radnor. Its aim was to grant relief or small interest free loans to the "deserving and industrious poor", to deter begging and to promote emigration in suitable cases. The committee was comprised predominantly of retired military men, Folkestone and Sandgate being popular residences for ex-army officers due to their associations with the nearby Shorncliffe barracks.[71]

Whilst the Society assisted poor workers, it offered no help to the able-bodied unemployed, who were generally considered to be responsible for their situation due to an unwillingness or inability to work. Cases were carefully selected, the sixth Earl of Radnor, for example, was particularly circumspect; [he] "did not think that one could insist too much on the need for full inquiry and careful investigation".[72] The sick and elderly were assisted if found to be deserving of relief. In March, 1895, it was recorded that, on average, the COS relieved about 44 sick and elderly individuals every week throughout the year.[73]

Begging was, of course, something to be discouraged in a fashionable health resort. An editorial in the *Folkestone News* of 1886 condemned the use of deformed children and children trained to beg by their parents:

> while relieving the simulated misery which dogs us in the streets, we are in reality turning a cold heart and a deaf ear to real sorrow and distress, and encouraging the very profitable trade of mendicancy.[74]

Cases were often specially recommended for subscribers to the Society, and relief was generally given in the form of vouchers for groceries and coal, or fees were paid to convalescent homes and hospitals. There were constant requests for letters of recommendation to Victoria Hospital and St. Andrew's Convalescent Home. Money contributed to the Society was divided between an emergency fund, a fund for chronically ill parishioners, and money for small loans to tide families over times of hardship until they found employment.[75]

---

[70] *Folkestone Up-to-Date*, 25th January, 1904
[71] Folkestone COS, Journals for Weekly Relief, 1910-1914, Fo/Z1/F2/2, EKAC
[72] COSAnnual General Meeting, 10th July, 1904
[73] *Folkestone Up-to-Date*, 21st March, 1896
[74] *Folkestone News*, 16th January, 1886
[75] COS Annual General Meeting, 10th July, 1904

The COS also funded an establishment in the town situated on Grace Hill called "The Travellers' Rest". Although accommodation was not provided moral instruction and religious guidance were available. One commentator in a local newspaper, however, considered it a misuse of funds, and:

> more ornamental than useful in relieving the destitute, and although it probably played an important part in obtaining subscriptions, it did not carry out the wishes of the benevolent subscribers so well as if it were open earlier in the morning and late at night, and provided a night's lodging…for to give a man a hot pint of coffee and a bit of bread , and then send him six miles through the frost and snow on a winter's night [to Elham workhouse], intensified his suffering and privations rather than relieving them.[76]

A major concern of the Society was teaching thrift and self-reliance to the working classes. Membership of a medical insurance club was often viewed by both the COS and the Poor Law Board as a prerequisite for being considered a "deserving case" and thus qualifying for relief.[77] From the early twentieth century, membership of provident clubs was taking over the role of subscribers' letters as a means for the working classes to secure access to medical treatment. By 1906 there were about seven million members of registered Friendly Societies nationally. Although club treatment was not dependent on patronage it remained selective, tending not to treat women, children or workers with a history or family history of chronic disease.[78]

In 1904, a particularly bad season in Folkestone with high unemployment, the COS initiated the Working Peoples' Benevolent Fund to help people save for the winter in order to pay rent and taxes. The scheme was limited to those earning 30 shillings a week or less, and money could not be drawn for other purposes. Despite the generous incentive of a two shilling bonus for every pound saved after £10 had been deposited, the fund closed in August 1905 after just over a year due to having attracted insufficient deposits. This episode indicates the extent of poverty amongst many local workers and the difficulty of saving for periods of unemployment and sickness.

Many cases assisted by the Society reveal the often protracted and unpredictable course of pulmonary tuberculosis invariably resulting in

---

[76] *Folkestone Up-to-Date*, 10th August, 1893, p.7

[77] B. Abel-Smith, *Hospitals 1800-1948*, 1964, p.101

[78] B. Abel-Smith, *Hospitals,* 1964, pp.218, 228

economic and physical collapse. The records of 31 year old Edward Jenkins who applied for help in June, 1897 also reflect the fear of disclosing a diagnosis of consumption. Jenkins, of James Street, was a van driver for the Corporation stores and was married with two children under three. He had been out of work for one month following an apparent attack of pneumonia, earned 22 shillings a week, had no relatives and received no aid from the parish. His rent was seven shillings and sixpence a week and he received four shillings a week from a lodger. The Society noted that Jenkins was an "abstainer", generally a precondition for receiving assistance, not in arrears with his rent, and his wife was judged to be respectable and kept the house clean and tidy. Jenkins did not belong to a Friendly Society, despite earning a relatively good wage, and doubted whether, as he had been ill in the past, any club would take him. He was also concerned that he could no longer afford to purchase medicines. The Society granted him two shillings worth of coal and groceries a week.

In October Jenkins was informed that relief would not to be continued unless a medical certificate was produced. Following some prevarication he brought the medical certificate, which certified consumption. Relief continued, together with visits and investigations from the Society, until the end of May 1898. In February, 1899 his wife applied for relief claiming that Jenkins was suffering from bronchitis. Relief was granted until June when she reported that her husband had found work. Jenkins apparently worked from July 1900 until he again became ill with consumption in August 1903. The couple insisted it was a seasonal complaint and that he would be able to work during the spring and summer. Relief was recommended until the spring, but in April 1904 Jenkins was transferred to the register of chronic cases and died shortly afterwards.[79]

From being reasonably well off Jenkins' situation would have deteriorated steadily, his employment became irregular and his wife was unable to work due to having infant children; perhaps his lodger moved out. He was also finding it difficult to afford medicine. Regular visits ascertained that the family were "respectable", nevertheless he delayed producing a medical certificate for three weeks after being informed that his relief would be terminated without one. He presented himself as suffering from pneumonia and bronchitis on the first two applications for relief which, while he may have been suffering from more than one illness, suggests that he was wary of disclosing his diagnosis. Both the husband and wife were at pains to assure the Society that his problem was only

[79] Folkestone COS, Journals for weekly relief, 1910-1914

temporary and related to the season, despite Jenkins twice applying for relief in the summer.

From the turn of the century much of the Society's funds were being used to prevent cases in receipt of Poor Law outdoor relief from being forced into the workhouse infirmary, which generally resulted in the break up of families and the loss of homes. Nevertheless, the Committee concluded that the practice of helping families to survive, rather than encouraging thrift and endeavour, created dependency:

> it is felt that too large a proportion of the money entrusted to the committee is disbursed in small doles to the aged and deserving and sick poor, to save them from going into the Union against their wishes; the outdoor relief of 2/6 to 3/6 per week given by the Guardians being insufficient for the support of those who have no relatives to help them, and in a place where such high rents have to be paid.[80]

The continuation of outdoor relief, supposedly discontinued under the 1834 Poor Law Act was obviously pragmatic; it could be more costly to put the breadwinner in the workhouse and support the family than to assist a large family on a small income. Outdoor relief was intended to supplement a low wage, charity or a pension; it was insufficient to subsist on, and recipients were forced to depend upon charity or theft.[81]

The Society felt that the Elham Board of Guardians should grant an increase of outdoor relief in particularly deserving cases to enable them to subsist without the Society relieving the Poor Rates. During 1904 the COS had relieved 950 cases for short periods, whilst five cases received grants for more than six months and 25 cases were granted relief throughout the year.

Nevertheless, the Guardians considered themselves unable to increase their rates of relief. In January, 1904, over 600 parishioners had been summonsed for non-payment of rates, and during the previous decade an average of 500 individuals a year had been summonsed. The majority of the Board were loath to sanction the spending of any more municipal funds when so many townsmen were unable to meet existing rate charges.[82] Indeed their primary function, and an important aim of the

---

[80] COS Annual General Meeting, 10th July, 1904, Folkestone COS minutes of monthly meetings, January 1886-September 1913, Fo/Z/1/A/M/1-4

[81] M. MacKinnon, Poor Law Policy, Unemployment and Pauperism, *Explorations in Economic History,* 23, 1986, p.302

[82] COS AGM, March 1st, 1906, Folkestone COS minutes of monthly meetings, January 1886-September 1913, Fo/Z/1/A/M/1-4

COS,[83] was considered to be curtailing outdoor relief and thus reducing pauperism through encouraging the self-sufficiency of the working classes.[84] Although the Elham Guardians did not accede to the Society's suggestion, they determined to examine individual cases more closely, and decided to involve more women to investigate and report on cases in order to elicit more information regarding their character and circumstances.[85]

The judgemental and selective nature of assistance offered by the Board of Guardians to the sick poor was remarked upon in a Folkestone newspaper in 1895.[86] On the other hand assistance that was not properly directed could, it was claimed, have a deleterious effect. In 1905 Lord Radnor, addressing a COS meeting, asserted that: "too much indiscriminate charity was a bad thing, and had a demoralising effect on poor people".[87] And Captain Bradshaw suggested that the number of cases given assistance should be subject to further discrimination:

> it is proved that liberal and adequate help given to a certain limited number of deserving cases is of greater value than small doles widely scattered.[88]

This process of selection appears to have operated according to quite narrow moral and economic criteria; those assessed as being able and willing to live in accord with middle class values of industriousness, self discipline, piety, cleanliness and sobriety being offered some assistance if they possessed no relatives capable of supporting them, and the remainder being assigned to the workhouse or left to fend for themselves.

Some cases were felt to be not worth assisting; fishermen and their families suffering from tuberculosis were regularly considered too fond of drink to warrant help despite recommendations by doctors or clergymen.[89] This antipathy to boatmen on the part of the civic elite may, in conjunction with recent deaths, casualties and financial losses sustained by them, have contributed to the formation of the Folkestone Fishing Boat Insurance Company, covering 35 boats, in 1884.[90]

---

[83] B. Abel-Smith, *The Hospitals*, 1964, p.101

[84] C. Bellamy, *Administering Central-Local Relations*, 1988, p. 180; B. Abel-Smith, *The Hospitals*, 1964, p. 93

[85] Elham Board of Guardians meeting, 26th March, 1904, quoed in Folkestone COS AGM, 10th July, 1904, EKAC G/EL/3/2

[86] *Folkestone Up To Date,* 22nd June, 1895, p.4

[87] Lord Radnor at COS AGM, 15th February, 1905, Folkestone COS Minute Book

[88] Lord Radnor at COS AGM, March 1st 1906, Folkestone COS Minute Book

[89] Folkestone COS, Journals for weekly relief, 1910-1914

[90] A. Nevill, *The Story of Folkestone*, 2009, p.143

Sexual impropriety was another reason cited for denying aid. Eliza Marks, a 66 year old widow and jobbing needleworker from Spring Cottages in Foord, living with a consumptive daughter of 26, was refused aid due to "the irregular way her house was kept". Following enquiries both the Guardians and the COS refused the woman relief because a married man was reported to be living with another woman in her house, and a daughter in the asylum had had two illegitimate children. Her records were marked "a case for the workhouse".[91]

Relief could also be denied if a house was overcrowded. In 1895 a young man living with his sister and her family was suffering "galloping consumption". Despite the house belonging to a member of the Hythe Board of Guardians, relief, it was claimed, would be seen as an encouragement to overcrowding. The young man was taken to the Union where he died. [92]

There is no record of the society providing food or coal for victims of tuberculosis at an early stage of the disease when it may have offered hope of recovery. Invariably cases were in an advanced condition and improvement was doubtful. Many had large families, and temporary grants of food would have been unlikely to restore them to a condition in which they were able to support themselves. Consequently the children would probably have remained undernourished.

For example, when Mrs Rainer, a mother of eight from Alexandra Street, was referred in January 1912 after having been discovered to be ill with consumption and having no work, one ticket for three shillings worth of groceries was granted with a visitor's comment: "Mrs Easton reports the family are almost starving and must go to the Union".[93] And in January 1904, Peter Barton, a 43 year old consumptive with ulcerated legs, living with his mother, had applied for outdoor relief. He was visited twice, but not taken to the workhouse as he was considered too ill to move. He was granted six shillings in February, and the COS provided milk, eggs and a nurse; he died the following month.[94]

In December 1912, 51 year old Thomas Wilshire, married with four young children, applied for relief. He was a labourer, but had been an invalid for three years suffering from tuberculosis of the hips, and his wife was suffering from tuberculosis of the throat and was unable to work. They were given the usual grocery and coal vouchers for three weeks. The vouchers were to be exchanged with nominated tradesmen, and were

---

[91] Folkestone COS, Journals for weekly relief, 1910-1914

[92] *Folkestone-Up-To-Date*, 22nd June, 1895, p. 4

[93] Folkestone COS, Journals for weekly relief, 1910-1914

[94] Ibid.

marked "not to be sold or exchanged for beer or tobacco".[95]

The Board of Guardians and the committee of the COS appear generally to have denied relief to consumptives if they judged them to be at all capable of working, removing them to the workhouse infirmary to die when their health broke down. In September 1902, Robert Horn, a 38 year old single labourer with no relations, applied for out relief. He was described as "wholly disabled" with consumption, and in receipt of two shillings and sixpence a week from a Friendly Society. He was granted one shilling medical relief a week to the end of the half year. However, in March 1903 it was reported that he was only partially disabled and that he was capable of working. He was struck off, applied for a continuance of out relief which was refused, and consequently he was forced to enter the workhouse.[96]

Despite the warnings and recommendations regarding the infectious nature of tuberculosis contained in Yunge-Bateman's report of 1899, little action appears to have been taken by the Council or local charities to control the spread of the disease. Throughout the records of the Society and the Board of Guardians no mention is made of any attempt to isolate consumptives from their children or other members of the family, to provide sputum flasks and handkerchiefs, to disinfect houses or to advise consumptives on hygienic practices such as sleeping separately and using separate cutlery. Occasionally a brief visit to a hospital or convalescent home was funded by the Society.

35 year old George Jefferson of Canterbury Road was married with two young children, he had been a carpenter but in 1908 was running a small sweet shop and letting lodgings. Jefferson was referred to by a visitor in December 1908 as being "very ill with consumption" and had not been able to work at his trade for a long time, subsisting on five shillings and threepence a week from the carpenter's union. The family could no longer let lodgings owing to Jefferson's illness. Following the usual investigations the Society paid £1 for him to go "to the country", and two guineas to visit a sanatorium at Ventnor. Jefferson continued to run his sweetshop and no mention was made of the dangers of infection.[97]

Similarly, in February, 1911, Thomas Vye, a 33 year old fish hawker of Marshall Street, living with his wife Esther and their four young children, applied to the Society. He suffered from consumption and his wife attended the hospital as an outpatient with the disease. They were given two shillings' worth of groceries and one shillings' worth of coal for three

---

[95] Folkestone COS, Journals for weekly relief, 1910-1914

[96] Elham Union Application and Report Book, September 1902 - October 1903

[97] Folkestone COS, Diary and Committee Report Books, 1895-1917, Z1/AD7

weeks, and Vye was encouraged to return to selling fish around the town. Unsurprisingly, all the cases relieved by the COS were from the overcrowded and insanitary north and east wards of the town.[98]

The COS pursued a system that was, perhaps, increasingly regarded by some as anachronistic during the first decade of the twentieth century. Despite a more sympathetic spirit of philanthropy and municipal welfare emerging at this time, manifested in the Guilds of Help and the more progressive urban Poor Law Unions, the persistence of evolutionist inspired attitudes to the poor remained common in the south of England. The COS 's primary aim of encouraging self reliance amongst the working classes was incompatible with proposals from the Society for Medical Officers of Health and other reformers for the early diagnosis and treatment of tuberculosis. Additionally, the COS were resented by the working classes due to their practice of closely investigating the private lives of applicants for aid. The conviction of many members of charities that the poor and sick were largely responsible for their own plight, and that they exhibited a natural tendency to laziness and deceit, was an attitude heavily influenced and sustained by social Darwinist ideas.

The COS and religious charities were, in general, concerned with altering the behaviour of the working classes, persuading them of the benefits to be derived from thrift, hard work, piety and independence, and encouraging middle class notions of respectability and cleanliness. Lists of donors and benefactors were published annually in Folkestone by the COS and by the Community of St. John the Baptist who managed St. Andrews convalescent home, thus contributing to the philanthropic reputation of aristocratic and middle class residents. Both organisations refrained, however, from advocating improvements to the living and working conditions of the poor, and no help was offered to the families of the unemployed, apart from the nuns' soup kitchen during the economic hardships of the 1890s and the pre-war years. Those suffering from pulmonary tuberculosis were only assisted by the COS if they lacked relatives able to support them and were positively unable to work. By this time, of course, only palliative care could be offered and the sufferer would either die at home or be removed to the workhouse.

The Clewer Sisters of St. Andrews

As overcrowding, unemployment and poverty increasingly affected working class districts of the town from the 1880s various convalescent

[98] Folkestone COS, Diary and Committee Report Books, 1895-1917, Z1/AD7

homes, many established and run along overtly religious lines, began to emerge in Folkestone. Inspired and funded through the mood of evangelicalism prevalent throughout the nineteenth century, the larger of these institutions, such as St. Andrew's, were governed by boards constituted from retired military officers, the local aristocracy and clergy.

It seems probable that many of these institutions, as well as some of the hundreds of lodging and boarding houses[99] established during this period emerged in order to take advantage of Folkestone's reputation as a health resort for the tubercular, particularly considering the ubiquity of the disease, the lack of provision for its treatment and the increasing optimism of the medical profession regarding its cure. Certainly more beds belonging to the largest of these institutions, the St. Andrew's Convalescent Home, were occupied by the tubercular than by those suffering from any other disease.

The founders of the institution, the Community of St. John the Baptist, were an order of High Anglican nuns founded in 1852 at Clewer, Berkshire by Harriet Monsell, the Irish aristocratic widow of an Anglican prebendary who had vowed to work for God on the death of her husband from consumption, and who retired to live on the Bayle in Folkestone in 1875. The sisterhood was originally founded to save fallen women, and church penitentiaries were established first at Clewer and, subsequently, in other parts of the southern counties.[100]

The Community, initially encouraged by the high Anglican parish priest Matthew Woodward, initiated missions in the parishes of St. Eanswyth in 1875 and later in St. Saviours in the north ward of the town. These endeavours were funded by the Church Commissioners in an attempt to counter the growth of nonconformity in working class districts.[101] Possibly the Community was attracted to Folkestone due to its demographic similarity to Windsor, where the Sisters had conducted a moral struggle in the 1860s that had contributed to the passing of the Contagious Diseases Act in 1866. Both were garrison towns with a sizeable population of Irish navvies who had worked on the construction of the railway, and as such certain areas were probably viewed as potential sites of vice and corruption.[102]

In 1880, on the invitation of the local vicar, the Reverend Claude

---

[99] In 1882 there were 345 lodging houses in Folkestone (not including boarding houses, public houses, hotels or apartments) according to Kelly's directory

[100] V. Bonham, *A Joyous Service: The Clewer sisters and their Work*, V. Bonham/CSJB, 1989

[101] A. Nevill, *The Story of Folkestone*, 2009, p.191

[102] V. Bonham, *A Joyous Service,* 1989

Hankey, two Sisters began a mission in the rapidly expanding district around the junction of the Folkestone to Dover railway where rows of artisans' dwellings had grown up to house railway workers. The Sisters and Hankey fostered various local institutions designed to provide spiritual aid, and an alternative to the overcrowded dwellings and public houses in the district. A temperance movement, a savings scheme, a working mens' society, mothers' meetings, bible classes, maternity societies and guilds were all introduced in the nascent parish of St. Saviours in the 1880s and 1890s, as well as a school and a chapel.

In 1885 the mission district became a separate parish under the patronage of Ewan Christian, the Archbishop of Canterbury, and the Earl of Radnor donated a site for the building of a parish church, that was consecrated in 1901. Gertrude Marryatt, the Sister Superior of the Home, acknowledged that impoverished districts were invariably to be found in coastal resorts:

> In Folkestone, as in other seaside towns, there must always be an obscure suburb in which poverty and sometimes distress are concentrated – a quarter which naturally tends to hide itself…Such a district is St. Saviours, acknowledged to be the poorest in the town, and, as regards population, one of the largest.[103]

Initially opened in two houses in Guildhall Street in May 1875, the St. Andrew's Convalescent Home appears to have been born from necessity rather than design.[104] The tubercular were excluded from general hospitals and there was an acute shortage of places to care for the many consumptives discharged from the few specialist London hospitals, such as the Brompton Hospital for Consumption. The biographer of the Community of St. John claims that many consumptives were forced to resort to tramping on being discharged from such institutions during this period.[105]

In 1880 Gertrude Marryat, succinctly characterised the function of convalescent homes:

> Every days' experience proves the value and indeed the absolute necessity of such an institution as this, in connection with, or as supplementary to general hospitals. These latter as a rule, discharge their patients, not in a condition of perfect cure, but only sufficiently convalescent to allow of

[103] G. Marryatt, Records of St Saviour's Mission, Folkestone, CSJB, March 1915, Berkshire Record Office D/EX1675/1/12/21/1

[104] V. Bonham, *A Joyous Service*, 1989

[105] Ibid.

> their being removed…and this consideration is the more important when it is remembered that such patients as it receives, mostly depend for their livelihood on their own labour. Such institutions consequently have rapidly increased in number, and are much sought after, and generally well supported.[106]

Although conditions varied, these institutions offered a higher standard of care than workhouse infirmaries. Apart from the problem of providing for the consumptive poor, there existed very little recourse for tradesmen, teachers and the lower middle class in general. St. Andrew's treated both sexes, paying as well as "free' patients", and initially accommodated people from a variety of social backgrounds. In 1884 a childrens' ward was also opened:

> the different classes of patients range[d] from the poor boy who sweeps a crossing to the certified schoolmistress, ladies in distressed circumstances …labouring people, both men and women, domestic servants, soldiers, sailors and persons of the middle class, all of whom have associated very pleasantly together, as there is no separate accommodation for the different classes.[107]

The Home received patients suffering mainly from tuberculosis of the lungs, other forms of tuberculosis, "debility", bronchitis, influenza and other respiratory disorders. Some were terminally ill and had been discharged from metropolitan hospitals as incurable.[108]

St. Andrew's purported to offer "kind nursing, wholesome nourishment, and pure air, with able medical attendance", and Folkestone was considered "a town peculiarly fitted by position and climate for such an institution".[109] The Home was funded by donations and subscriptions; annual subscriptions of one guinea entitled the subscriber to a letter of recommendation providing the holder with a bed for three weeks on payment of two shillings and sixpence per week, thereafter the charge per bed was nine shillings. An annual subscription of twenty guineas entitled the subscriber to have a patient in a bed throughout the year at the cost of two shillings and sixpence per week in 1875. A list of subscribers and

---

[106] Medical reports of St. Andrew's Convalescent Home, Folkestone, 1875-1935, Records of the Community of St. John the Baptist, Clewer, Berkshire Record Office, D/EX 1675/14/2/1

[107] Medical reports of St. Andrew's Convalescent Home, 1896

[108] Records of the Community of St. John the Baptist, Clewer, Berkshire Record Office, D/EX 1675/14/2/1

[109] Ibid.

donors was published annually, contributed to by many of the local aristocracy and clergy.

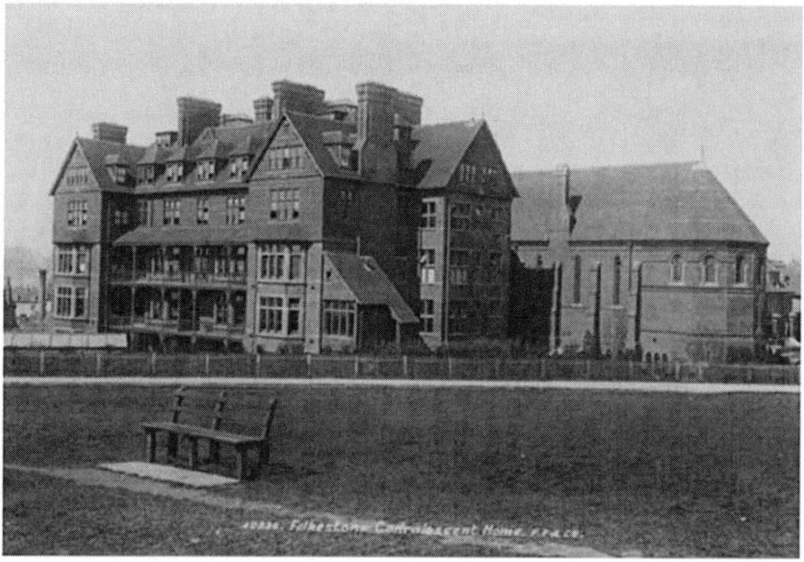

Illustration 7.1: St Andrew's Convalescent Home and chapel, 1898.

Treatment consisted of rest and exercise, where appropriate, both in and beyond the limited grounds of the Home. Diet was also viewed as being of fundamental importance. Patients were given four meals a day and weighed regularly. Medical supervision, however, seems to have been restricted to twice weekly rounds by the medical officer.[110]

Such sporadic medical care by physicians of convalescent homes appears to have been the norm in the late nineteenth century. In 1890 William Chubb, physician to the *Beach Rocks* Convalescent Home in the neighbouring town of Sandgate, responded to a letter in the *BMJ* suggesting that the medical supervisors of convalescent homes should examine each case and maintain temperature charts and notes of their progress. He explained that it was not generally possible for doctors who relied on their private practice for a livelihood to devote such time to supposedly convalescent patients even when, as was often the case, they

---

[110] Records of the Community of St. John the Baptist, Clewer, Berkshire Record Office

were in need of medical care:

> The Home with which I am acquainted takes in about eight hundred cases annually, a considerable number being chest cases from the Brompton Hospital and often the work takes more time than I can spare.[111]

During the 1880s and 1890s both institutions were treating about 100 patients at any one time who were suffering from a variety of chronic ailments, mostly consumption, but also cases of typhoid fever, pneumonia and influenza, and one is left with the impression that the work of the untrained nursing staff may often have been extremely demanding. But if the care given to the tubercular poor was limited, convalescent homes were nevertheless a valuable resource in the late nineteenth and early twentieth centuries. As well as treating members of Friendly Societies and Trades Unions they provided an alternative for some Boards of Guardians, who sent their chronically sick from workhouse infirmaries for short periods.

By 1884 a larger building capable of accommodating more than 100 patients had been completed with the help of legacies and donations at the cost of £16,000. The foundation stone was laid by the Duchess of Edinburgh, and the Home benefited from the special patronage of Queen Victoria's daughter, Princess Christina of Schleswig-Holstein, as did the later Benenden Sanatorium.

The suitability of prospective entrants to St. Andrew's was scrutinised prior to their admission and discipline was strict. Subscribers and donors to the Home were requested to restrict their letters of recommendation to patients who exhibited "cleanliness of persons and clothes…moral character and temperate habits". The rules for subscribers also reflected the Sisters' concern for fallen women:

> women who are known to have at any time lost their respectability of character, can not be sent to the Home without a special statement of their case sent to the Sister Superior.

Any patient known to have visited a public house or to have indulged in "gambling, swearing or immoral conversation" was removed, and all patients not entirely bedridden were expected to attend services at the large High Anglican chapel attached to the Home.[112]

---

[111] W. L. Chubb, *BMJ*, 3rd May, 1890, p.1055

[112] *Instructions to Subscribers and Donors*, St. Andrew's records, 1895, Records of the CSJB, D/EX 1675/14/2/2

Patients were nursed by the Clewer Sisters, who were mainly daughters of the aristocracy and clergy, and medical supervision was provided by staff from the Victoria Hospital on an honorary basis, primarily by Robert Leamon Bowles between 1875 and 1902. Bowles was consultant physician at the Victoria Hospital from its inception in 1890, and donated £1,000 towards its construction; he was also Medical Officer of the Folkestone Charity Organisation Society from 1885 to 1904, and sat on the committee of St. Andrew's. From the 1890s the staff included about twelve nursing Sisters and sixteen servants as well as a physician, assistant physician and surgeon practising on a part time basis. In 1876 St. Andrew's treated 290 patients, in 1887 1,428 and in 1899 2,241.[113]

From the medical reports of the Home it would appear that the mid-1880s signalled the onset of an extended period of economic deprivation. Admissions increased and the Committee appealed for more funds:

> The circumstances which have reduced the comforts and luxuries of the wealthier classes, have deprived the Poor of absolute necessaries, and it is to avert and remedy the ill effects of increased hardship, privation and insanitary conditions generally among the Poor, that the Home pleads for increased help.[114]

Local subscribers to the Home began to recommend deserving cases from around Folkestone, and in 1885 it was stated in the minutes of the Society's committee meeting that:

> the increased application for the admission of cases from the neighbourhood, show that the Home is proving a blessing in its community.[115]

However, the majority of patients came from outside the area. In 1881 patients were received from eight metropolitan Union infirmaries, six cottage hospitals, twelve provincial hospitals (including Dover, Canterbury and West Kent), and from 25 London hospitals. In 1885 1,325 patients were treated in the Home, but in the Committee minutes for that year they found it necessary to state that St. Andrew's was:

> not intended as an asylum for acute and incurable cases. It is the more needful to use these words of caution, on account of the growing custom of sending patients in an advanced stage of illness (more especially

---

[113] Medical reports of St. Andrew's Convalescent Home, Folkestone, 1875-1935

[114] Minutes of Committee Meeting, St Andrew's Convalescent Home, 1886

[115] Medical reports of St. Andrew's Convalescent Home, 1885

> consumptive cases), requiring an amount of nursing and attention, which the institution does not undertake to give and is not prepared to provide.[116]

Critically ill cases, generally those who relapsed shortly after admission, were dispatched to the town's Victoria Hospital.[117]

In 1886 a medical referee was appointed in London to certify the suitability of proposed admissions, nevertheless the problem persisted. In the following year 33 cases were rejected by him, fifteen described as being "in the third stage of *phthisis*" and ten as being "very advanced *phthisis* and failing much". Subsequently about 50 applicants a year were found to be ineligible.[118]

During the 1890s continuing reference was made in the committee minutes and annual reports of the Home to the number of advanced cases of consumption being sent from Poor Law Unions and hospitals for consumption:

> The medical officers also note the fact that an increasing number of *phthisical* patients has been sent to the home in a stage of the disease which makes them a possible source of danger to the other inmates. Such cases should not be recommended for admission, as no arrangements exist at the home for their separation. In the instances to which allusion is made the certificates have been so drawn up as to give the impression that the illness is not sufficiently grave to require the opinion of our medical referee.[119]

It can be imagined that some sponsors would have found it hard to refuse the tubercular letters of recommendation on the grounds that their disease was too far advanced. In 1899 the Committee concluded that if the practice of sending advanced cases continued consumptives would have to be excluded altogether. In the following year they announced:

> It is with deep regret that this course has to be taken, in the interest of other patients, as it has entailed the rejection of, and consequent great disappointment to, many who were pining for the refreshing sea breezes.[120]

---

116 Medical reports of St. Andrew's Convalescent Home, 1885
117 Ibid, 1890
118 Ibid, 1885
119 Ibid, 1899
120 Ibid, 1900

The Committee of St. Andrew's considered the possibility of providing separate accommodation for consumptives, but donations were apparently unforthcoming, and nothing came of it. From 1901 patients registered as suffering from *phthisis*, *haemoptysis* or *diarrhoea* (both common symptoms of consumption) were no longer recorded as being admitted, and the Committee minutes noted:

> There has been a most marked decline in the severity of the cases admitted into the House during this year, owing, doubtless in a great measure, to the new rule which, regretfully, had to be enforced, excluding *phthisical* cases; of late years these had been in such excess that they had become a source of considerable anxiety, and additional expense for nursing etc., besides being injurious to their fellow patients…[121]

The reason for Bowles and the Sisters' anxiety is not overtly stated, and the threat of infection is never specifically mentioned in the Community's records. Indeed in 1901 cases suffering from typhoid fever were accepted in the Home. It may have been that consumptives in an advanced and febrile state were increasingly difficult to care for and their presence may have alarmed fellow patients. It is more likely, however, that the Committee's decision to exclude further cases of consumption was primarily due to local residents' complaints and adverse publicity regarding the number of pauper consumptives admitted to convalescent homes and sanatoria in neighbouring Sandgate. During the 1890s an increasing number of destitute consumptives from London had been sent to the Home, and members of the Committee, themselves prominent local residents, would have been aware of the threat their admission at St Andrews could have posed for Folkestone's reputation as a health resort.

Discouraging Sickness: Etchinghill Infirmary and Elham Guardians

Despite victims of consumption, together with their wives and children, being particularly vulnerable to destitution and to being thrown on the mercy of the parish, there was a strong aversion to entering the Elham workhouse and its infirmary. Often no other affordable means of medical relief, or even of subsistence, apart from the charity of the leisured classes, was available to most consumptives prior to the National Insurance Act. Being unable to join a Friendly Society, as was Robert Jenkins, and being denied access to treatment at a voluntary hospital, a

[121] St Andrew's, Committee Minutes, 1901

respectable working family could easily be reduced to pauperism by the disease.

The extended debates of the Royal Commission on the Poor Law, which sat from 1905 to 1909, highlight, in particular, conflicting attitudes towards the sick poor, and conflicting responses to the perceived infectiousness of consumption. It was still rare for separate accommodation to be provided for the tubercular in provincial workhouse infirmaries at this time. Although Medical Officers of Health were trained in preventive medicine the Poor Law Medical Service was generally more concerned with discouraging the admission of the sick to workhouse infirmaries.[122]

The operation of the Poor Law was seen as inefficient and brutal by some, but was regarded as a necessary deterrent by others, and the ethos of discriminating between the deserving sick and malingerers was well entrenched. Poor Law medical officers were unlikely to classify consumptives as other than able-bodied paupers until the latter stages of the disease. This put Poor Law officials at odds with the preventive ideals of the Medical Officers of Health, who viewed the deterrent ethos underlying the Poor Law system as a barrier to any unified medical service.[123]

According to the investigations of Sidney and Beatrice Webb, who were advised by Arthur Newsholme and George Newman, both influential Medical Officers of Health and advocates of reform in the treatment of consumption, not only did there exist no treatment for consumption under the Poor Law, but in general no action was taken to inhibit infection:

> Under the Poor Law there is practically no sanitary supervision of *phthisis* in the home of the patient…*Phthisis* cases are maintained in crowded, unventilated houses.[124]

Nor were cases isolated from the community until they were *in extremis:*

> It was given in evidence on high authority that the very great mortality from *phthisis* – a disease to which no less than one-seventh of the total cost of the Poor Law is said to be directly or indirectly due – is to be attributed in no small degree to the fact that sufferers are not encouraged to present

---

[122] J. Brand, The Parish Doctor: England's Poor Law Medical Officers and Medical Reform, 1870-1900, *Bulletin of the History of Medicine*, 35, 1961, p.106

[123] B. & S. Webb, *The State and the Doctor*, London: Longmans, 1910

[124] S. & B. Webb, eds., *The Break-Up of the Poor Law: Being Part One of the Minority Report of the Poor Law Commission*, London: Longmans, Green & Co, 1909, p.221

> themselves for treatment in the early stages of the disease, when it is often curable, but when they are still capable of going to work, and are not regarded as destitute and thus not technically eligible for a Medical Order. Under the present arrangements of the Poor Law Medical Service, such cases are left outside its ken, until in due course the ravages of the disease have reached a stage at which the sufferer, having in the meantime perhaps infected other members of his family, becomes simultaneously eligible for Poor Law medical relief and incapable of deriving from it any real advantage. In fact the Poor Law doctor seldom knows *phthisis* in any but its incurable stage, shortly before the sufferer enters the Workhouse to die. In some places, we were informed, one-third, and even one-half, of the deaths from *phthisis* take place in the Poor Law institutions.[125]

By the first decade of the twentieth century some urban workhouse infirmaries had improved their treatment of consumptives. Reformist Boards of Guardians began to provide drugs and trained nurses, and even offered some form of open-air therapy. However, provincial and rural workhouses remained notoriously inhospitable, guided by the principle of "less eligibility".[126]

The Local Government Board also appeared reluctant to adopt the principles of preventive medicine. When the Bradford Poor Law Guardians attempted to encourage early cases of pulmonary tuberculosis to enter their infirmary, endeavouring to treat them before they became destitute and moribund, the LGB felt obliged to remind them that their function was to deter, not attract, those seeking relief, and that their actions could be construed as encouraging pauperism.[127]

Significantly, F. H. Bentham, chairman of the Bradford Board of Guardians, was also a founder member of the "new philanthropy", the Guild of Help, which was committed to combating poverty locally, and was less concerned with the personal failings of the destitute.[128] The ideology of the Guilds, however, had little impact in the south of England. In Folkestone the principle of deterrence was maintained into the twentieth century. In 1893 councillor Logan, an east end shopkeeper and proprietor and founder of *Folkestone Up to Date* described the Poor Law as being designed:

---

[125] S. & B. Webb, eds., *The Break-Up of the Poor Law*, 1909, p.230

[126] S & B Webb, eds., *The Break-Up of the Poor Law,* 1909; H. T. Bulstrode, *Report on Sanatoria,* 1905-6

[127] S & B Webb, eds., *The Break-Up of the Poor Law*, 1909, p.243

[128] K. Laybourn, *Modern Britain Since 1906*, London: Tauris & Co., 1999, p.8

> to make everything so uncomfortable that people often prefer death, or the prison cell, rather than avail themselves of assistance for which they have paid all their lifetime.[129]

The Elham Union affords a prime example of the operation of the principle of "less eligibility". In July, 1891 Folkestone Borough Council had sold the Sessions House, underneath which casual workers had traditionally been accommodated, and had provided no alternative for the homeless and itinerants in the town. During 1892 7,300 "casuals" had sought accommodation in the workhouse, and, in August 1893, it was reported that 445 individuals, including 46 children and 34 women, had been admitted to the workhouse during the previous fortnight compared with 267 for the same period in 1892. The workhouse was built to house 293, and the number of paupers admitted had doubled in ten years, due mainly to unemployment.[130]

The *labour test*, hard and monotonous work that had to be undertaken in return for Poor Law relief, was intended to deter applicants. Applied more in rural workhouses in the south of England[131] the test had been repealed in January 1893 at Elham. It was, however, reinstated in July by James Stewart Davy, Local Government Board Inspector and, by 1905, the head of the Board's Poor Law Division. Davy considered Elham Union to be "one of the worst workhouses in Kent", but was determined that paupers should be encouraged to be more self-sufficient in these times of increasing unemployment:

> Here we have a class of people who will tramp about and if possible live without work, and all experience has shown us that the only way to deal with them is by some sort of deterrent punishment. They can never be got rid of. Death will not rid us of them, neither will whipping of the cat tail. But if you abolish the task of work in the Union, you bring not only twice the number of casuals into your own Union, but also into that of your neighbours.[132]

---

[129] *Folkestone Up-to-Date,* 25th March, 1893, p.3. The *Folkestone Up-to-Date* was a '*new*' Liberal newspaper published in support of the Municipal Reform League.
[130] *Folkestone Up-to-Date*, 20th July, 1893
[131] J. J. & A. J. Bagley, *The English Poor Law*, London: Macmillan, 1966, p.52
[132] J. S. Davy, quoted in *Folkestone Up-to-Date*, 20th July, 1893, p.5; Davy was an important witness for the Royal Commission on the Poor Law. He argued for removal of the sick from the Poor Law as a means of reverting to a more deterrent regime for able-bodied paupers. Beatrice Webb considered him '*intent on reaction'* – S&B Webb, *English Local Government: English Poor Law History,* Pt. II, volume II, 1929, p.470, quoted in B. Abel-Smith, *Hospitals 1800-1948*, 1964

At a meeting of the Board of Guardians in September 1893 the Congregationalist minister, the Reverend A. J. Palmer, proposed relaxing the labour test for casuals and improving the diet and accommodation. Each inmate was daily required to sledgehammer four hundredweight of granite in an iron cage until it was small enough to be forced through a metal grille; this had recently been reduced from eleven hundredweight.[133] Palmer condemned stone breaking as "unremunerative, barbarous and degrading" for men (many of whom were physically unfit) existing largely on bread and gruel. The motion was voted down with all the notoriously conservative rural Guardians voting against it.[134] This attitude towards the destitute still prevailed in 1895 when Guardians voted against using "casuals" to cultivate the land or to extend the workhouse as they felt that such labour would have constituted less of a deterrent than stone breaking.[135]

In July 1893, Dr. Fuller, the Medical Officer of the Local Government Board visited the Elham Union following complaints from the Folkestone branch of the Municipal Reform League, which had been formed in November 1892. Fuller's report concluded that there existed insufficient accommodation for the sick, that the nursing wards were "very unsuitable", and that special dietary requirements (such as broth or beef tea) were routinely ignored. Dr Bishop, the Union Medical Officer, denounced the report as "infamous lies", but considering his low income and the poor regard in which the inmates were held locally his lack of supervision is not surprising. Bishop was paid £90 a year in 1893, out of which he was obliged to purchase drugs and appliances.[136]

The report was forwarded to a Committee of the Elham Guardians in October, when a recommendation that Dr. Bishop should visit the infirmary on a daily basis was voted down, chiefly by the rural Guardians. There would certainly appear to have been a need for some form of regular medical attendance in the infirmary as there was no trained nurse. Even in the workhouse one Guardian noted that there was not one able bodied person, describing it in 1893 as "nothing but a hospital".[137] At this time the evidence indicates that about 150 individuals at any one time may have

---

[133] In 1895 the Elham Guardians were reported as voting to purchase the *toughest* granite available, Kentish ragstone from Hythe. *Folkestone Up-to-Date*, 19th January, p.5

[134] *Folkestone Up-to-Date*, 28th September, 1893

[135] *Folkestone Up-to-Date*, 2nd September, 1895

[136] *Folkestone Up-to-Date*, 23rd December, 1893

[137] Mr Swoffer of the Elham Board of Guardians, *Folkestone Up-to-Date*, 12th October, 1893

been suffering from some illness in the workhouse.

In response to the adverse publicity surrounding the Union[138] a movement developed in the town, publicised by the Folkestone branch of the Municipal Reform League and supported by the Local Government Board, to build a workhouse nearer to Folkestone.[139] This would have obviated the need for paupers and their visitors to walk the six miles across country to Etchinghill, and could have provided adequate accommodation for the local destitute. A characteristically melodramatic, though essentially accurate, impression of the Union's accommodation at this time was recounted in an editorial of the *Folkestone-Up-to-Date*:

> frost and snow is on the ground and the people dropping exhausted on the road or contracting consumption and rheumatics by being placed in a stable between a dead house and a pigsty.[140]

The more conservative attitude towards the proposed Folkestone workhouse, which eventually prevailed, was articulated in the editorial column of the Conservative weekly *The Folkestone Herald*:

> In every tramp – too often synonymous with scamp – we were asked to see a man and a brother, and we were invited to build a casual ward for his accommodation in this town. Good and bad, clean and unclean, diseased or healthy, honest men or thieves – all were to be gathered into a tramps' paradise in Folkestone-on the-Sea. Had the scheme been successful, the town of Folkestone would have been infested with these people, and there would be a constant overflow into Sandgate and Hythe.[141]

In *The Herald*'s report the metaphor of the spreading infestation of the sick and destitute suggests that their proximity posed a very real threat of social contagion to the local establishment.

Considering the Union's recent infamy it could, perhaps, be considered disingenuous of Captain A. H. Bradshaw, addressing the Folkestone Charity Organisation Society in 1904, to remark upon the:

---

[138] The reformist newspaper *The Star* had adopted the case of the administration of the Poor Law in Folkestone, publishing an article entitled '*The Black Hole of Etchinghill*', on 22nd August, and 8th & 11th September, 1893, which prompted an enquiry in the House of Commons, reported in *Folkestone-Up-to-Date*, 17th August, 1893

[139] *Folkestone-Up-to-Date*, 10th August, 1893

[140] *Folkestone Up-to-Date*, 28th September, 1893 p.6

[141] *Folkestone Herald*, 12th August, 1893

> strange objection that some had to go into the infirmary. They had many cases that ought to go into the infirmary, but the families looked upon it as a disgrace, though they saw no disgrace in begging, or even in getting money by trickery.[142]

Nevertheless, as the town prospered it attracted more casual workers, causing unemployment to rise. The Mayor's Distress Fund Committee of 1904 concluded that the problem was created by the early marriages of the working classes, the decline of the building trade, drinking, gambling and a refusal to save. The working classes were "drawn to the glamour of town life" from the countryside, initially to find work, but they rarely returned home.[143]

In 1910, the COS reported:

> a large amount of unemployment as in previous years, mostly among general labourers [and] an abnormal amount of sickness of various kinds.

In addition many skilled workmen were experiencing difficulty in finding regular employment due to being undercut by itinerant workers, and temporary employment was being taken by school leavers who subsequently failed to learn a trade. Lord Radnor observed that there were "many young men in the town who could not hope to find a future here", and the Society resolved to continue assisting suitable individuals to emigrate.[144]

The case histories in the records of the Board of Guardians and the Charity Organisation Society show how easily, due to an absence of any other provision, even quite well off tradesmen and their families came to be totally dependant on charity after having been afflicted with consumption. Assistance from charity and the Poor Law was invariably insufficient to support the victim's struggle against the disease, and the principle of deterrence ensured that the privations leading to the onset of the active disease were in no way reduced. During the 1890s both applications for relief and deaths in the workhouse infirmary rose,[145] as did the incidence of consumption and infant mortality.

---

142 Folkestone COS Annual Meeting, 10th July, 1904, FCOS minute books, EKACFo/Z/1/A/M/2

143 Elham Board of Guardians, April 1904, quoted in *Hythe and Sandgate Standard*, 9th April, 1904

144 COS Annual General Meeting, 9th March, 1910, FCOS minute book of monthly meetings, 1902-10, Fo/Z1/AM3

145 Death rates in Folkestone District Institutions from General Registry Office, Poor Law relief statistics published fortnightly in *Folkestone-Up-To-Date*.

CHAPTER EIGHT

OPEN-AIR TREATMENT FOR THE WORKING CLASSES, 1890-1912

Although the open-air treatment for consumption had been promoted in popular and medical publications in England from the 1850s,[1] it remained the preserve of the well-to-do. It was not until the mid-1880s that elements of the medical profession, inspired by Koch's discovery of the *tubercle bacillus* and a steady decline in the death rate from consumption,[2] appealed for a broader, more systematic application of the therapy to include the less affluent.

This was not the only response to the problem of the tubercular poor. Due to the growth of unemployment from the 1890s, the influence of social evolutionism and the perceived benefits of dryer climates and sea voyages, working class consumptives were still encouraged by doctors and charitable organisations to emigrate to the colonies, often with tragic results.[3]

Hermann Weber, house physician to the German Hospital in Dalston, London, was one of the earliest and most influential proponents of the benefits of fresh air for the entire population, his lectures on open-air treatment having been published in the *British Medical Journal* of 1885. Drawing on his familiarity with Brehmer and Dettweiler's sanatorium work, which had been established in Germany since the mid-1850s, Weber

---

[1] B. W. Richardson, *The Hygienic Treatment of Pulmonary Consumption*, London: John Churchill, 1857; J. H. Bennet, *On the Treatment of Pulmonary Consumption by Hygiene, Climate and Medicine*, London: John Churchill, 1866

[2] According to O. R. McCarthy, The Key to the Sanatoria, *Journal of the Royal Society of Medicine*, volume 94, August, 2001, the mortality rate dropped from 3,239 per million in 1861-70 to 2,429 per million in 1881-90

[3] F. Parkes Weber, A Change of Air in young adult life and early middle age, *The Practitioner* no. 481, volume 81, no.1, July, 1908; L. Bryder, "A Health Resort for Consumptives":Tuberculosis and Immigration to New Zealand 1880-1914, *Medical History*, 40, 1996

chided the British for their temerity with regard to the outdoors:[4]

> Fear of the inclemency of the weather is far too great amongst the public as well as the profession. Patients affected with chronic consumption …ought to spend the greater part of most days in the open air, and ought not to be deterred by a little rain, or mud, or low temperature.[5]

In a dry climate the fear of chills was irrational, he claimed, and the open air was invaluable for strengthening the appetite, the digestion and in relieving night sweats, restlessness and depression. Weber claimed to have achieved great benefits from placing his patients in the open air, even acute or febrile cases, in summer or winter for weeks or even months as long as they were sheltered from the wind.

The prospect of a solitary and cold existence separated from their families must have filled many tuberculosis sufferers with misgiving. English doctors commonly referred to the "fear of air" prevalent amongst the working classes,[6] and from the 1890s evangelical campaigns by Medical Officers of Health and organisations such as the NAPT attempted to inculcate a middle-class fondness for the open air into the lower social orders.

Weber urged physicians to educate the general public in the necessity of sleeping with open windows and of spending as much time as possible in the open air. He advocated the establishment of small, separate hospitals for the tubercular poor, suggesting Sandgate, amongst other sites, as a suitable location. His prescription of open, revolving shelters and pavilions with verandas and balconies was to be generally adopted within the next ten or fifteen years. Also his recommendation of pulmonary gymnastics anticipated the popularity of physical exercises designed to strengthen the lungs in the 1920s and 1930s.[7]

The publication of Weber's articles in the *British Medical Journal* eventually led to Malcolm Morris, editor of *The Practitioner*, devoting the June 1898, July 1899 and July 1901 issues of his journal to the climatological treatment of tuberculosis. These publications included

---

[4] Contradicting Weber's perception G.V. Poore, *The Practitioner,* July, 1901, p.453, states: "In foreign countries, where all classes dread open windows and insist on stagnant rooms for living and sleeping in, consumption is much more prevalent than in England".

[5] H. Weber, The Croonian Lectures on The Hygienic and Climatic Treatment of Chronic Pulmonary Phthisis, *BMJ*, 28th March, 4th & 11th April, 1885

[6] Unidentified author, The Fight Against Consumption, *The Practitioner*, July, 1901, p.453; see also Larking, *Notes on Folkestone*, p.76

[7] H. Weber, The Croonian Lectures, 1885, p.642

contributions from all leading exponents of the therapy, and led to the founding of the National Association for the Prevention of Consumption in 1898.

Sanatorium treatment was widely publicised as an effective therapy for tuberculosis in the 1890s, and increasingly appeals were made in medical journals for the open-air treatment of the poorer classes.[8] Dr. Burton-Fanning's experimental open-air regime for working class consumptives at Cromer in the mid-1890s indicated that English winters were no barrier to the treatment of the disease, and he consequently urged the construction of sanatoria for "the humbler *phthisical* patient".[9]

In the early 1890s some London Boards of Guardians, such as Poplar and Lambeth, acquired members more sympathetic to the plight of destitute consumptives and began sending them to coastal convalescent homes such as *Beach Rocks* at Sandgate and St. Andrew's at Folkestone in order for them to benefit from the air.[10] Friendly Societies also sent consumptive members to seaside institutions, some of which, like *Beach Rocks* in 1900, they purchased and managed.

By the turn of the century an ideological shift from the Poor Law ethos of deterrence, and the selective patronage of deserving sick individuals – as epitomised by letters of recommendation to voluntary hospitals and convalescent homes – to a broader vision of social reform and universal treatment for the tubercular was becoming evident in some urban districts. A movement towards municipal socialism[11] had in certain towns and boroughs extended into the domain of public health, and by 1905 the notification of tuberculosis had become compulsory in Brighton, Liverpool, Manchester, Sheffield and Bolton. These towns had either built sanatoria or converted existing Poor Law institutions for the treatment of consumption.

As had been recognised in the Report of the Royal Commission on the Poor Laws in 1909:

---

[8] H. Weber, Thje Croonian Lectures, 1885; J. A. Lindsay, The Problem of the Consumptive Poor, *The Lancet*, 4th December, 1897; L. S. Beale, The open-air treatment of tuberculosis, *The Lancet*, 10th December, 1898; F. W. Burton-Fanning, The Open-Air Treatment of Phthisis in England, *The Lancet*, 26th March, 1898

[9] F. W. Burton-Fanning, The Open-Air Treatment of Phthisis in England, *The Lancet*, 26th March, 1898, pp. 854-857

[10] *Folkestone Herald,* 7th April, 1900, p. 13, quoted in *Truth,* 19th April, 1900

[11] T. D. A. Cockerell, Municipal Activity in Britain, *American Journal of Sociology*, volume ii, no.6, May, 1906

> The more enlightened and the more progressive Guardians of today find themselves, not merely administering "relief" under deterrent conditions, but building and equipping hospitals for the sick, lying-in homes for young mothers, institutions for the epileptic, sanatoria for the *phthisical* and farm colonies for the unemployed...[12]

At Lambeth in December 1905, for example, where between 100 to 120 workhouse infirmary beds were regularly occupied by consumptives, the great majority of whom were in an advanced condition of the disease, MOH Marcus Quarry had initiated a new system. Previously cases, unaccompanied by medical records, had been continuously transferred between District Medical Officers and Poor Law Medical Officers resulting in overcrowding and the inevitable deterioration of patients. Now the dying and the less serious cases were cared for at home. The Union Medical Officer and his assistants were employed full time, the assistants living at the infirmary, and a trained nursing staff was being recruited for home treatment. Balconies had been added to the infirmary and windows were kept wide open in accordance with the prescriptions of open-air therapy.[13]

The reformist impulse exhibited by public health professionals in some poor urban districts at the start of the twentieth century was in contrast to the antipathy to state intervention that still characterised rural southern England. Largely reflecting the tradition of liberal government wherein private philanthropy was encouraged and the action of public officials in social affairs kept to a minimum, Britain was one of the last nations to adopt an interventionist policy regarding tuberculosis. This liberal approach contrasted with Germany's vigorous state control, epitomised by Bismarck's workers' insurance scheme which had been introduced as early as 1889.

British administrations would also have been wary of public resistance to coercive public health measures, following reactions against the implementation of the Contagious Diseases Act of 1866, whereby women could be taken off the street and forcibly treated and isolated if suspected of having contracted venereal disease.[14] This reluctance to enforce the isolation of individuals would have been heightened by increased middle

---

[12] Report of RCPL, Cd.4499, p.1004

[13] Report of RCPL, appendix volume ii, 26th June, 1906, Cd.21253, 21271-3, 21290, 4499, p.1004

[14] D. Cheney, *The Hateful Ordeal at Seven Star Street – The Operation of the Contagious Diseases Acts in Dover 1870-1886,* MA dissertation, University of Kent, 1990

class fears of socialist inspired unrest amongst sections of the working classes.

Further state intervention in the lives of the sick and destitute was also viewed as an encroachment on the moral crusade of middle class Church and voluntary organisations. The railway magnate and M.P. for Hythe and Folkestone, Sir Edward Watkin, expressed the belief that state charity could undermine Christian charitable institutions, remarking in a speech delivered at the opening of the refurbished *Beach Rocks* at Sandgate in 1892:

> [I have] been somewhat alarmed with the everlasting calling upon Parliament to assist everyone…Where would have been the Christianity of their country if such opinions had always prevailed.[15]

The 6th Lord Radnor echoed these paternalist sentiments in 1921. Contemplating the waning influence of Church and aristocracy in the sphere of local charity he called for an end to moves towards the centralisation of power, claiming that public hospitals would never win the trust of the people to the same degree as had the system of voluntary hospitals and honorary staff.[16]

It was not only the Poor Law, funded by local ratepayers, that bore the social cost of tuberculosis prior to its treatment under the National Insurance Act of 1911. In addition to the action of local public health authorities, Friendly Societies and Trade Unions supported consumptive workers at home as well as administering various institutions for treating the disease.[17]

There is evidence that by the turn of the century institutional treatment was being provided in the Folkestone area for tubercular members by working class organisations as well as by reformist urban Boards of Guardians. At least two convalescent homes were managed by Friendly Societies within five miles of Folkestone. In 1900 *Beach Rocks* was sold to the committee of the Morley Convalescent Homes, who also maintained an institution at St. Margarets Bay near Dover.

Due largely to artisans and the better off workers seeking to avoid the operation of the hated Poor Law, Friendly Societies were expanding at this time. Between 1897 and 1910 membership increased at a rate of 140,000 annually.[18]

---

[15] *Sandgate Visitors List*, 2nd July, 1892
[16] *The Folkestone Health Congress, Folkestone Express*, 25th June, 1921
[17] H. T. Bulstrode, *Report on Sanatoria for Consumption*, 1905-6, p.236
[18] D. Green, *Working Class Patients*, 1985, pp.100, 179

Many workers' organisations had begun to send their members for sanatorium treatment as they considered it a more cost effective way of treating tuberculosis. Because of the chronic nature of the disease Friendly Societies in England often paid two and even three times as much in sick pay to consumptives as the average sick pay to members dying from other causes,[19] and one seventh of all Friendly Society deaths were reportedly due to consumption.[20]

Confronted with this haemorrhaging of their funds, Friendly Societies arrived at the conclusion that the cost of treating tuberculosis in sanatoria would be less than that incurred in the payment of sickness benefit to consumptive members if no effective treatment were provided.[21]

In November 1902 the committee of the National Conference of Friendly Societies sent a deputation to Germany to investigate the sanatorium treatment of tuberculosis. Following this, in May 1903, a committee was formed under the auspices of the Hospital Saturday Fund, an organisation that supported hospitals through the contributions of working people, with the object of forming an association of Friendly Societies and Trade Unions to build and maintain sanatoria for their members. This was to become the National Association for the Establishment and Maintenance of Sanatoria for Workers Suffering from Tuberculosis. Founded on 16th October, 1905, the Association bought 250 acres of land, including a church and a working farm, near the village of Benenden in the Weald of Kent at the cost of £20 an acre. In July 1906 Princess Christian of Schleswig-Holstein, the late Queen's daughter, laid the foundation stone to the sanatorium.[22]

Dr. Thomas Lister, advisory physician to the Benenden sanatorium, emphasised that the aim of sanatorium treatment for the working classes in England was, as in Germany, primarily economic:

> to restore the economic value of the afflicted working man for a sufficiently long period to make his treatment a paying proposition for the Friendly Society in which he was insured.[23]

Friendly societies were not philanthropic organisations. The moving force

---

[19] South London District of the Ancient Order of Foresters, quoted in *The Englishman*, 12th January, 1910

[20] *Daily Telegraph*, 3rd June, 1909, p.11

[21] B. McPate, *Benenden, The History of the Benenden Healthcare Society 1905-2005,* York: W. Sessions Ltd., 2006, p.44

[22] B. McPate, *Benenden*, 2006, pp.1-9

[23] Dr. T. D. Lister, quoted in *The Morning Post*, 13th May, 1912.

to provide sanatorium treatment for workers was the economic interest of societies and a concern with the cost effectiveness of members' contributions. Nevertheless, as the anti-tuberculosis movement gained momentum, some doctors and workers were beginning to view sanatorium treatment as a therapy that should be available to all as a right.

Charles Garland, a former telegraphist, who by 1904 had founded and been elected chairman of the Post Office branch of the National Sanatorium Association, stated that he began the organisation "in order to give to the impecunious sufferer in the Post Office the rich man's remedy for his disease".[24] In 1910 only 5% of the population could afford the estimated £400 a year it would cost to be treated at a sanatorium, whilst 13,000,000 – the bottom third of the working classes – were entirely dependant on the Poor Law or charity to sustain them during episodes of chronic sickness.[25]

Similarly, Arthur Latham, physician at the Brompton Hospital for Consumption and co-founder of the sanatorium at Benenden, believed that every man had a right to be protected from the adverse effects of industrial capitalism:

> The working man…has begun to realise that consumption and other forms of tuberculosis are products of civilisation and that they can be prevented. Shortly he will demand with no uncertain voice that he has a citizen's right to be protected from this product of civilisation, and that he shall be assisted when he falls a victim, not only in his own interests, but in the interests of the community at large.[26]

In 1910 Latham estimated that between 10,000 and 11,000 victims of pulmonary tuberculosis languished in Poor Law infirmaries each year with little hope of recovery, 4,000 of these being in London.[27] Moreover, Latham claimed, outdoor relief under the Poor Law as a direct result of illness and destitution caused by consumption would be greatly in excess of the amount expended on indoor treatment.[28]

The development of a coordinated system of sanatorium treatment created by workers' mutual aid organisations would, however, have been inimical to emerging "new" Liberal conceptions of the role of the state. Government action to create a more egalitarian society and improve the health, education and living conditions of the working classes was the

[24] C. Garland, 1927, quoted in McPate, *Benenden*, 2006, p.7
[25] A. Latham & C. Garland, *The Conquest of Consumption*, 1911, p.107
[26] Ibid, p.15
[27] Ibid, p.66
[28] Ibid, p.93

essence of "new" Liberalism promoted by Lloyd George and other prominent Liberals.

These reforms required a strong interventionist state in order to inculcate a new sense of duty and sacrifice for the greater good of the nation. This ideology represented a fundamental shift from the Liberal philosophy of limited government and *laissez-faire* economics practised in the mid-nineteenth century.[29] The growing influence of workers' organisations may also have been perceived as a potential threat to national stability, and Lloyd George, having travelled to Germany to investigate the financing of invalidity pensions in 1908,[30] would have been aware that Bismarck had successfully initiated a state run workers' insurance scheme in order to defuse the power of socialist organisations.[31]

In 1906 LGB inspector Timbrell Bulstrode had remarked that the National Sanatorium Association lacked co-ordination:

> The nearest approach to this condition of affairs [the German system of sanatorium treatment] in Great Britain is to be found in the Friendly Societies and the Trades Unions, but there is not about these organisations anything approaching the centralisation and co-operation which is to be found in the Workmen's Insurance System in Germany.[32]

After the National Insurance Act was passed in 1911 this attempted amalgamation of workers mutual aid societies was fatally undermined. Benenden's annual report of December, 1917 commented that support for the sanatorium from workers' organisations was poor.[33]

Before the introduction of this legislation, however, both Friendly Societies and some progressive urban Boards of Guardians were sending tubercular patients for open-air treatment at coastal convalescent homes and sanatoria, particularly in the south of England. The introduction of working class consumptives to select and conservative health resorts was, at least in the case of Folkestone and Sandgate, to have considerable social

---

[29] J. Gehrke, *Georgist Thought and the Emergence of Municipal Socialism in Britain, 1870-1914*, p.23, http://schalkenbach.org/on-line-library/scholars-forum/municipal-socialism-in-britain/

[30] K. O. Morgan, Lloyd George and Germany*, The Historical Journal*, volume 39, no.3, September, 1996, p.757

[31] M. Pelling, V. Berridge, M. Harrison & P. Weindling, chapter 4, p.136, C. Webster, ed., *Caring for Health: History and Diversity,* Oxford University Press, 2001, p.122

[32] H. T. Bulstrode, *Report on Sanatoria for Consumption*, 1905-6, p.236

[33] LGB correspondence with Benenden sanatorium, 1912-1919, NA MH 48/77

repercussions that would contribute to highlighting the perceived poor health of the working classes and influence government responses to the problem of tuberculosis.

In Folkestone, particularly from 1898, concerns over infection and a lowering of the "social tone" were aggravated as the number of consumptives sent chiefly from East London to John James Jones' sanatoria in neighbouring Sandgate continued to increase. In the summer of 1907 *The Lancet*'s reporter caught the mood of anxiety prevalent amongst local residents, who appeared to be chiefly concerned with the apparent lack of discipline and order exhibited by the sick and destitute Londoners:

> From the Jones's homes of Sandgate the undisciplined patients who, for the most part, are suffering from pulmonary tuberculosis, can easily stroll up to the Leas, mingle with the fashionable crowd that gathers on this favoured spot, and listen to the Folkestone band. Doubtless these pauper patients behave as well as can be expected in the circumstances; but there are some rough elements among them…and from notably such poor districts of London as are represented by the Poplar Union. Nor are the inhabitants, who treat their own paupers in a very different manner, inclined to believe that the ratepayers of London and other centres would approve of the manner in which their money is spent at Sandgate. If patients are sent to the seaside at the public expense this is done so that they may be cured by undergoing regular treatment. It is true that in most cases listening to music on the Leas does the patients more good than loitering about the public houses at Sandgate. The ratepayers of Folkestone, however, are not animated with such loving kindness as to tax themselves to provide bands for the benefit of paupers from Poplar and other such places. Thus, at Folkestone, as well as at Sandgate, there was a joyful anticipation that, after an Act of Parliament had been obtained, something more like order and discipline would prevail at the Jones's homes.[34]

The Lancet's account of rough and undisciplined consumptive paupers from the poorest London Boroughs mixing with Folkestone's fashionable health seekers by the Leas bandstand reveals the sense of social disorder felt by the town's residents in 1907.[35] This emerging system of treatment according to need was in stark contrast to the paternalist structures through which access was granted to health care or to the receipt of charitable or Poor Law relief in Folkestone, and demonstrates differing approaches to

---

[34] The Renewal of the Sandgate Sanatoria Scandal, *The Lancet,* 29th June, 1907, p.1606

[35] Ibid, p.1809

poverty, chronic disease and social conformity.

Only by convincing members of charities, Boards of Guardians and sponsors of their industriousness and moral respectability could a family in Folkestone hope to avoid destitution and the workhouse in the event of the breadwinner developing chronic disease leading to unemployment. The desolate experiences of the tubercular poor were, at best, only potentially alleviated as a result.

The stated function of the local Board of Guardians and the Charity Organisation Society was to deter pauperism, reliance on the state and charity, to eliminate the practice of begging and to encourage self-reliance. This well established individualist ethic can, however, be seen as conflicting with the newly emergent public health imperative of preventive medicine whereby consumptive workers were encouraged to seek treatment at an early stage of the disease.

There is some evidence that Friendly Societies encouraged the early institutional treatment of consumption as a more economic option than merely providing sickness benefit.[36] However, at least before the implementation of the state tuberculosis scheme, the tubercular were encouraged to work if they were at all able by Boards of Guardians, particularly in rural workhouses in the south of England. This was also the attitude of COS members and many public health officials.

Although the more affluent sufferer from tuberculosis continued to be encouraged to visit Folkestone and Sandgate, indeed the towns' economies depended on attracting the wealthy invalid, paupers sent to Sandgate by Boards of Guardians from the east end of London were objected to as posing a particular threat to the health of residents.[37]

Nevertheless, consumptives were not separated from other inmates at the Elham union infirmary until 1904, neither had they been provided with separate accommodation at St. Andrews or in any other institution in the town. This local controversy, which will be explored in the following chapter, highlights the anomaly of contrasting local attitudes to two distinct social classes receiving treatment for tuberculosis within two miles of each other. It also provided one of the earliest forums in England where the infectiousness of tuberculosis and the problems it posed to society were debated.

---

[36] B. McPate, *Benenden, The History of the Benenden Healthcare Society 1905-2005,* York: W. Sessions Ltd., 2006, p.44; J. C. Riley, Ill Health During the Mortality Decline: The Friendly Societies' Experience, *Bulletin of the History of Medicine*, 1987, p.583

[37] The Renewal of the Sandgate Sanatoria Scandal, *The Lancet,* 29th June, 1907, p.1808

CHAPTER NINE

A PAUPERS' PARADISE BY THE SEA: THE SANDGATE SANATORIA CONTROVERSY 1884-1915

Residents of Sandgate at the end of the nineteenth century would have been well aware not only of the personal tragedy wrought by epidemics of disease, but of the consequent harm to the town's reputation as a health resort and the disastrous effects on the local economy. As the example of Folkestone has demonstrated, during the nineteenth century major threats to the health of towns were posed by rapid population growth. Profit-driven private utility companies often failed to provide regular supplies of water which were also at risk of contamination by inefficient or non-existent sewage systems. Such conditions resulted in epidemics of cholera and typhoid, lethal water borne diseases unknown in England before the nineteenth century that could prostrate and kill victims in a matter of hours.[1]

At Sandgate both the rise of population and an absence of local authority powers to raise rates to improve sanitation contributed to chronic health problems in the late 1840s and 1850s. Edwin Chadwick's sanitary inspection of the town in 1848 recognised that its demise in salubrity and prosperity had occurred as a result of its initial popularity as a health resort:

> with the increase of population, no further provision having been made for the removal of excrementitious matter, it has accumulated in the substratum to an extent that nearly every well in the present town is polluted by its percolation...The consequence of this state of things has been that visitors who, from its advantages of position, climate, and site, had been in the habit of frequenting the town, have been driven from it to other places of resort, where a purer atmosphere and purer water can be had, and that others have been deterred from coming to it by its reputation

---

[1] S. Szreter, *A Central Role for Local Government? The Example of Late Victorian Britain*, www.historyandpolicy.org, 16.10.08., p.3

> for unhealthiness. A heavy pecuniary loss has thus fallen upon the population.[2]

As a consequence of Chadwick's report, Sandgate was constituted a Local Board of Health in 1849. In 1852 the water supply and drainage of the town were improved, and a water supply of 20,000 gallons per day was contracted from the Folkestone Waterworks Company requiring the levying of a one shilling rate from householders.

Local surgeon George Moseley promoting the benefits of Sandgate in his 1853 publication *Sandgate as a Residence for Invalids*, still felt the need to reassure potential visitors that *diarrhoea* was no longer a problem in the town:

> I cannot say that the complaint is by any means common, nor does it attack so often visitors on their first arriving, as it does in the Isle of Wight, Brighton, or Torquay.[3]

However, in the autumn of 1854, only one year after Moseley's promotion of Sandgate's particular qualities as a health resort for the tubercular, fever and *diarrhoea* preceded an outbreak of cholera in the town in which 94 inhabitants contracted the disease and 48 cases proved fatal. This was at the height of the cholera epidemic of 1853-55 during which 23,000 deaths occurred in Britain in 1854 alone. Despite having escaped the epidemics of 1826-1838 and 1848-1850 Sandgate, together with Canterbury and Tonbridge, provided the main focus of the disease in Kent at this time. The adjacent Shorncliffe barracks also suffered 41 deaths from cholera in the following year.[4]

A report by a General Board of Health inspector in 1855 concluded that the construction of the public drainage by the Local Board of Health had been defective and that the water supplies remained contaminated.[5] A further inquiry by the General Board of Health in 1856 reported on the continued foul state of the beach and the necessity of re-laying the leaking and improperly connected sewage pipes:

---

[2] E. Chadwick, *Report to the General Board of Health on the town of Sandgate*, 1849, p.22

[3] G. Moseley, *Sandgate as a Resort for Invalids*, London, John Churchill, 1853, p.43

[4] C. Collins, *Cholera and Typhoid Fever in Kent,* Paper no.004, www.kentarchaeology.ac.

[5] T. E. Blackwell, *Report to the General Board of Health on the Drainage and Water Supply of Sandgate, in connexion with the late Outbreak of Cholera in that Town*, 21st February, 1855

> Until the drainage is rendered complete, and the public are assured that such is the case, it is impossible that Sandgate can regain its old position, even now it is notorious that had it not been for the establishment of the [military] camp in the neighbourhood of the town the shopkeepers would have been almost ruined. Scarcely a lodging house was let last season, and it will be the same again and again until the evils which are now so dangerously apparent are grappled with and effectually removed.[6]

To counter the impression that the local authorities were reactionary or inept it should be borne in mind that these sanitary undertakings were then in their infancy. The glazed earthenware sewage pipes prescribed by Chadwick, for example, were a recent innovation, and the problems posed by laying pipes along the precipitous and variable incline from the cliffs to the coast were largely unprecedented. As would be expected from communities depending to such a great degree on a reputation for health, these sanitary undertakings were generally entered into enthusiastically by members of the local authorities.

In Sandgate, as in Folkestone, the livelihood of all sectors of the population from hotel owners to fishermen, laundrymaids and haberdashers depended on the towns' reputation as health resorts. The unexpected arrival of diseases such as cholera and typhoid, together with a growing popular awareness of the dangers resulting from poor sanitation, would, however, have made local authorities wary of creating any public anxiety over the dangers posed to the health of visitors and residents. In the event of any crisis, meetings of the local authorities regarding health issues were generally closed to the press and public.

One positive consequence of the cholera epidemics of the 1850s and 1860s was that subsequent improvements to sanitation were probably responsible for a decline in deaths from tuberculosis. Chadwick's reforms, it was claimed, reduced the incidence of "sanitation diseases" such as cholera and typhoid, and consequently improved resistance to the *tubercle bacillus* amongst the population.[7]

Despite the catastrophe of the cholera epidemic Sandgate eventually recovered its reputation as a prestigious health resort ideally suited for the open-air treatment of consumption and scrofula. This would have been enhanced by the publication of Moseley's book, as well as by its proximity

---

[6] A. L. Dickens, *Report to the General Board of Health on an Inquiry with respect to the proceedings of the Local Board of Health, the state of the public works of water supply and drainage &c. of Sandgate*, 30th May, 1856

[7] S. Szreter, The Importance of Social Intervention, 1988, p.17; Folkestone Public Health Congress and the Sandgate Scandal, *The Lancet*, 2nd July, 1904, p.48; C. Bellamy, *Administering Central-Local Relations*, 1988, p.140

to the rapidly developing elite health resort of Folkestone, of which it was virtually a suburb. And in 1885 the influential and widely published Hermann Weber suggested Sandgate as a climatologically suitable location in an article advocating the establishment of small hospitals for the tubercular poor.[8]

It is possible that John James Jones, the owner and manager of Sanatoria in Sandgate from the late-1880s, was influenced by Weber to specialise in the treatment of consumption in the town. Jones recounted how he had been inspired to devote his energies to helping the sick and needy after attending a sermon delivered by the founder of the Bristol orphanages, the Reverend George Muller, at the Bethesda Chapel.[9] In 1874 he founded the Homerton Mission, an evangelical charity to assist the poor, through which he also promoted the emigration of London paupers to the colonies.[10]

Having briefly managed a smaller convalescent home in Dover, Jones first arrived in Sandgate in 1889 to manage *Beach Rocks.* He had been instrumental in arranging the purchase of this property for the London Samaritan Society and Homerton Mission. At this time he was 35 years old. From a relatively humble, evangelical background, he had received a commercial education and, according to *The Times,* by 1888 he was earning £312 annually for managing the Homerton Mission, and between £400-£700 a year as a travel and shipping agent. Presumably this was for arranging the emigration of poor, and possibly chronically sick, individuals to the colonies. Jones was thus a relatively well-off man when he arrived at Sandgate.[11]

The Samaritan Society also ran another convalescent home, Shaftsbury Lodge, in Bournemouth. Both institutions charged roughly the same rates of admission and operated the same system of subscription letters and medical certificates as obtained at the St. Andrew's Convalescent Home in Folkestone. In 1892 patients recommended by guinea subscribers were charged five shillings per week, private patients paid ten shillings or

---

[8] H. Weber, The Croonian Lectures on the Hygienic and Climatic Treatment of Chronic Pulmonary Phthisis, *BMJ*, 28th March, 4th & 11th April, 1885

[9] *Christian Herald*, 19th December, 1883, Fynmore Collection, Folkestone Library, 942.23 FOLK

[10] J. J. Jones, *Advantages of the Dominion of Canada*, December, 1883, British Library, rare books section

[11] J. J. Jones, *Advantages of the Dominion of Canada*, 1883; *The Lancet* 22nd August, 1903, p.565; *The Times, 22nd* November, 1888, p.13; L. Bryder, A Health Resort for Consumptives, 1996

twelve shillings, and "cases of extreme need" were admitted free.[12]

Purchased in 1882 by the London Samaritan Society, *Beach Rocks,* a large house situated on the shingled Sandgate seafront, originally accommodated 60 patients. By 1888 the acquisition of two more properties provided a further 82 beds, and in 1891-2 the main building was demolished, rebuilt and furnished at a cost of £20,000 to accommodate 250 patients. Many local dignitaries attended the opening, and the work of the Society was initially perceived as a great philanthropic undertaking. Sir Edward Watkin, owner of the South Eastern Railway and M.P. for Hythe and Folkestone, announced that 12,610 people had already been received into the Society's Homes in Sandgate, over 3,000 had been helped to emigrate, and a "large number" of the poor and destitute had been given food, clothes and lodging.[13]

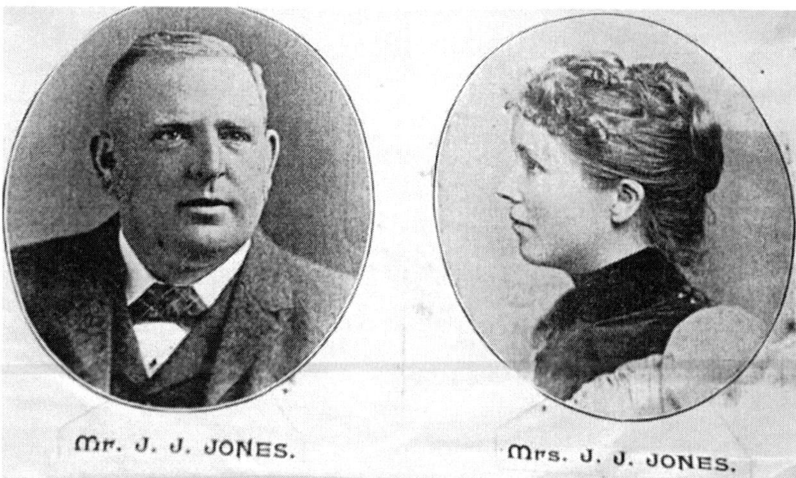

Illustration 9.1: John James Jones and his second wife c.1892.

Jones' evangelical pragmatism initially attracted charitable donations for the Society and civic recognition for himself. He was elected

[12] Unidentified cutting in Fynmore Collection dated 30th June, 1892, Folkestone Library, 942.23 FOLK

[13] *Sandgate Visitors' List*, 2nd July, 1892. Interestingly Sir Edward Watkin, M.P. for Hythe, on opening the home, proudly compared the British tradition of private Christian philanthropy with the French practice of state financed medical institutions.

councillor for Hythe shortly after his arrival at Sandgate, councillor for the Sandgate Local Board of Health in 1891, although he declined to stand, and was a member of the Elham Board of Guardians in the 1890s.[14] In 1892 Mr. Horton, the Mayor of Hythe, was reported in a local newspaper as saying:

> he thought it was a toss up whether the Sandgate Local Board had Mr. Jones or whether Hythe did, and said they would like to have him Mayor of Hythe some day. Mr. Holden (ex-Mayor of Folkestone) said he did not think Hythe would catch Mr. Jones, but that Folkestone would at some time.[15]

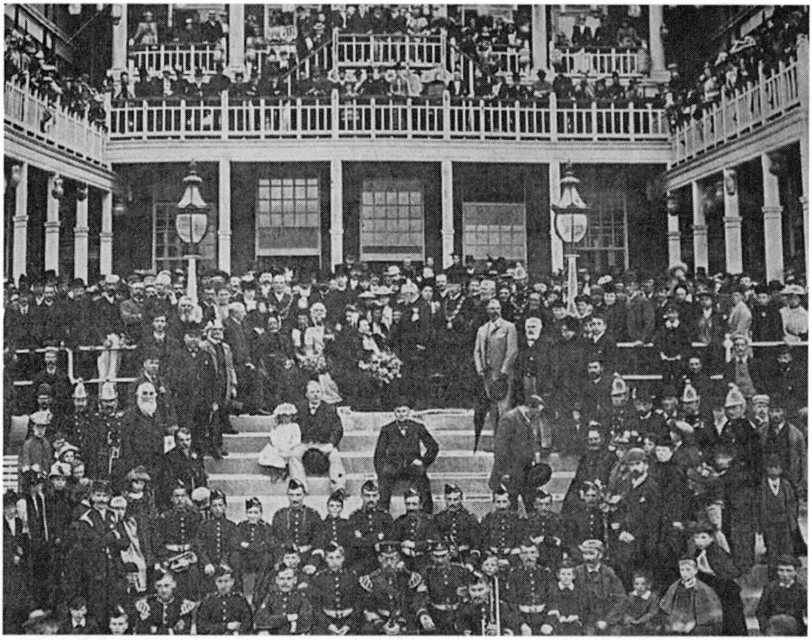

Illustration 9.2: The Opening of *Beach Rocks* Convalescent Home at Sandgate in 1892.

[14] Evidence of Dr. Kirkby Robinson, Minutes of Proceedings before the House of Lords' Select Committee on Sandgate Urban District Council. Bill, May 1905; Sandgate LBH & UDC Minutes 1885-90, 1890-93

[15] Unidentified local newspaper cutting, 1892, in the Fynmore Collection, Folkestone Library, 942.23 FOLK

Jones' social ascendancy was checked from April 1893 when Henry Labouchère's crusading weekly journal, *Truth*, accused him of appropriating donations to the Samaritan Society. The paper had allegedly uncovered a previous denunciation by the Charity Organisation Society, and charged Jones with being a "professional charity monger" and a "successor of Mr. Squeers".[16] This was always denied by the Society, whose committee publicly supported Jones and published annual audited accounts.[17] Nevertheless, this demonstrates that Dickens' caricature had obviously alerted the crusading press to the potential abuses practised by charitable fundraisers.

The effect of these attacks on Jones' public image were somewhat mitigated by the organisation of benevolent gestures to both poor, disabled children from London and to local children.[18] For example, in January 1896, 188 sick and disabled children were selected from the Ragged Schools of east London and escorted by fourteen nurses down to Sandgate by train:

> These children…are for a whole fortnight to be accommodated at that well known depot of benevolent kindness, the Beach Rocks Convalescent Home and Hospital…[to] enjoy the transformation from the slums of London to the picturesque environs of the Home in which they are to be sheltered and, indeed, feted.[19]

Following the publication of more defamatory articles in *Truth,* the trustees of the London Samaritan Society investigated Jones' management of *Beach Rocks* and the accounts of the Society but apparently discovered no financial improprieties. According to the Society's bi-annual report of 1893 a management committee had taken over the running of the Home after Jones' health had failed. This was, ostensibly, as a result of helping to launch the Sandgate lifeboat in a strong gale in an attempt to save the crew of the cutter *Bienvenue*, in addition to the anxiety caused by the trustees' report.[20] However, it would appear from J. S. Davy's report for the Local Government Board on the Sandgate Homes of 1898 that Jones had taken poison and narrowly escaped with his life.[21] Possibly as a form of

---

[16] *Truth,* 7th November, 1901

[17] Letter from London Samaritan Society in *The Christian World*, 24th September, 1896; *Folkestone Herald*, 19th August, 1893

[18] *Folkestone Herald*, 11th January, 1896; 5th July, 1902

[19] *Folkestone Herald*, 4th January, 1896

[20] Bi-annual report of London Samaritan Society ending 31st May, 1893, quoted in *Folkestone Herald*, 19th August, 1893

[21] Marginalia, J. S. Davy, Report for LGB, 23rd December, 1898, MH 12/5051

insurance in the event of his death, Jones took the opportunity of acquiring further property in the town at a much reduced rate following the Sandgate landslip of March 1893. The property was registered in the names of his wife and children, and by 1898 Jones and his family were in possession of eight further properties in the town, some of which they employed as homes for sick pauper children sent by metropolitan Boards of Guardians.

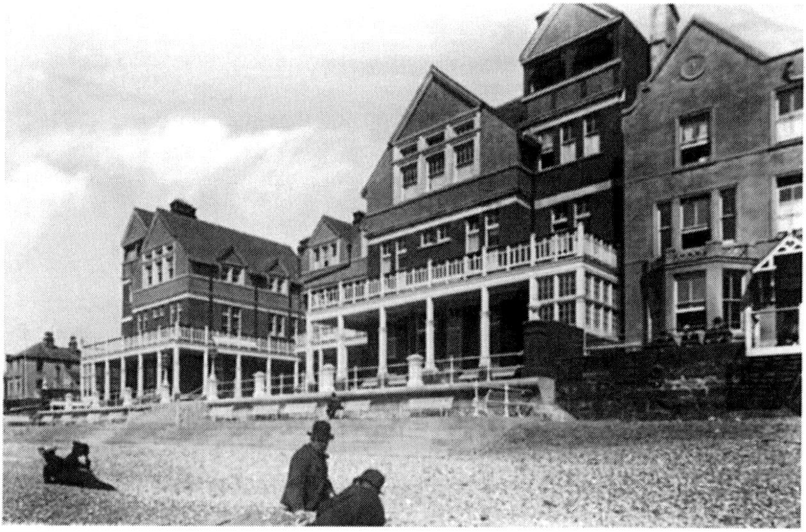

Illustration 9.3: Beach Rocks Convalescent Home, Sandgate, 1891.

This course of action led to further opposition from local residents and the town Council, who sent two "memorials" to the Local Government Board in 1898. These petitions claimed that Jones was turning the town into a *lazaret*, that he was responsible for a rise in the death rate, and complained of the threat to Sandgate's future as a health resort due to the increasing numbers of invalids to be found in the town and on the seafront.[22]

[22] One of the 78 signatories was H.G. Wells, then recuperating in Arnold House, Sandgate after his health had failed due to consumption.

By this time it was evident that the town was becoming less supportive of Jones' enterprise. Many residents were openly antagonistic, some who had moved to Sandgate for their health were leaving, and even that aspect of it carried out under the charitable auspices of the London Samaritan Society did not escape criticism. It was claimed by one Sandgate resident that "Beach Rocks, though nominally a convalescent home, is largely used as a hospital for consumptive persons".[23]

As we have seen in the case of St Andrew's, although convalescent homes were differentiated from "hospitals for disease" in the legislation, due to patients being considered to be free from active disease, consumption was such a protean complaint that patients were liable to relapse and become febrile at any time. In addition those suffering from the disease were rarely admitted to voluntary hospitals and metropolitan Poor Law infirmaries became overwhelmed with the tubercular, at least until public sanatoria became available after World War One.

For example, in 1904 Lambeth Infirmary alone was stated to be admitting between 300 and 400 consumptive cases a year. In 1899 it was so overcrowded that Guardians felt compelled to send 100 consumptives to Jones' sanatoria, it being the only institution available that provided nursing for a fee that was considered affordable.[24] Jones had discovered a niche market for treating destitute consumptives, chiefly from the east end of London, who were surviving longer and resorting to the workhouse when no longer able to support themselves or their families.

One of Jones' immediate neighbours, the popular novelist Florence Warden, was an ardent opponent of his Homes, having written various letters of complaint to the Local Government Board and the Urban District Council, as well as to the local and national press. Her husband, Councillor James, and J. J. Jones had each brought charges against the other for assault following a violent public affray in the streets of Sandgate in early September 1899; both parties being ordered to pay court costs. In a letter to the Local Government Board of November that year Miss Warden furnished them with a lurid account of life in Sandgate:

> The town is now in a disgusting state, with crippled men dragging themselves in and out of the public houses, filling the seats on the Parade, and standing about in their shirt-sleeves smoking and expectorating onto

---

[23] Memorial of Sandgate Urban District Council to Local Government Board, Records of Local Government Board, Elham Union, 9th June, 1898

[24] Evidence of Dr. Marcus Quarry, M.O. Lambeth Union, Minutes of proceedings before the Select Committee of the House of Lords on the SUDC Bill, 22nd March, 1905, p. 245

> the neighbours' gardens from the steps of the Jones' Homes. Many of the patients brought down here by Jones are entirely helpless, and are simply carried into the houses to their beds. Many of them seem to be so ill as to have been wholly unfit to make the journey.[25]

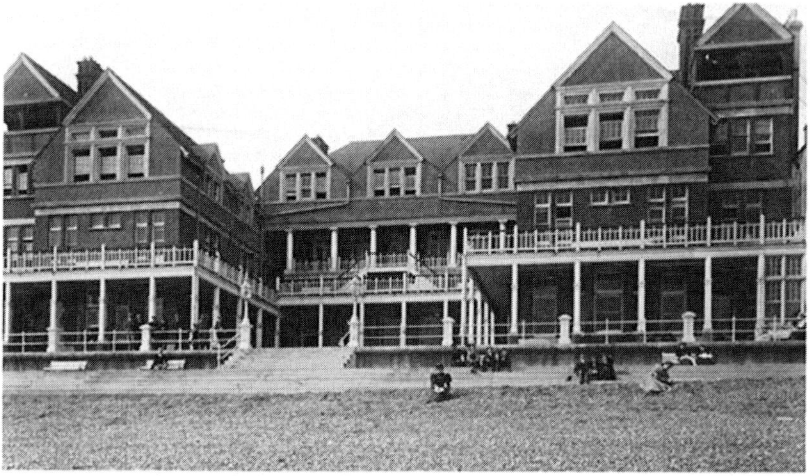

Illustration 9.4: Beach Rocks, Sandgate, 1896.

In his defence Jones had, throughout the 1890s and early years of the next century, sent repeated complaints to London Boards of Guardians concerning the advanced condition of consumptives being sent to his homes. However, as becomes clear in the parliamentary debates surrounding the 1905 Sandgate Bill, at this time working men and women only tended to apply for relief when they became physically incapacitated. As Professor W. R. Smith explained to the Select Committee of the House of Lords reading of the Sandgate Bill:

> no person applies to the Poor Law medical authorities for medical treatment in connection with *phthisis* unless it has come to such a stage that the man is rendered incapable of discharging his ordinary duties…it is only when their health breaks down that they seek relief from the Boards of Guardians.[26]

---

[25] Letter from Florence Warden to the LGB, 7th November, 1899, LGB correspondence, NA MH 12/5051

[26] Evidence of Professor William R. Smith, Minutes of proceedings before the Select Committee of the House of Lords on the SUDC Bill, 22nd March, 1905

In the same letter Florence Warden further accused Jones of planning to acquire the proceeds from the proposed sale of *Beach Rocks*, an institution built and maintained from charitable donations. This charge was soon to be adopted in Labouchère's *Truth*.

Meanwhile, the treatment of workhouse children was proving particularly troublesome and potentially dangerous due to the risk of epidemics from such complaints as measles, diphtheria, ophthalmia and ringworm. Despite the opinion of the LGB that his establishments were valuable resources for the children, Jones decided to discontinue their treatment and to focus exclusively on the treatment of consumption, which was not then subject to notification or to any legal regulation.[27]

Sandgate residents were quick to employ the contagion argument in appealing to the LGB for support in closing the Homes. The Board decided that this was a matter over which they were unable to take any action due to the fact that consumption was not considered an infectious disease under the Infectious Diseases Notification Act of 1889. Neither was it classified as a "dangerous infectious disorder" as prescribed under section 126 of the Public Health Act of 1875. The LGB advised the residents of Sandgate that this was an issue for the Local Board of Health and its Sanitary Authority. However, Charles Perry, the MOH for Sandgate, could find no contravention of the existing public health regulations under which he could prosecute the management of the Homes.

Further adverse publicity was generated when, from 1896, the 42 roomed Grosvenor House was opened. Operating as an hotel in the summer months, when it received tour parties from London arranged by Thomas Cook & Sons, it served as an institution for consumptives for the remainder of the year.[28] As there existed no legal restrictions or regulations for the treatment of consumption in institutions no action was taken other than Jones' son, Frederick Board-Jones, being refused a liquor license for the establishment by local magistrates.[29]

Many residents and local Councillors became progressively frustrated with the inability or unwillingness, as they perceived it, of the LGB to act on their behalf. Jones had come to be regarded by many in the town as a commercial speculator exploiting sick paupers for a profit, although he operated the same financial system as the Sisters of St. John the Baptist at St. Andrew's. He charged slightly less per bed and managed his institutions

---

[27] J. S. Davy, Memorandum, Report for LGB, 1st June, 1899, MH 12/5051

[28] *Truth 18th* May, 1899; *Daily Express* 27th July, 1900

[29] *Folkestone Herald*, 26th September, 1896; Board-Jones was also refused permission to build a pier at Sandgate.

efficiently through the provision of his own meat, dairy products, bread and other essentials, in addition to providing his own laundries, dispensary and transport.[30]

Jones was unabashed in public and decided to use the controversy to his own advantage:

> Our homes are increasing in number every month or so, and such foolish conduct does not injure us, but rather aids us in our enterprise, inasmuch as the criticisms I refer to have frightened the persons who would come to live in Sandgate, and frightened those who already were living in Sandgate, by telling them there is a likelihood of disease being conveyed to them or their children. The result is that those who hold property either sell it to us, or rent it to us, at a comparatively low figure. Therefore I think you will see very clearly that the authors of such criticisms are only playing our game to a financial extent they have never dreamt of…today we probably hold about one sixth or one eighth of the whole town. If the adverse criticism goes on sufficiently long, and our success is as great in the future as it has been in the past, we shall probably have one half of Sandgate within a year or two.[31]

Jones' financial opportunism and increasing notoriety made his Homes subject to more scrutiny than many other such enterprises. They were visited regularly by representatives of Boards of Guardians and their Medical Officers, LGB inspectors, journalists and churchmen.[32] In 1898 Jones, whilst still managing *Beach Rocks* under the auspices of the London Samaritan Society, announced that his other Homes would henceforth be run as a private family concern.[33]

This move from the management of a charitable organisation to the operation of a commercial business was largely unprecedented, and viewed with suspicion by many residents. Running the Homes on a professional basis may, however, have resulted in improved care for the patients. The medical supervisor, William Chubb, was placed on an annual salary of 100 guineas a year for daily attendance on patients at *Beach Rocks*, and £100 to visit the other Homes every day. In addition about 40 other members of staff were employed by 1898.[34] In 1900 Jones was claiming that, despite adverse criticism, his Homes had grown to be

---

[30] *Folkestone Herald*, 23rd April, 1900, p.13

[31] J.J. Jones, interviewed in *Folkestone Herald,* quoted in *Truth,* 19th April, 1900

[32] In his LGB report of December 1898 J. S. Davy remarked that visits by church ministers provided a very useful form of inspection, NA MH 12/5051

[33] *Truth*, 9th February, 1899, pp. 335-339; 9th March, 1889

[34] Dr. Stephenson's report, LGB Records, December, 1898, NA MH 12/5051

"probably the largest establishment of their kind in the United Kingdom".[35]

Unusually for charitable institutions Jones' Homes were run on non-sectarian lines and patients were permitted to worship where they chose or not at all. Jones' expressed intention was to avoid the routine and regulations common in institutions of the time and to organise patients into "families" enjoying the atmosphere of an "English Home".[36] This was patently at odds with the Poor Law ethic of deterrence which, as described in chapter seven, was rigorously upheld locally, and was applied equally to the aged, children and to the sick.[37] The one regulation that Jones claimed commanded instant dismissal from his Homes if not adhered to was a prohibition against expectoration inside or out of the sanatoria.[38]

This comparatively relaxed management of paupers in a select coastal health resort unused to the proximity of the working classes was perhaps as disturbing for residents as the fear of infection. Pauperism referred to a condition that had come to be seen as biological as much as economic. For much of the middle classes the term represented a degenerate residuum of flawed humanity that posed a threat for civilised society whether or not they were overtly diseased.[39] In mitigation Jones maintained that many consumptives sent by Poor Law authorities should not be termed "paupers":

> though in the legal sense they undoubtedly are paupers, in the social sense they are of a somewhat better class than what is generally understood by the term "pauper".[40]

Jones' observation reveals the social cost of tuberculosis on many who were not the poorest in society, skilled artisans and clerks for example, who were reduced to destitution by this chronic wasting disease. The good behaviour of these destitute urban consumptives was endorsed by a correspondent from *The Lancet*, who visited Sandgate in 1903, staying in lodgings next to one of Jones' sanatoria. He considered them to be clean, tidy and quiet, and could find nothing in their behaviour to object to:

---

[35] *Folkestone-Up-to-Date*, 7th April, 1900, p. 13
[36] *Folkestone Herald*, 23rd April, 1900, p.13
[37] G. Slater, *Poverty and the State,* London, Constable & Co., 1930, p.97
[38] *Councillor & Guardian,* 20th December, 1902;
[39] G. Jones, *Social Hygiene*, 1986, p.81
[40] *The Lancet*, 22nd August, 1903, p.566

> I doubt whether patients belonging to some more prosperous class would behave better and create less trouble than these paupers. The cry against them at Sandgate is loud and strong, but as far as it is directed against them as paupers it is uncharitable.[41]

Regardless of their good behaviour, it was the social class of consumptives treated in the town that appears to have been the prime concern of Sandgate residents. As John Huntley, deputy chairman of Sandgate Urban District Council, remarked "it did not excite the same attention when the patients were of a higher class socially".[42]

As both the Urban District Council and the LGB found themselves unable to remedy the situation, so the fortunes of the town deteriorated with falling property values and a shortage of seasonal visitors. A comment from one ex-resident typifies the feeling in Sandgate at the time. He felt compelled to leave the town:

> due to the very frequent funerals, and the number of unfortunate patients, many in the last stage of their suffering, permitted to lie about exposed to public view were truly appalling and most disastrous to the welfare of Sandgate. Should not isolation be the first consideration?[43]

Jones was now operating a private business in ten properties in Sandgate,[44] and was no longer dependent on attracting charitable subscriptions, which may have been less readily forthcoming than previously. J. S. Davy, the LGB inspector, although concerned with the lack of accountability of private institutions, realised that the Board possessed no powers to prohibit them receiving sick paupers from Boards of Guardians or Friendly Societies:

> It is to my mind a question as to whether Guardians should be allowed to board out paupers at establishments which are run for profit and as a business. The Board as it is incur a heavy responsibility in certifying the ordinary Houses which are ostensibly managed for charity; for it is impossible to really supervise establishments where there is no responsible

---

[41] Ibid, p.566

[42] Minutes of Proceedings before the Select Committee of the House of Lords on SUDC Sanitary Powers Bill, May, 1905, HL/PO/PB/5/71/23

[43] Letter from H. J. Portington Perry of Tunbridge Wells, quoted in *Minutes of Proceedings before the Select Committee of the House of Lords on SUDC Sanitary Powers Bill*, May, 1905, HL/PO/PB/5/71/23

[44] The *Daily Express* of 27th July, 1900 reported that Jones owned 23 properties in Sandgate.

> Medical Officer, no dietary table, and no audit. But in the case of Charitable Homes the Board have a guarantee for good management in the social position or charitable zeal of the Committees. Committees however well intentioned are apt to be negligent or ignorant of their duties, but generally speaking in the case of charitable institutions they are some protection to the inmates and to the Board. In the case of institutions which are managed by professional philanthropists there is little cause to fear, for the manager must court the utmost publicity and freedom of inspection in order to draw the subscriptions of the public, and his livelihood in a measure depends on the efficiency of his establishment. But when there are no subscriptions and the institution is simply run for profit there are none of these guarantees and checks, and the Board have to depend on the casual visits of the Guardians and the annual visit of their inspector…Yet looking to the powers conferred upon the Board by statute, I do not see how they could except by legislation prohibit the reception of paupers into the establishments now existing. If Sandgate is to be closed to paupers it must be done on general principles, and these principles would also apply to Margate and to Rottingdean.[45]

Again there is no mention of any perceived threat of infection. Davy appears chiefly concerned that an institution operating outside of a charitable framework may be motivationally suspect, indeed he comments on "the dislike that everyone must feel for the methods employed by men of Mr. Jones' profession".[46]

Yet, equally, he realised that the accommodation and management were at least as good as any obtainable elsewhere, and was wary of the consequences of prohibiting the treatment of patients of Union infirmaries in private institutions, particularly as there existed very few beds anywhere for the treatment of consumptives at this time. Jones claimed in 1900 that he had treated thousands of consumptive patients sent by Friendly Societies as well as by Boards of Guardians:

> over 3,000 *phthisical* patients from the Brompton and other hospitals since 1874, and also The Spurstowe Charity, Hackney have sent us at least 5,000 patients, the Hearts of Oak Society have sent us over 2,000, and the Hospital Saturday fund over 3,000.[47]

In January 1900 the Sandgate Urban District Council, the successor to the Local Board of Health, applied to the LGB for an inquiry into the

---

45 J. S. Davy, Report for the LGB on the Sandgate Homes, 23rd December, 1898, MH 12/5051

46 Ibid.

47 *Folkestone Herald*, 7th April, 1900, p.13, quoted in *Truth,* 19th April, 1900

management of the Jones' Homes following the publication of their Medical Officer's report for the year 1899. Out of 55 deaths in the town 31 had occurred in the Homes, 13 being diagnosed as due to consumption.[48] The LGB were of the opinion that there were insufficient grounds for an inquiry; cases of diphtheria, originating at the Homerton Fever Hospital, had been removed to the Folkestone sanatorium and the Board was satisfied that every precaution had been taken to prevent infection. They advised the SUDC that if the Homes were managed in such a way as to constitute a threat to public health, the Council should itself take proceedings against Jones.[49]

From 1899 to 1903 Labouchère continued to devote many pages of *Truth* to attacking Jones' "charitymongering" and his "curious trade in diseased paupers", as well as to castigating the LGB and the Sandgate UDC for their ineffectiveness in regulating the Homes. He was also critical of the editor of the *Folkestone Herald* for publishing verbatim an interview with Jones, whilst denying space to his detractors.[50] Even *Truth,* however, was aware of the hugely overcrowded condition of metropolitan Poor Law and charitable infirmaries, and of the urgent need felt by their Medical Officers to offer hope to the sick and to provide space for those awaiting admission:

> All the infirmary officers practically tell the same story, namely, that it is often of great importance for the benefit of patients in the infirmaries that they should be sent to the country or seaside for change of air; that the desirability of sending them away is further enhanced by the greatly overcrowded state of the Metropolitan infirmaries; and that the Jones' homes are practically the only places where the requisite accommodation is provided at a price which the Guardians are prepared to pay.[51]

Compounding the problem, from 1901 consumptives were no longer admitted to St. Andrew's Convalescent Home in Folkestone which had treated about 100 such patients annually, mostly from urban Unions.

---

[48] Letter from L. D. Brockman, clerk to SUDC to LGB, 6th February, 1900, LGB correspondence, MH 12/5051

[49] Letter from H. J. Parsons to SUDC, 19th February, 1900, LGB correspondence, MH 12/5051

[50] *Truth*, 9th February, 9th March, 18th May, 1st June, 8th June, 15th June, 24th August, 1899, 11th January, 1st March, 15th March, 5th April, 19th April, 10th May, 12th July, 18th October, 8th November, 22nd November, 1900, 7th March, 20th June, 7th November, 1901, 1st May, 4th December, 1902, 1st January, 9th January, 5th February, 1903

[51] *Truth,* 7th November, 1901

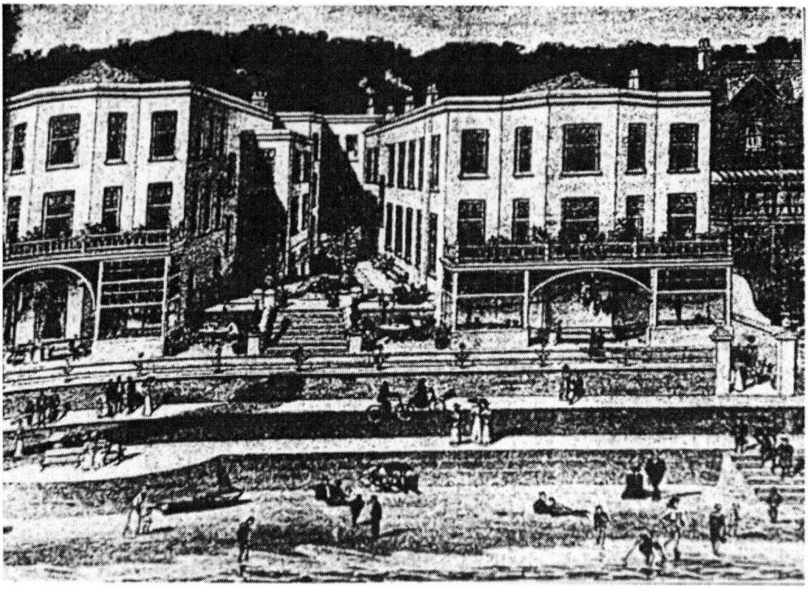

Illustration 9.5: A copy of a sketch of Grosvenor House Sanatorium, Sandgate taken from a letterhead of the Seaside Convalescent Homes and Hospitals, Sandgate, November 1899.

By 1902 Jones was circulating leaflets to Boards of Guardians throughout the country entitled *Particulars of the Homes for the open-air treatment of Consumption and other Diseases of the Chest.* These stated:

> In consequence of our having recently visited 23 sanatoria for consumptive patients on the continent, including those at Nordrach (Germany), Davos Platz and Leysin (Switzerland), and the improvements now being carried out to make our treatment, &c., as near as possible similar to the methods adopted on the continent we have decided to make our places known as Sanatoria instead of Seaside Homes.[52]

Having 126 beds in five properties in the centre of Sandgate used exclusively for the treatment of consumptive patients, Jones was now predominantly receiving cases from workhouse infirmaries and operating as a private entrepreneur. As such he attracted more scrutiny; specifically criticism relating to the lack of suitable grounds for the exercise of

[52] *The Lancet*, 22nd August, 1903

patients, and the lack of supervision by a resident doctor. Jones himself was not medically qualified, and Dr. Chubb had resigned his position in about 1901. More responsibility for Jones' patients fell on Dr. Perry, Medical Officer of Health for the town, and in 1900 the Urban District Council was forced to apply to the LGB to increase his salary due to his growing duties at the Homes. Perry was subsequently granted an extra £15 a year.[53]

As well as receiving pauper patients from urban Unions, private consumptive patients were also treated at Sandgate; first class patients were charged 35 shillings, and 45 shillings with a private bedroom, second class 25 shillings or 33 shillings, and patients from workhouse infirmaries one guinea per week. As an anonymous consultant physician at Folkestone remarked to the *Lancet* correspondent:

> Mr. Jones is a very clever administrator. By taking charge of paupers for £1 1s. a week he is doing a work that many hospitals would not care to undertake.[54]

From the point of view of Boards of Guardians and the LGB Jones was providing a useful service, but 1903 proved to be a particularly bad year for Sandgate. Out of a population of 1,955, 64 deaths were recorded as against 37 births, 45 of the deaths being due to pulmonary tuberculosis. During the course of the year 897 patients known to be suffering from consumption had been treated in sanatoria in the town for periods of between three weeks and a few months. The situation received extensive exposure in the *Lancet*, which criticised the Homes for having insufficient medical supervision, exhibiting a lack of discipline, permitting diseased persons to frequent public places, and for callously making a profit from disease. "Can we afford to sanction such speculation in human misery?" the journal appealed.[55]

The sense of a potential threat posed to the health of respectable families by the introduction of the sick and destitute to seaside towns spread as the story was developed in the popular press and by medical journals. In 1904 a letter was published in the *Lancet* from Arthur J. Harries, one of the examining medical officers to the Alfred Bevan Memorial Convalescent Home in Sandgate, warning "against the dangers necessarily arising from indiscriminate contact with these unfortunate tuberculous patients and their *dejecta*", and applauding the journal for their

[53] *Sandgate Sanitary Papers 1897-1900*, LGB correspondence, NA MH 12/5051
[54] *The Lancet*, 22nd August, 1903, p.569
[55] *The Lancet, 18th* June, 1904, p.1752

advocacy of reform in a matter:

> of such serious importance not only to the ordinary inhabitants of Sandgate but to convalescents in various stages of susceptibility and to the swarms of young soldiers from the neighbouring Shorncliffe camp.[56]

The Lancet's reporter went on to suggest that:

> those who make a trade of collecting together and catering for persons suffering from pulmonary tuberculosis should be classified as carrying on an unwholesome industry... they should, like soap-boilers and guano manufacturers, be placed under certain restrictions.[57]

As Davy was aware, tuberculosis was not legally classified as an infectious disease, and there appeared to be no means of regulating the Homes other than through legislation. The local authorities found themselves powerless in the face of plummeting property values, declining seasonal trade and fears of infection.

The Sandgate (Sanitary Powers) Bill

On May 19th 1904, Sir Edward Sassoon, Member of Parliament for Hythe and Folkestone, appealed in the House of Commons for the provision of more powers for local authorities to enforce precautions which, he claimed, were considered necessary by the medical profession for public safety. The President of the LGB, Walter Long, replied that a consumptive patient posed less danger when in a Home than when not in a Home, when there were no constraints on his movements. For Long, the dangers of infection in metropolitan Boroughs, experiencing in some cases a doubling of claimants of Poor Law relief at this time of industrial depression, were apparently seen as paramount.

In the House of Lords on the following day Sassoon again drew the attention of Mr. Long to the lack of regulations to restrict the growth of "consumptive homes or so-called sanatoria" in populous districts of health resorts. Local authorities, he stated, were being forced to consider resorting to costly litigation in order to remedy "this grave evil". Tuberculosis, he claimed, was "one of the most infectious diseases that medical science had to contend against", and he requested greater parliamentary powers to combat the problem or practical advice from the

---

[56] *The Lancet* 25th June, 1904, p.1821
[57] *The Lancet*, 2nd July, 1904, p.48

Board on how to remedy the situation in the case of Sandgate.[58] Long rebuffed Sassoon's appeal, claiming that no sufficient cause for action had been shown, and stating that a district could not be protected from infection by regulations.

The LGB had no resources to implement or affect policy, its inspectorate having been reduced from the 1850s due to resistance to central interference.[59] It had for decades been chiefly occupied with mediating tensions arising between local government and property owners on the one hand and national policy and collective action on the other.[60] The Board has been described as "a byword for compromise, pragmatism and conservatism"[61] and, in the absence of any evidence that tuberculosis had increased amongst the residents of Sandgate, Long's main concern would have been to support Boards of Guardians in their attempts to restore consumptives to a state of self-sufficiency, thereby reducing pauperism.[62]

In Folkestone the situation was discussed further by municipal dignitaries, local physicians and various specialists on public health and the treatment of tuberculosis at the Congress of the Royal Institute of Public Health, which was held in the town in July 1904.[63] Subsequently a public meeting was held at Sandgate in January 1905, when it was decided by 70 votes to 11 to promote a private Bill to gain powers to license and regulate hospitals for consumption, and to provide for the compulsory notification of consumption in the town.

A Bill was introduced in the House of Lords later in the year:

> to provide for the licensing and control of hospitals for disease, for the notification of tuberculosis and to make other provisions for the health of the Sandgate urban district and for other purposes.

The object of this Bill was to prevent the establishment of sanatoria for the treatment of tuberculous patients unless a special license was granted for this purpose. *The Lancet* commented:

---

[58] Reported in *The Times*, 26th May, 1904

[59] C. Bellamy, *Administering Central-Local Relations,* 1988, p.148

[60] Ibid, p.111

[61] Ibid, p.233

[62] Ibid, p.180

[63] One of the most eminent contributors, Professor Ferdinand Hueppe of Prague, argued that research on 30,000 consumptives at a German sanatorium demonstrated that an inherited or acquired predisposition, through ill health or adverse working conditions, was a precondition to acquiring the disease. *Journal of State Medicine*, volume xii, January, 1904, p.589

> To Sandgate appertained the honour of having become the pioneer town of Great Britain …This very small community has spent £3,000 to get a special Act of Parliament which, as an example, was to prove of great benefit to all towns in general and to Folkestone in particular.[64]

In fact the Infectious Diseases Act of 1898, a seminal and controversial piece of public health legislation, had been initiated as a private and local Act,[65] and so the Sandgate Bill was viewed as possibly the precursor of another piece of social legislation; as *The Lancet* declared "this is at once a local and a national question".[66]

The situation at Sandgate would undoubtedly have contributed to calls for the regulation of hospitals for the treatment of consumption. Whilst England at the time boasted the lowest mortality rate for tuberculosis in Europe, there existed no government legislation for its control, and beliefs concerning its infectiousness were divided.[67] *The Lancet* considered that the government should prohibit the operation of such hospitals in towns:

> If in a town one out of every five inhabitants is afflicted with tuberculosis the four healthy persons are placed in a precarious position. Though the law does not require the isolation of cases of pulmonary tuberculosis, and in fact does not in any way deal with this disease, most persons would approve of regulations that would prevent the wholesale accumulation of such cases in populous centres. Public opinion and medical opinion may not approve of the compulsory notification of pulmonary tuberculosis; but regulations forbidding the creation of hospitals for the outdoor treatment of consumption in the centre of a town seem to follow naturally upon the recognition that tuberculosis is to a certain extent an infectious disease.[68]

This perspective of the problem was endorsed by the House of Lords. They did, however, add amendments to the Sandgate Bill requiring compensation to be paid to the owners of hospitals for consumption for structural alterations incurred in putting the building to some other use. The Lords also added a clause requiring compensation for disturbance of a business in the case of a licence being refused. The significance of these

---

[64] *The Lancet,* 8th June, 1907, p.1606

[65] Evidence of Prof. Henry Kenwood, MOH Stoke Newington, Minutes of Proceedings before Select Committee of the House of Lords, May 1905

[66] *The Lancet*, 13th August, 1904, p.482

[67] Report of SUDC advice from Dr. Kenwood in 1900, evidence of R. J. Fynmore, Minutes of Proceedings before Select Committee of the House of Lords, May 1905

[68] *The Lancet*, 13th August, 1904, p.482

amendments was not immediately apparent and will be discussed later in the chapter.

The passing of this Act was seen, at least by *The Lancet,* as a precedent that could prevent the wholesale, unregulated importation of consumptive paupers into health resorts by unscrupulous opportunists intent on exploiting Boards of Guardians struggling to cope with overcrowding in urban workhouses. On the other hand at least one MP was concerned that the proposed legislation could provide a license for social exclusion at health resorts. At the reading of the Bill in the House of Commons Mr. H. J. Wilson, member for Holmfirth, argued that the sick poor should not be denied the therapeutic benefits of sea air, and urged:

> the undesirability of allowing the powers granted in this case to be used as a precedent, with the results of shutting out the poorer classes from the smaller health resorts on our coast and elsewhere. All alike were entitled to the benefit of fresh air, and local authorities ought not, except under extraordinary circumstances, to be allowed to exclude sick people from their districts.[69]

But the fundamental point at issue in considering whether this legislation was warranted was to what extent tuberculosis posed a threat of infection.

The records of the House of Lords' Select Committee reviewing the Sandgate Bill reveal the evidence of a succession of experts introduced both in support of and in opposition to these proposed reforms. Marcus Yunge-Bateman, MOH for Folkestone and medical referee for the Royal Hospital for Consumption at Ventnor, considered that the health of Folkestone was directly affected by conditions in Sandgate, particularly as a consequence of schools in Sandgate being frequented by children from Folkestone. In his opinion visitors to Sandgate could not avoid contact with consumptive patients, and he had advised Folkestone Council to include the compulsory notification of tuberculosis in a parliamentary bill they planned to promote.

Adopting a contrasting position, the Council representing the Jones family quoted from Dr. Rufenacht Walters' recent book on consumption, which was generally accepted as being authoritative during the proceedings, "it is perfectly certain that under ordinary hygienic conditions the danger of infection from a *phthisis* patient is purely imaginary".[70] Dr.

---

[69] H. J. Wilson, Parliamentary Debates House of Commons, Returns of Commons, 1905, p.51, Hansard, 4th series: volume 1-199, 1886-1908, UKC library

[70] F. Rufenacht Walters, *Sanatoria for Consumptives*, 3rd edition, London: Swan Sonnesnschien, 1905

Kirkby Robinson, MOH for the East Kent district for over 30 years, accepted that this was so, but only if the proper precautions were taken.

John Huntley, the deputy chairman of Sandgate UDC, admitted that it was largely the deteriorating class of patients at Sandgate that had caused unrest amongst local residents.[71] Likewise, Dr. Alfred Gore, Medical Officer for the Sandgate Homes since September 1903, agreed that it was the appearance of the patients that provoked objections to them:

> I do not think it is the slightest menace to the health of Sandgate, the only thing I admit is that the patients are not beautiful. They are in evidence and it is very nasty to see them about.[72]

Gore claimed to have taken advice from the Folkestone Medical Society before accepting the position, and assured the Committee that the Homes were of great benefit to poor Londoners, and that a very large number of them improved.

Dr. Marcus Quarry, Medical Officer for the Lambeth Union during the past ten years, provided a perspective from the capital, where consumption was "very prevalent". A third of all deaths from consumption occurred in Poor Law infirmaries, and between 300 and 400 consumptives a year were admitted to Lambeth Infirmary; "as a rule they come to us when the hospitals have done with them, when they cannot attend to them any longer as they are hopeless".[73]

Quarry explained that, because of their need to work, the poor only attended hospital when their health was "broken down". There were tens of thousands of consumptives at large in London streets without any form of regulation. In 1904, for example, 27,451 outpatients had attended the Royal Hospital for Diseases of the Chest in the City Road.

In 1899, due to extreme overcrowding in their infirmary, the Lambeth Guardians had appointed a committee to find suitable homes in the south east. Over twenty institutions had been visited around the Kentish coast, many of which did not provide nursing, and the few that would accept consumptives were charging three guineas per week. Quarry regarded the risk of infection as "very remote", whilst conceding that "these people are not pleasant to look upon". Quarry quoted Koch, "our greatest authority",

---

[71] J. Huntley, Minutes of Proceedings before the Select Committee of the House of Lords on SUDC Sanitary Powers Bill, May, 1905

[72] A. Gore, Minutes of Proceedings before the Select Committee of the House of Lords on SUDC Sanitary Powers Bill, May, 1905, p.212

[73] M. Quarry, Minutes of Proceedings before the Select Committee of the House of Lords on SUDC Sanitary Powers Bill, May, 1905, p.236

in claiming that infection from coughing only occurred indoors, and thus would not affect the residents of Sandgate:

> sunlight rapidly kills the *bacillus* of *tubercle*…those patients [in Sandgate] are exposed to more sunlight than is possible in Lambeth, so that the risk in Sandgate is enormously less than it is in Lambeth.[74]

Despite his conviction that the risks were negligible, Quarry agreed that regulation by the LGB could help to avoid the dispatching of cases that were too far advanced, and claimed that he only selected for treatment the 8-10% of consumptive cases entering Lambeth Infirmary whom he considered had a prospect of having their disease arrested and returning to work to support their families. Quarry concluded by arguing that the patients gained real benefit from their stay in Sandgate, and that there existed no other alternative to Lambeth's overcrowded infirmary:

> There does not exist any Home or Institution for the reception of Poor Law patients of the London Unions, and the only place we have at present are these Sandgate Homes. Therefore I have no doubt in my own mind whatever that the benefit of residing at a seaside place like Sandgate is infinitely preferable for these patients to keeping them within our overcrowded infirmary.[75]

Arthur Larking had practised for eight years at Folkestone, published a book on Folkestone as a health resort for consumptives, and possessed a diploma in Public Health from Cambridge. He testified that he had always found the Jones' Homes well managed and clean with a good standard of nursing, the windows were always open and the buildings were well ventilated. Larking emphasised that the death rate at Sandgate was low, despite the recent unavoidable deaths of advanced cases at the Homes. There was, he said, only one doctor in Sandgate and not much illness, and as far as he knew there had been no increase in cases of consumption amongst residents. The Medical Officer of Shorncliffe military camp had informed him that the rate of consumption there was half that existing at other home stations.

Larking was of the opinion that consumption was engendered by inheritance as well as infection, and that the current "phthisophobia", or fear of infection, constituted a great injustice to consumptives. The

[74] Ibid, p.245

[75] M. Quarry, Minutes of Proceedings before the Select Committee of the House of Lords on SUDC Sanitary Powers Bill, May, 1905, p.242

recently instituted system of voluntary notification at Folkestone had been introduced only to identify and educate cases against infection in the home. There was, he claimed, no danger of infection in the street. Larking considered that, even if consumptives did "spit about", it had been proven that the bacteria would be rendered harmless in a few hours due to the effects of sunshine and fresh air.[76] Indeed he ventured so far as to claim that:

> I think you might flood Shorncliffe Camp and Sandgate with consumptives and if they were in the open air and under the regulations that are carried on by Mr. Jones I do not believe there would be any danger to anybody.[77]

Larking was persuaded by the claims of the Brompton Hospital for Consumption and other institutions for consumptives that hospital staff had never been infected. He asserted:

> I think it has been greatly exaggerated, the infectivity of *phthisis*, and it is calculated to cause a great injustice to consumptives in this country – to make them out as subjects worse than smallpox [sufferers] and lead them to be ostracised and persecuted.[78]

Professor William R. Smith had been president of the Royal Institute of Public Health for the past ten years, was professor of forensic medicine at Kings College, and formerly MOH for Woolwich and house physician at the Brompton Hospital for Consumption. He was also chairman of the Public Health Committee of Holborn, and vice-chairman of St. Giles Board of Guardians, thus possessing a broad experience of tuberculosis. Professor Smith felt that it would present serious problems for Boards of Guardians in London if there were no provisions for consumptives such as existed at Sandgate. He insisted, "the homes in themselves are no menace whatever".[79]

---

[76] A. E. Larking, Minutes of the Proceedings before the Select Committee of the House of Lords on SUDC Bill, May 1905, p.9

[77] Ibid, p.31

[78] A. E. Larking, Minutes of the Proceedings before the Select Committee of the House of Lords on SUDC Bill, May 1905 p.5

[79] W. R. Smith, Minutes of the Proceedings before the Select Committee of the House of Lords on SUDC Bill, May 1905, p.48

Smith referred to the tens of thousands of consumptive outpatients who visited the Brompton Hospital and Victoria Park Hospital at Hampstead each year with no adverse effects on the populations resident there, according to MOH reports from these districts.

> The conditions in Sandgate are absolutely superior to what we who live in London have to suffer from the thousands of cases which are passing through our streets[80]...I cannot conceive for the life of me why some evidence cannot be adduced of injury to the people [of Sandgate] if for these twenty years any has been produced.[81]

Had there been any infection of the troops at Shorncliffe, Smith observed, the Sandgate Urban District Council would certainly have heard from the War Office by now. This evidence again reflects contemporary medical opinion that the *tubercle bacillus* only presented a threat when not exposed to sunlight. Thus pulmonary tuberculosis was perceived as a disease transmitted from infected buildings rather than directly from person to person.

It is significant that even witnesses in support of the Bill regarded Ransome and Walters, who both argued against the interpersonal contagiousness of consumption, as being the most advanced medical authorities on the subject. Professor Henry Kenwood, for example, MOH for Stoke Newington and co-author of a book on hygiene and public health, agreed that Ransome and Walters were "the two greatest authorities on the subject".[82] From the responses of medical experts both for and against the Bill it becomes evident that medical opinion at this time continued to regard environmental factors, chiefly insanitary slum areas, as posing a greater threat for the spread of tuberculosis than did the person of the consumptive. Ventilation, space and domestic cleanliness were generally considered to be sufficient to prevent infection.

Even Charles Perry, Medical Officer of Health for Sandgate since 1879, and a witness in support of the Bill, did not seek the closure of the Jones' Homes. Whilst he was embarrassed by Sandgate's increasing notoriety, and was in favour of stricter medical supervision in the Homes, he felt that their closure would drive consumptives to exist in unhygienic

---

[80] Ibid, p.51

[81] Ibid, p.53

[82] H. Kenwood, Minutes of the Proceedings before the Select Committee of the House of Lords on SUDC Bill, May 1905, p.65

places where basic sanitary precautions were not followed.[83]

For many doctors at this time, and particularly the more mature practitioner, polluted environments - dark, damp and overcrowded courtyards and alleys – were seen as the repositories of disease rather than infected individuals. As a consequence of this perspective the disease was particularly associated with inhabitants of the poorest districts, as were programmes of disinfection and hygienic instruction. Tuberculosis was by this time generally established as a disease of the working classes and was not viewed as posing a threat of infection amongst the more educated, civilised and hygienic, or within their well-ventilated and increasingly sanitised suburbs. Nor were the tubercular regarded as infectious when under medical supervision and being made to use pocket spittoons.[84]

This evidence demonstrates that in the early twentieth century the English medical profession had, in general, not adopted a focus directed solely at the transmission of germs through interpersonal relationships. Ransome's perception of the infectivity of buildings due to contaminated dust, the expectoration of consumptives and inadequate ventilation was common at least until the 1930s. The *bacillus* was generally understood as being capable of retaining its virulence in house dust for up to six months, but was considered to be rendered harmless following exposure to light, air or water.[85] In 1920 H. Hyslop Thomson, MOH and Tuberculosis Officer for Hertfordshire, continued to stress that consumption was spread through infected housing:

> The term "contact" is now used in relation to tuberculosis, and is no doubt responsible to some extent for the mistaken views held by the public with regard to the infectious nature of the disease. Further, the term is misleading as it conveys the impression of infection by personal contact with the patient, whereas the chief danger lies in house or dust infection, and individuals may be, and frequently are, attacked by *tubercle bacilli* who have never been in actual contact with any case of the disease.[86]

---

[83] C. E. Perry, Minutes of the Proceedings before the Select Committee of the House of Lords on SUDC Bill, 18th May, 1905, p.10

[84] J. Tyndall, *New Fragments,* London: Longmans, 1892, p.416; H. T. Bulstrode, *Report on Sanatoria for Consumption*, 1905-6, p.56

[85] J. Tyndall, *New Fragments*, London: Longmans, 1892; Georg Cornet, *The Diffusion of Tubercle Bacilli Exterior to the Body*, 1888; M. Worboys, Was There a Bacteriological Revolution in Late Nineteenth Century Britain?, *Studies in History, Philosophy, Biology & Biomedical Science,* 38, 2007, pp. 20–42

[86] H. H. Thomson, *Tuberculosis and Public Health*, Longmans: London, 1920, pp. 14-15

As a consequence of this focus on the dangers attached to dust, germ theory came to be grafted onto pre-existing conceptions of *miasma* and filth as constituting the source of disease. Koch's discovery of the *tubercle bacillus* did not lead to a medical revolution, but rather germ theory was adopted syncretically, adapting to contemporary medical theories rather than initiating "a series of conflicts between incommensurable paradigms".[87] Ransome, in company with a majority of the English medical profession at the time, did not view transmission of the disease directly from person to person as a threat and attempted to allay fears of the possibility of direct contagion: "I believe that in temperate climates direct infection from patients is one of the rarest events".[88]

Dr. Alfred Hillier, visiting physician to the London open-air sanatorium, and co-author with Robert Koch of *The Prevention of Consumption*, published in 1903, was also convinced that houses constituted the main source of infection. The prevalence of this perspective and the widespread belief in the disinfecting properties of fresh air and sunlight suggests the persistence of ideas underlying Chadwickian sanitary science that focused on the eradication of sources of infection from the physical environment.

This body of evidence surrounding the Sandgate Bill and the Select Committees' discussion of the epidemiology of tuberculosis is significant in that it demonstrates that medical experts consistently argued that the problem of tuberculosis be confronted through the reform of working class housing. This advice was rejected by successive administrations in favour of a focus on isolation, public education, and conformity to an infection model of disease control.

This view of the environmental reform of working class districts as constituting the most effective means of reducing cases of tuberculosis, together with improving the resistance of individuals to the disease, continued to be advocated by the medical profession in England until the major housing reforms of the 1930s. In 1921 John Robertson, MOH for Birmingham, observed that such reforms were still sadly lacking:

---

[87] M. Worboys, Spreading Germs, *Medical Innovations in Historical Perspective*, ed. J. V. Pickstone, 1992, p.109; an account of how germ theory adapted to fit popular miasmatic models of infection in the United States is given in Nancy Tomes, *The Private Side of Public Health: Sanitary Science, Domestic Hygiene and Germ Theory 1870-1900, Bulletin of the History of Medicine*, volume 64, 1990

[88] A. Ransome, Consumption, A 'Filth Disease', 1898, p.16

> I am more convinced than ever that the way of improving the health and morality of the people is to give the great mass of them living in our large towns decent conditions of housing. This has never yet been attempted for the old parts of any of our towns.[89]

It is evident from a review of the six days of deliberations in the House of Lords, as well as the further two days in the Commons, that the aetiology of tuberculosis was disputed by the experts. However, the majority of them, even at this early date, and the two key works referred to during the proceedings, viewed insanitary environments as the chief danger, being of the opinion that consumptives did not pose a serious danger to others, but that tuberculosis was engendered in, and spread due to dark, inadequately ventilated, overcrowded and insanitary housing.[90]

During the debate at the House of Lords the evidence of experts, who were described by *The Lancet* as having been introduced by the LGB, ensured that the Jones' Homes were not summarily closed and would for some time remain as a valuable resource both for the Board and for urban Guardians.[91]

Although the Bill was passed, permitting the Homes to be regulated by the SUDC, they could not be closed without the payment of substantial compensation. Following lengthy debate it was decided that a system of licences would be initiated. Licences would only be issued for the management of sanatoria if regulations drawn up by the SUDC and approved by the LGB were met. However, if licences were refused the Homes could not be closed without the payment of compensation, and neither could they be bought out by the Council unless this was with the mutual consent of both parties.

After the passing of the Act it became apparent that, should any of the Homes be refused a licence for the treatment of consumptives, they were perfectly at liberty to accept "convalescents", a class of patient not treated under the Act. As *The Lancet* correspondent observed:

> The object of not a few property owners is to get rid of the homes altogether, and this because of their pauper inmates. The allegation that many of the paupers are dangerous neighbours, because they might spit in the streets and spread tuberculosis, was utilised as a strong argument against the homes. Nevertheless, if no more tuberculous patients were received at the homes the fact that some 200 paupers…are crowded

---

[89] J. Robertson, *Journal of the Royal Sanitary Institute*, volume xli, no.4, March, 1921

[90] A. Ransome, Consumption, 1898, p.14

[91] *The Lancet*, 29th June, 1907, p.1808

together in a small town of less than 2,000 inhabitants is their principal grievance.[92]

The LGB was concerned that if applied generally the Act may have resulted in the abolition of at least half of the establishments used to treat working class tuberculous patients in the country. Accordingly they delayed the sanctioning of regulations drawn up by the Council to the point where there would have been insufficient time to assess applications for licensing the Homes before the deadline for licences to be issued. Consequently the applications could not be refused by the Council without the payment of substantial compensation, and thus licences for five sanatoria for the treatment of consumption were issued from March 1st, 1906 to March 1st, 1907.[93]

The 26 year old Percy Harold Jones, who had taken over the management of the sanatoria in 1903, following the death of his father in March of that year, now took advantage of the situation by sending letters to Boards of Guardians throughout the country implying that they had received the sanction of the local authority:

> Our Sanatoria for Consumptives are now licensed by the Local Sanitary Authority, under Act of Parliament 5, Edw. 7th, xxx., Ch. Clxxxvii., and are also subject to inspection by the Medical Officer of Health for Sandgate…We believe that our homes are the only establishments of the kind which have been licensed by a local authority under an Act of Parliament.[94]

An attempt was then made by the clerk of the Sandgate Council, L. D. Brockman, who had been responsible for guiding the Act through Parliament, to persuade the Council to buy out the sanatoria in order to restore the town's reputation as an elite health resort:

> When once the stigma of Sandgate as a colony for consumptive patients is removed there is no reason why the value of properties [which had been reduced by more than 50%] should not increase…I know, and I may well tell you, that until you make it impossible for any such establishments…to exist in Sandgate the place will be avoided as if it were plague-stricken by the class of visitor whom you desire to attract to the town.[95]

---

[92] *The Lancet*, June 29th, 1907, p.1808
[93] Ibid, p.1809
[94] *The Lancet,* June 29th, 1907, p.1809
[95] Ibid, p.1808

The offer to purchase of £12,000 made in January 1906 was refused and Brockman, claiming that the Council lacked the courage of their convictions in not withholding the licences, was forced to resign. Brockman blamed "the political and partisan constitution of the Local Government Board" for the "departmentally stifled law".[96] And in fact the LGB had succeeded in maintaining the Sandgate Homes as a resource for overcrowded London Unions. The real beneficiaries were the Boards of Guardians of London's East End and the impoverished consumptives of those districts who were subsequently able to continue resorting to Sandgate, despite the reactionary political constitution of Sandgate and Folkestone's local authorities.

By 1907 the Sandgate Urban District Council finally got its regulations for the licensing of hospitals for consumption sanctioned by the LGB, the regulations now being such that the management of the Homes was quite able to conform to them, and thus avoid risk of closure. Five sanatoria were now licensed to accommodate a total of 123 consumptives.

On January 10th, 1914 Sandgate Council eventually received the sanction of the LGB to purchase the sanatoria, and for a loan of £9,500 to be repaid over a period of 60 years. The delay of eight years, which must have affected the economic fortunes of Sandgate considerably, would appear to have been engineered by the LGB in order to assure the provision of treatment and accommodation for urban working class consumptives until alternative sanatoria were available. In fact the sanction for the purchase of the Homes was not granted by the LGB until Jones had acquired a 265 acre site about fifteen miles distant at Bockhanger, near Ashford, on which he had erected two pavilions to accommodate 200 consumptives. The Jones' enterprise was further facilitated by an agreement to rent five sanatoria from the Sandgate Council at a cost of £465 annually until March 31st, 1915, presumably to facilitate the transition of patients and equipment from one establishment to the other.[97]

The Sandgate Bill was one of the first instances when the infectiousness of pulmonary tuberculosis had been debated in Parliament. Although there existed a popular fear of infection from the tubercular at the turn of the century amongst the educated classes, and particularly a deep-seated and complex fear of contagion from the *social residuum,* tuberculosis experts in England largely resisted an unqualified view of the disease as infectious. The expert testimony presented to parliamentary

---

[96] *The Lancet,* 13th July, 1907, p.111

[97] Minutes of SUDC 1914-17, EKAC, Ud/Sg/AM1/15

committees debating the Sandgate Bill downplayed the dangers of infection, reflecting the general opinion of the English medical profession in the early twentieth century that the *tubercle bacillus* only posed a danger of infection in dark, dusty, poorly ventilated and overcrowded conditions.

Pulmonary tuberculosis was not generally perceived as a disease transmitted by the spread of germs directly from one person to another through talking or being otherwise in close proximity. Consumptive patients were transported to convalescent homes in Folkestone and Sandgate from London and beyond by train at concessionary rates on a regular basis, being sent and received by doctors.[98] And, in contrast to the emotive response to the presence of consumptives in Sandgate, Folkestone Borough Council actively promoted itself as a health resort particularly suitable for the treatment of tuberculosis. It also regularly invested in advertising its climatological advantages and facilities for the tubercular invalid. In 1905 as much as £25 per week was invested in advertising,[99] and as late as 1919 health guides were promoting Folkestone as a town where open-air cures for consumption could be carried out unsupervised and throughout the winter.[100]

An exclusive concern with the threat posed by consumptive paupers in Sandgate, together with a continued interest in attracting affluent consumptives to the town, suggests that residents' anxieties were more complex and deeply rooted than can be explained by a fear of infection. The dismissal by public health professionals of the dangers of infection was unlikely to have been voiced merely in order, as has been suggested,[101] to allay panic amongst the general population. As one expert indicated, due to the proximity of the Shorncliffe barracks to Jones' sanatoria, the War Office would have had no compunction in insisting on precautionary measures if infection had been understood as posing a danger.

In conclusion, it must be acknowledged that it was the presence of paupers in Sandgate rather than a fear of infection that precipitated the outcry against the Jones' Homes. There is little evidence of public or

---

[98] *Particulars of Beach Rocks Convalescent Home*, London Samaritan Society, 1894; Minutes of Committee of St Andrew's Convalescent Home, D/EX1675/14/1/1

[99] Folkestone Borough Council Minutes of Special Committees, p.56, Fo/AMc 23/1

[100] T. D. Luke, *Spas and Health Resorts of the British Isles*, A&C Black: London, 1919; Neville Wood, *Health Resorts of the British Isles*, 1919

[101] A. Hardy, *The Epidemic Streets*, 1993, pp.258-263

professional concern over the behaviour of consumptives at Folkestone. Patients from St. Andrew's Convalescent Home were permitted to walk around Folkestone due to their grounds being very limited. However, the nuns' admissions criteria were more restrictive and discipline more rigid. And, perhaps most importantly for the public perception of their convalescent home, despite having little more medical supervision than Jones' sanatoria, St. Andrews was managed and run by a religious community rather than by a private entrepreneur.

The Parliamentary records relating to the Sandgate Bill suggest that from the late 1890s an emphasis on restoring the health of the tubercular was adopted by some Poor Law Unions. Following the 1894 reforms abolishing property owning as a qualification for membership of Boards of Guardians, and the subsequent representation of men and women with a more reformist ideology,[102] attempts were made by Boards of Guardians in some London boroughs and industrial northern towns to provide working class consumptives with some form of open-air therapy and an improved diet.

Institutions that admitted consumptives existed in most coastal towns in the south-east of England[103] to which some Boards of Guardians and Friendly Societies had been sending cases of tuberculosis since the mid-1880s. Although many were ostensibly convalescent homes and not subject to certification or inspection by the LGB,[104] institutions such as those at Sandgate were regularly utilised by the more progressive urban Unions who were convinced of the benefits of fresh air for the tubercular.

[102] G. Slater, *Poverty and the State,* 1930, p.165

[103] W. R. Smith, SUDC Bill, House of Lords, 17th May 1905, p.53; L.D. Brockman, ibid. 17th May, p.27

[104] J. S. Davy, Head of Poor Law Division, Royal Commission on the Poor Laws, 1909, appendix volume i, 19th February, 1906, Cd. 4625, 3808

PART III:

EARLY SANATORIUM TREATMENT

CHAPTER TEN

TUBERCULOSIS AND THE BEGINNING OF A STATE HEALTH SYSTEM: THE NATIONAL INSURANCE ACT, 1911

Although the Sandgate Bill was essentially an attempt to resolve a conflict between local and central interests, much of its significance lies in the fact that it drew attention to the extent of pulmonary tuberculosis, particularly in certain London Poor Law Unions. Through the evidence of medical experts it identified a need for the open-air treatment of destitute consumptives, both in the hope of restoring them to an employable condition and in order to relieve overcrowding in urban infirmaries.

The Sandgate controversy also served to highlight the scarcity of institutions where the lower classes could be treated in the open-air and heralded the end of an era of largely unregulated institutional treatment for destitute consumptives. As tuberculosis had been identified as a major cause of destitution it was to become central to plans for the development of health insurance schemes by both workers' organisations and the government.

This chapter identifies the factors that determined this unprecedented expansion of public health structures in Britain during the early twentieth century. It also examines the political and ideological arguments surrounding the introduction of sanatorium treatment for the working classes and the beginnings of a more integrated conception of the health of society.

As described in the previous chapter, and as acknowledged in the Report on the Royal Commission on the Poor Laws, an ideological movement away from the Poor Law principle of deterrence was under way in some urban centres in the first decade of the twentieth century.[1] At the same time, as was also noted in the Report, there existed "an extraordinary

[1] T. D. A. Cockerell, Municipal Activity in Britain, *American Journal of Sociology*, volume ii, no.6, May, 1906; Report of RCPL, Cd.4499, 1906, p.1004

variation in Poor Law administration in different districts",[2] and the LGB had completely failed to secure any national uniformity of provision for the destitute between local authorities.[3]

Although in some urban Unions tubercular patients received a better standard of care, spending a few weeks in one of a handful of specialised institutions, such as the Brompton Hospital for Consumption, or in convalescent homes, others were parsimonious or corrupt and medical supervision was minimal. Also, particularly in rural districts, consumptives were, as described in chapter seven, left to subsist at home on a meagre supplement of groceries and coal provided by charities or the Poor Law or, more commonly, were supported by relatives, neighbours or friends.[4]

At this time of high unemployment and widespread poverty it was becoming increasingly apparent that existing charitable and local authority resources were inadequate for coping with the related issues of poverty and sickness. The destitute and consumptive were widely evident in the slums of towns and cities, in workhouse infirmaries and tramping the countryside.[5]

Due to the difficulties of diagnosing tuberculosis until the advanced stage of the disease and the reluctance or financial inability of sufferers to consult doctors whilst they were still able to work, estimates of the number of people suffering from the disease varied widely. In 1897 the number of consumptives in Britain was conservatively estimated at not less than 200,000. Only 1,160 beds were then available in hospitals for consumption and sanatoria, a meagre resource of one bed for every 200 cases.[6] However, in 1909 the number of people suffering from the active form of the disease in England alone was assessed as being 500,000 with only 1,500 beds being affordable to "moderately thrifty workers" and less than 500 beds provided free of charge.[7] This anomaly in gauging the extent of tuberculosis may, however, be accounted for by the introduction of compulsory notification for cases of pulmonary tuberculosis under the care of the Poor Law or the Asylums Board from 1908.

Of prime concern for twentieth century administrations was the fact that tuberculosis predominantly affected the youth of the nation; young

---

[2] Report of RCPL, Cd.4499, 1906, p.1013

[3] Ibid, p.993

[4] Report of R.C.P.L., 1906, volume xlii, p.92

[5] V. Bonham, *A Joyous Service – The Clewer Sisters and their Work,* 1989

[6] J. A. Lindsay, The Problem of the Consumptive Poor, *The Lancet*, 4th December, 1897, p. 1435

[7] A. Latham & C. H. Garland, *The Conquest of Consumption*, London: T. Fisher Unwin, 1911, p.52

parents and workers. In 1898 consumption was reported as being the cause of more than one third of deaths occurring between the ages of fifteen and 45 and nearly half of all annual deaths between the ages of fifteen and 35.[8] Increasingly it was coming to be viewed by politicians as a threat to the economic health of the nation and a barrier to achieving "national efficiency". Apart from disabling wage earners and young mothers tuberculosis was an enormous drain on charities and the Poor Law.

In 1911 John Burns, President of the LGB, stated that one third of deaths from consumption in London occurred in Poor Law infirmaries and that 30-50% of the cost of pauperism was attributable to sickness, of which consumption was the chief factor.[9] And in the same year Dr Christopher Addison, MP for Hoxton, Shoreditch, claimed:

> I believe about a million and a half annually of Poor Law expenditure goes on persons suffering from tuberculosis. If we can prevent the spread of tuberculosis amongst the people who are to be insured we should prevent them coming within the ambit of the Poor Law, and in that way we should indirectly, but none the less effectually, be reducing the burden upon the Poor Law with regard to this disease.[10]

Addison was one of the architects of the state tuberculosis scheme which was largely modelled on the German system of sanatorium treatment. In contrast to the parsimonious and *ad hoc* provision of the Poor Law and local charitable organisations, Germany's massive state investment in public sanatoria and national insurance appeared to represent a model of social and economic efficiency. Compulsory insurance had been introduced in Germany in July 1889 for workers whose income did not exceed £100 per year. This so-called "economic cure", it was claimed, saved the nation about £1,000,000 annually by 1900, both through the prevention of chronic invalidism and by restoring the tubercular to work, even if only for a few years.[11]

Sanatoria were seen as a crucial adjunct to this national insurance system. Pensions paid to chronic tuberculosis sufferers created an insupportable drain on the insurance fund, and the prime function of the sanatorium was to treat selected cases in an early stage of the disease so

---

[8] C. E. Fitzgerald, The Prevention of Tuberculosis, 1898, p.933

[9] J. Burns, *Transactions of the NAPT*, Annual Conference, Caxton Hall, Westminster, July 19-21, 1911, London: Adlard & Son, p.25, p.28

[10] Dr. C. Addison, House of Commons debate, 12th July 1911, Hansard volume 28, cc398

[11] M. Smith, The Renewal of the Sandgate Sanatoriums Scandal, *The Lancet*, June 18th, 1904, p. 1752

that they could be returned to work. It was claimed at the International Congress of Hygiene at Brussels in 1899 that German sanatoria permanently restored 7,000 workers to their occupations annually and prolonged the working capacity of another 20,000 for at least two years.[12]

In 1904 *The Lancet* questioned whether the claimed "extinction of pauperism" in Germany, as a consequence of the insurance system, had not achieved more in reducing tuberculosis than the provision of sanatoria.[13] This focus on poverty as a cause of ill health was, however, seen as politically radical. The German insurance scheme was conceived as a means of reducing chronic sickness in order to maximise productivity.

Whilst disease was understood as being a cause of poverty, the disproportionate incidence of disease amongst the working classes was, in both Britain and Germany before 1914, more generally ascribed to their immorality or ignorance than to economic hardship. Poverty and unemployment, predominantly seen by theorists and policy makers before the First World War as being due to the failings of the workforce or the temporary result of fluctuating trade cycles,[14] were seldom acknowledged as being a direct cause of disease at this time.[15]

Despite the conclusions of the 1904 Report on Physical Deterioration that the health of the working classes had deteriorated to such an extent that it posed a threat to the security of the nation that could only be averted by legislation, Balfour's Conservative government was opposed to any expenditure designed to improve the living conditions of the working classes.[16] Although this administration did initiate a Royal Commission on the overburdened and inefficient Poor Laws before resigning in 1905, their failure to respond to calls from elements of the medical profession and other middle class reformist groups, such as the Fabians, for major administrative and social reform provided an opportunity for the Liberals to assume the initiative. In 1906 they were overwhelmingly elected on the promise of improving conditions for the working classes.

Campbell-Bannerman and Asquith's administrations launched a series

---

[12] M. Smith, The Renewal of the Sandgate Sanatoriums Scandal, *The Lancet*, June 18th, 1904, p. 1752

[13] Ibid.

[14] G. Sutherland, Social Policy in the Inter-War Years, *Historical Journal*, volume 16, no.2, June, 1973, p.426

[15] J. M. Eyler, Poverty, Disease, Responsibility: Arthur Newsholme and the Public Health Dilemmas of British Liberalism, *The Millbank Quarterly*, volume 67, Supplement 1, 1989, pp.113-116

[16] B. B. Gilbert, Health and Politics: The British Physical Deterioration Report of 1904, *Bulletin of the History of Medicine*, 39, 1965 p.150

of Acts designed to, or at least designed to appear to, protect the health of the most vulnerable members of society, the previously neglected mothers, children and the elderly, and to ensure the improved economic efficiency of the nation. The Liberal Party could not be said to have an organised programme of social reform, but rather responded to a growing awareness of social problems.[17]

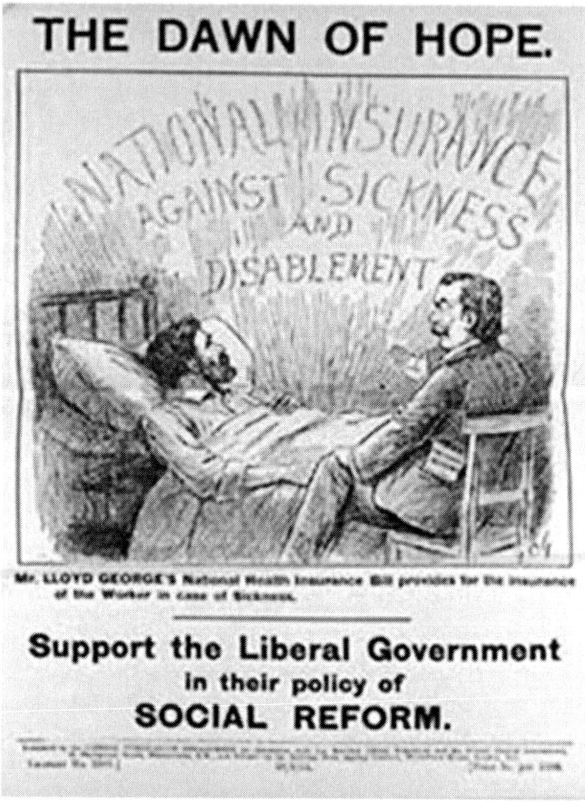
THE DAWN OF HOPE.
NATIONAL INSURANCE
AGAINST SICKNESS
AND
DISABLEMENT
Support the Liberal Government
in their policy of
SOCIAL REFORM.

Illustration 10.1: Cover of a pamphlet published by the Liberal Party in June, 1911 to promote the National Insurance Bill.

---

[17] B. B. Gilbert, David Lloyd George: Land, The Budget and Social Reform, *The American Historical Review*, volume 81, no.5, December, 1976, p.1061; G. R. Searle, *The Liberal Party: Triumph and Disintegration,* London: MacMillan, 1992, pp. 108-110.

Asquith and Lloyd George, as well as reacting to calls for "national efficiency" and the amelioration of social problems that threatened the health of the nation, also felt the need to accommodate at least some of the aspirations of working class voters.[18] Whilst party politics were not strictly divided along lines of class at this time, the Labour party not being a serious political force until 1920,[19] the New Liberals deliberately courted working class votes from 1906.[20]

Although the popular association of state intervention with the imposition of the unpopular 1834 Poor Law reforms made many workers suspicious of government reforms, Lloyd George had identified the lack of provision for the chronically sick and their families as an issue that the Party could address in order to garner support from the working classes.

As Asquith's Chancellor of the Exchequer he repeatedly promised that the Liberals would assist the thousands who were suffering financial distress through "ill health, premature breakdown or death of the breadwinner", by the introduction of a disability pension.[21] These plans were, however, frustrated by the continued resistance of the House of Lords to the passage of the socially redistributive budget of 1909. This led to a financial crisis for the government in the following year that necessitated two general elections.

The Liberals were also intent on relieving the Poor Law system of the large financial drain caused by tuberculosis and were attracted to the German system of workers' insurance. When Timbrell Bulstrode's Report on Sanatoria, commissioned by the Local Government Board, was published in 1905-06 it promised to extend the working lives of thousands of consumptives, to relieve the cost on the Poor Rates of treating them, as well as to ease the congestion in infirmaries and hospitals for the disease.

Bulstrode's attitude towards the management of those afflicted with tuberculosis, reflecting the perceptions of many English middle class professionals at this time, was influenced by a eugenic ideal of biological advancement as well as by a belief in the efficacy of sanatorium treatment.

---

[18] G. R. Searle, *The Liberal Party,* 1992, pp. 108-110; K. Laybourn, *Modern Britain Since 1906,* London: Taurus, 1999, p.12

[19] P. Williamson, The Conservative Party 1900-1939: From Crisis to Ascendancy in *A Companion to Early Twentieth-century Britain,* ed. C. Wrigley , Oxford University Press, 2003, p.3

[20] P. Clarke, *Lancashire and the New Liberals,* Cambridge University Press, 1971; M. Bentley, The Liberal Party 1900-1939: Summit and Descent, *A Comparison to Early Twentieth-century Britain,* ed. C. Wrigley, Oxford University Press, 2003, pp.28-9

[21] B. B. Gilbert, David Lloyd George, 1976, p.1061

He felt that the adoption of something similar to the German model could provide a system of control of the tubercular that would greatly benefit society:

> Were there in operation in this country some great social organisation such as the Compulsory Insurance System in Germany there would by this fact alone be set up a machinery having such an intimate touch with the industrial wage earner that the selection of early cases, the continued observation of cases discharged from sanatoria, and the provision of suitable employment would be enormously facilitated.[22]

He did not accept that tuberculosis was, considering its prevalence, "in any degree personally communicable",[23] and argued that the slow national decrease in the incidence of the disease had not improved in towns such as Brighton, Manchester and Sheffield where consumptives had been isolated in institutions.[24] He was also concerned that notions of the contagiousness of the disease would result in "the weakening of family ties, loss of employment, and the creation of a leper class".[25]

Bulstrode was of the opinion that heredity was the predominant factor in contracting consumption and was known to have been influenced by the eugenicist Karl Pearson,[26] Professor of Eugenics at the Galton Institute from 1911-1933, who argued that inferior stock should not be permitted to reproduce.[27] Whilst accepting the effectiveness of open-air treatment for the tubercular, Bulstrode believed that their reproduction would be detrimental to the national stock. Although he proposed treatment in sanatoria as a means of restoring consumptives to working capacity Bulstrode was convinced that the marriage of "tuberculous stock" would be detrimental to the future health of society.[28]

This conviction undoubtedly influenced his decision to emphasise the necessity for containment, isolation and the continued supervision of consumptives, the majority of whom were then in an advanced condition of the disease, as being of greater importance than therapy.[29] It seems

---

[22] H. T. Bulstrode, *Report on Sanatoria for Consumption*, 1905-6, p.236
[23] Ibid, p.56
[24] Ibid, p.62
[25] H. T. Bulstrode, On the Causes, Prevalence and Control of Pulmonary Tuberculosis, *The Lancet*, 1903, ii, pp. 76, 206, 304-5
[26] D. Watkins, *The English Revolution in Scientific Medicine*, 1984, p. 223
[27] K. Pearson, *A First Study of the Statistics of Pulmonary Tuberculosis*, London: Dulau & Co., 1907; *Second Study etc,* 1908
[28] H. T. Bulstrode, *Report on Sanatoria for Consumption,* 1905-6, p.55
[29] Ibid, p.5

evident that Bulstrode considered the containment and supervision of consumptives to be of importance not in order to prevent infection, although he did acknowledge that there existed a slight danger of infection from advanced cases, but rather to restrict the possibility of the disease being transmitted to future generations.

At the same time as Bulstrode was compiling his report on sanatoria a Royal Commission was considering a reform of the Poor Law system that had become overburdened with the chronically sick and those perceived as unemployable. These were individuals categorised as epileptic, "feeble-minded" and the tubercular, sections of the population that workhouse infirmaries were poorly equipped to cope with. However, as no consensus was achieved, two conflicting reports were eventually published.

The proposals of the Minority Report authored by Beatrice and Sidney Webb and supported by the SMOH were based on the conviction that much disease, and particularly tuberculosis, would be preventable if programmes of hygienic instruction and moral reform directed at the working classes were implemented. Although, like the COS, the Webbs were concerned to maintain social and economic control of working class behaviour, they saw the Poor Law system as fundamentally incompatible with the bacteriologically informed principles of preventive medicine promulgated by the SMOH. They favoured an interventionist public health approach which they saw as capable of producing results through the inculcation of "better habits of life", in contrast to the palliative "bottle of physic" dispensed by the Poor Law Medical Officer.[30] These proposals for the dissolution of the Poor Law system were supported by the Labour movement who were concerned to eradicate the stigmatisation associated with parish relief and the workhouse.[31]

Beatrice Webb's arguments for controlling the spread of tuberculosis emphasised the importance of morality – the avoidance of alcohol and sexual promiscuity - and both herself and Arthur Newsholme, by 1908 promoted to Chief Medical Officer of the Local Government Board, maintained that it was possible and necessary to reform the behaviour of the working classes. They believed that a community health service, directed at the community rather than the individual, was capable of instilling a sense of social responsibility and, in the case of tuberculosis in particular, a sense of duty and obligation to one's family and to the wider community. Newsholme, reflecting the zealous Methodism of his

---

[30] J. M. Eyler, *Sir Arthur Newsholme and State Medicine 1885-1935*, Cambridge University Press, 1997, p.209

[31] G. Sutherland, Social Policy in the Inter-War Years, *Historical Journal*, volume 16, no.2, June, 1973, p.425

upbringing, stressed that sacrifices would be demanded in this new era of "social evolution", and that a "new standard of physical self-control" would be expected of society.[32]

The ideology underpinning the Majority Report was fundamentally that of the COS. They were convinced that there existed a section of the population who were morally unfit and irredeemable, and that charity undermined the moral development of the poorer classes by discouraging them from work and thrift.[33] By voting to retain the treatment of consumption under the Poor Law Sidney Webb argued that the Majority Report was electing "to thus exclude the disease in England from the sphere of Public Health".[34]

The proposal of labour colonies for the unemployed contained in the Webbs' Minority Report does, however, indicate that the management of a *residuum* of the idle, irresponsible and degenerate was, at least in part, the object of all strands of opinion in the early English public health movement.[35] Practically all contributors to the Royal Commission on the Poor Laws, including the COS and the Webbs, considered that there existed an underclass that was unemployable, irredeemable and in need of institutionalisation of one form or another.[36] The groups targeted for isolation in colonies, labour camps and other institutions were the mentally ill, the epileptic, the disabled, the tubercular and the chronically unemployed.

In the first decades of the twentieth century eugenic arguments influenced the thinking of many Fabians, socialists and left wing New Liberals. Indeed Karl Pearson styled himself a socialist, championing eugenics as a rational programme designed to achieve the greatest potential for society. Signatories to the Majority Report of the Poor Law Commission, of whom six were members of the Charity Organisation Society, also displayed a social evolutionist approach to problems of

---

[32] Minority Report, Part I, p.282; J. M. Eyler, *Sir Arthur Newsholme,* 1997, pp.205-207

[33] G. Jones, *Social Darwinism and English Thought*, Brighton: Harvester Press, 1980, p.52

[34] S. Webb, *Public Health*, 23, 1909-10, 65, quoted in J. M. Eyler, *Sir Arthur Newsholme,* 1997, p.211

[35] D. Porter, Enemies of the Race: Biologism, Environmentalism & Public Health, in Edwardian England, *Victorian Studies*, 34:2, 1991; J. M. Winter, Public Health and the Political Economy of War, 1914-18*, History Workshop*, 26, 1988; G. Himmelfarb, *The Idea of Poverty: England in the early industrial age*, New York: Random House, 1985

[36] J. Harris, *Private Lives and Public Spirit: Britain 1870-1914*, London: Penguin, 1993; G. Sutherland, Social Policy in the Inter-War Years, 1973, p.426

health and poverty. They viewed the Poor Law as subsidising the reproduction of the "lowest social types", and recommended their detention and segregation. In fact it was clearly the aim of various upper middle class associations, including the Moral Education League, the Society for the Care of the Feeble Minded and the Eugenics Education Society, to eradicate the *residuum* – a proposal supported by H. G. Wells, Sir James Barr and others - through compulsory segregation in labour colonies and workhouses.[37]

The Minority Report's proposals for disbanding the Poor Law and instituting a universal system of behavioural and environmental reform were not, however, implemented. It has been argued that the Liberals had no intention of reforming the Poor Law. That John Burns, supported by the bureaucratic inertia of the LGB, of which he was President until 1914, and with Asquith's approval, was instrumental in frustrating the passage of the Minority Report proposals, which he felt were too radical. And that Lloyd George's decision to opt for national health insurance and the provision of public sanatoria had been signalled by his visit to Germany in 1908.[38]

Whilst the reports on the Poor Law succeeded in highlighting the system's inadequacies in preventing and curing disease, some of Lloyd George's comments regarding his proposed alternative for the sick poor reveal the extent of his distrust and lack of sympathy for elements of the working classes at this time. These remarks imply that the future treatment of the chronically sick and destitute was, perhaps, not intended to be any less harsh than under the workhouse regime. Lloyd George was particularly concerned that the scheme should not be taken advantage of by the "malingering" poor:

> no plan which human ingenuity can devise will succeed in stamping it out...a purely state scheme would inevitably lead to unlimited shamming and deception...

He was, nevertheless, reassured that money defrauded from workers' contributions rather than the Exchequer would be policed by the Insurance Committees who regulated the scheme, and that losses would be made good through reduced benefits or increased subscriptions.[39]

---

[37] P. M. H. Mazumdar, The Eugenists and the Residuum: the Problem of the Urban Poor, *Bulletin of the History of Medicine*, volume 54, 1980

[38] J. M. Eyler, *Sir Arthur Newsholme and State Medicine 1885-1935*, Cambridge University Press, 1997, pp.225-226

[39] D. Lloyd George, *Memorandum Explanatory of National Insurance Bill,* London: HMSO, May 1911, p.15

Both reports on the Poor Laws were rejected in favour of Lloyd George's 1911 National Insurance Act. Nevertheless the expanded role of preventive medicine and public health education espoused in the Minority Report - a schema which Dorothy Porter aptly refers to as "the panoptic overseer of communal life"[40] – remains in essence the model for the treatment of chronic contagious disease today.[41] However, the Webbs, the National Campaign for the Prevention of Destitution (organised by the Fabian Society to promote the Minority Report) and the SMOH all felt that the National Insurance Act had sidelined preventive medicine, an approach to public health which, they considered, Lloyd George had not fully comprehended.

In their opinion the Act had failed to implement preventive measures due to not instituting universal treatment and by demanding compulsory contributions from low wage earners.[42] In addition, they claimed, it encouraged malingering by leaving the choice of doctor to the patient, which they felt would perpetuate the working class preference for prescription medicine over hygienic instruction.[43]

Bulstrode's recommendations, providing for the open-air treatment of tuberculosis for the working classes, were largely accepted by the government as a blueprint for sanatorium treatment. And Lloyd George's system of insurance funded by workers, employers and the government appeared to offer a solution to the burden placed on Friendly Societies, Poor Rates and urban workhouse infirmaries by destitute consumptives.

More significantly, despite health provision under the National Insurance Act being restricted to sanatorium and maternity benefits, for the first time government intervention was moving beyond preventive measures such as the removal of insanitary "nuisances" and the isolation of acute infectious diseases.

Benenden sanatorium, developed largely from the contributions of working men, was used as an example and inspiration for Lloyd George's inclusion of sanatorium treatment in the National Insurance Act. On 12th

---

[40] D. Porter, Enemies of the Race: Biologism, Environmentalism & Public Health in Edwardian England, *Victorian Studies*, 34:2, 1991, p.171

[41] G. Mooney, Public health versus private practice: The contested development of compulsory infectious disease notification in late nineteenth century Britain, *Bulletin of the History of Medicine*, 1998

[42] Report of Royal Commission on the Poor Laws 1905-9, (Minority), p, 873, quoted in B. Abel-Smith, *Hospitals*, 1964, p.228

[43] D. Watkins, *The English Revolution in Scientific Medicine*, 1984, p. 237; The Preventive Provisions of the Insurance Bill, *Public Health*, volume 25, 1911-12, pp. 41-42

July 1911, in the Committee stages of the debate for the introduction of the Bill, Lloyd George quoted statistics for the treatment of consumption at Benenden. Of 168 cases treated in the previous year it was claimed that the disease had been arrested in 48.8% of patients, improved in 36.3%, whilst 14.2% were unimproved. This, claimed the Chancellor, represented a considerable success.[44]

Lloyd George's National Insurance Act provided medical treatment by a doctor chosen by the contributor from a local panel. Those initially eligible for medical cover were the employed earning less than £160 a year and aged between sixteen and 65. The scheme was funded by contributions of four pence per week from the insured (three pence for women), three pence from the employer and two pence from the state.

Admission to hospital was not covered but sanatorium treatment, the main health provision under the Act, was available with sanatorium benefit of ten shillings a week for men and seven shillings and sixpence for women for the first thirteen weeks of sickness, subject to strict compliance with doctor's regulations. Thereafter a pension of five shillings a week was paid during sickness or disability. This disability pension was entirely inadequate, being no more than had been available under Poor Law relief,[45] and many families with breadwinners invalided through tuberculosis would have felt that Lloyd George had reneged on his promise to improve their desperate situation.[46]

The prime intention of the 1911 National Insurance Act was to extend the principle of health insurance from the estimated one third of the working classes already covered by Friendly Societies, sick clubs and Trade Unions to all employees with an income of less than £160 a year. The sanatorium benefit of one shilling and threepence per week was to be administered by approved Local Insurance Committees who were empowered to send cases of tuberculosis to any institution registered by the LGB. Newsholme estimated that there existed about 45,000 consumptives among insured patients in England and Wales in 1911, requiring the provision of at least 7,500 beds. Although about 2,000 beds could be found in private and local authority institutions this left a shortfall of about 5,500 beds for which £1.5 million was provided by the

---

44 B. McPate, *Benenden,* 2006, p.9

45 Ellie Jackson, in M. Arthur, *Lost Voices of the Edwardians,* London: Harper Collins, 2006, pp.213-4. Her experience of Poor Law relief in Folkestone relates to the period 1900-1910.

46 D. Lloyd George, *Memorandum Explanatory of National Insurance Bill,* London: HMSO, May 1911, pp.2, 5, 10; K. Laybourn, *Modern Britain Since 1906,* 1999, p.17

Treasury for the building of public sanatoria, dispensaries and institutions for advanced cases.

The National Insurance Act was soon under criticism from all shades of political opinion. Both for failing to sufficiently acknowledge the role of poor environmental conditions in the spread of tuberculosis, and for creating a culture of dependency on the state that would exacerbate the trend towards degeneracy.

James Barr, the President of the British Medical Association, felt that the race would be better improved by allowing the individual to adapt to the environment rather than the reverse. He considered, along with other prominent social commentators, doctors and biologists influenced by eugenics, that the race would more efficiently be improved through the development of a strain of city dwellers who had become resistant to the *tubercle bacillus*.[47] Individuals from the lower classes who remained susceptible to the disease should be allowed to die out and discouraged from breeding. From Barr's perspective only some form of social engineering could prevent the propagation of tuberculosis amongst future generations:

> the long, narrow, flat chest and delicate lungs, and feeble resisting power to the *tubercle bacillus*, and to many other germs, is undoubtedly inherited, just as much so as the shape of our nose or the colour of our hair. Medical men who are shutting their eyes to the truth, and encouraging matrimony and the propagation of the species by mental and physical weaklings, are incurring a fearful racial responsibility, and their action should be condemned in no uncertain language.[48]

The Act was also criticised as "ludicrously costly and cumbersome", with 25% of contributions being used in the cost of their collection.[49] Another major effect of the 1911 Insurance Act was that, by acting to discourage charitable donations and subscriptions, it heralded the demise or metamorphosis of many institutions that already provided rest and recuperation for the tubercular. Nevertheless, charitable organisations were to remain essential to the health services. This 1912 report from St. Andrews Convalescent Home illustrates the frustration felt in the voluntary sector at the time:

---

[47] A discussion of the development of resistance to tuberculosis amongst urban Europeans is included in a debate of the Sociological Society in May, 1904. Eugenics: Its Definition, Scope and Aims, *The American Journal of Sociology,* volume 10, no. 1, 1904, pp.1-25

[48] J. Barr, *BMJ*, December 30th, 1911, pp.1714-1715

[49] H. de Carle Woodcock, *The Doctor and the People,* 1912, p. 170

> This is a time of special anxiety to institutions relying on public voluntary help. The subscribing power of the nation has been crippled by legislation and other causes. The fact that the income of the King Edward VII Hospital Fund was less in 1912 by £54,000 proves this. The progressive rise in the price of provisions and all commodities necessary to the maintenance of large institutions also causes concern for the future.[50]

A further criticism of the Act was its restricted application to the problem of tuberculosis. The unemployed, casual workers and the majority of women were still not covered by health insurance, and neither were the dependants of consumptives. This failing ensured that there was little incentive for early cases to quit employment and seek treatment. In order to remedy these shortcomings and to seek further professional advice the government commissioned the Departmental Committee on Tuberculosis of 1912-13.

The Committee, comprised largely of experienced MOHs and specialists in the disease,[51] recommended that the scheme should be available to all victims of tuberculosis, whether insured or not, and that it should be administered by local and County Council authorities. The scheme was based around a system of dispensaries, the idea of Robert Philip who had initiated the first dispensary in Edinburgh in 1887. Medical practitioners would recommend patients diagnosed with, or suspected of having, tuberculosis to a local dispensary, from where they would be assigned to a hospital, sanatorium or recommended for domiciliary treatment. Lloyd George acted on these recommendations, extending sanatorium benefit to the dependants of insured patients undergoing treatment and empowering local authorities to treat the uninsured, half the cost of which was to be met by the Treasury.[52]

The Committee went on to consider specialist opinion on how best to prevent, as well as cure, the disease. Although recommending the compulsory isolation of certain advanced cases of consumption who might pose a risk to their families through inhabiting particularly overcrowded or insanitary environments, the report emphasised the importance of

---

[50] Minutes of St Andrews Convalescent Home Committee, 1912

[51] The Committee included MOHs George Newman, Arthur Newsholme, James Niven, Arthur Latham and Robert Philip, in addition to pioneer sanatorium supervisors Noel Bardswell, Marcus Paterson and Jane Walker.

[52] N. McFarlane, Hospitals, Housing and Tuberculosis in Glasgow, 1911-1951, *Social History of Medicine*, 2 (1), 1988, p.66; A. S. MacNalty, Tuberculosis Work in England, *The Lancet*, January 26th, 1924, p.166

education and supervision for the control of infection.[53] The Committee also acknowledged that consumption was a disease largely determined by social and economic factors; "an advance in material prosperity of the community as a whole will be reflected in a decreased incidence of tuberculosis".[54] It also recognised that "the well-to-do classes", although less affected by the disease, still contracted tuberculosis due to:

> constitution, habits and methods of life, the nature of an individual's occupation, and the diseases and accidents to which he may have been subjected.[55]

The Committee demonstrated the conviction of the medical profession, and particularly specialists in tuberculosis, that the disease could at least be significantly reduced by environmental reform, and recommended improved housing, town planning and garden cities, open-air schools and research into the "social and economic causes of tuberculosis". They reiterated:

> any measures which result in a general improvement in the standard and condition of life are of the greatest importance in the preventing of tuberculosis.[56]

Although the 1913 Public Health (Prevention and Treatment) Act empowered local authorities to treat the uninsured the majority of recommendations contained in the Astor Report were not acted on. Government provisions to finance the universal treatment of tuberculosis were to prove "wholly inadequate", although the war was to intervene before such shortcomings could be exposed.[57] The National Insurance Act failed to provide a coordinated public health system due, initially, to a shortage of beds, inadequate funding and, later, the war.

The construction of sanatoria was generally halted during the war, and by 1919 the majority of beds for open-air treatment were occupied by tuberculous ex-servicemen, of whom it was estimated that 58,000 had contracted active tuberculosis due to war service.[58] In addition the

---

[53] *Final Report of the Departmental Committee on Tuberculosis*, volume I, 1913, pp.7-8

[54] Ibid, p.8

[55] Ibid, p.9

[56] Ibid.

[57] N. McFarlane, Hospitals, Housing and Tuberculosis, 1988, p.66; Abel-Smith, *Hospitals*, 1964, p.281

[58] L. Bryder, *Below the Magic Mountain*, 1988, p.70

economic downturn of the early 1920s restricted the sanatorium treatment of civilian workers to a small minority of those diagnosed with consumption. In fact there was hardly any provision for their treatment until the 1920s when it is estimated that only about 2% were admitted to sanatoria.[59]

Both the expansion of the state and the organisation of labour were hastened by the War. This exceptionally communal experience led to a more interventionist approach to public life.[60] The working classes were also becoming more active in civic life. Between 1914 and 1920 the membership of Trades Unions doubled[61] and, although there had been no previous Labour Party influence on health reform, at the 1918 party conference Dr. Marion Phillips, a member of the Womens' Labour League, carried a proposal for a unified health service incorporating the Ministry of Housing and the abolition of the Poor Law.[62]

Although a Ministry of Health was established in 1919, resources remained under the control of local authorities and the work of Medical Officers continued to be inhibited by the interests of local government.[63] Despite the Labour Party gaining control of 12 London boroughs in the 1919 election, a post-war retrenchment by the Treasury and taxation, supported by business and the middle classes, resulted in the Geddes cuts of 1921-2 and a disengagement of the state in the early 1920s.[64] The short-lived Labour Government of 1924 produced John Wheatley's Housing Act in that year which provided subsidies for local authorities to build homes for the working classes. This initiative was later suspended by successive Conservative administrations.[65]

Sanatorium benefit was discontinued in 1921 under the National Health Insurance Act of 1920, and thereafter local authorities became wholly responsible for the treatment of tuberculosis. An annual £300,000 grant from the Exchequer replaced contributions from the Insurance

---

[59] F. B. Smith, *The Retreat of Tuberculosis*, 1988, p.47

[60] A. Marwick, The Deluge: British Society and the Great War, London: Bodley Head, 1965

[61] J. E. Cronin, The British State and the Structure of Political Opportunity, *Journal of British Studies*, volume 27, no.3, 1988, p.219

[62] A. Marwick, The Labour Party and the Welfare State in Britain, 1900-1948, *American History Review*, volume 73, no.2, 1967, p.389

[63] Ibid.

[64] J. E. Cronin, The British State, pp.222-3

[65] A. Marwick, The Labour Party and the Welfare State, p.393

Committees which were disbanded.[66] The National Insurance fund was in deficit by 1921, and throughout the 1920s contributions from the Treasury were reduced as successive governments refused to extend health care.[67]

State intervention in the support and treatment of the tubercular has generally been interpreted by historians as a process of social improvement due to an increased concern on the part of reformers for the health and well-being of the working classes, facilitated by advances in medical science and sociology. It was, in fact, more the result of a haphazard dynamic of political conflict and short-term economic expediency. At the beginning of the twentieth century there existed little enthusiasm for an expansion of the state's responsibilities by the working classes or the Labour movement. The re-emergence of the "social question" was more a consequence of middle class anxieties. Calls for greater control and supervision of elements of the chronically sick working classes were voiced almost exclusively by health professionals and social reformers, who were often responding to a social evolutionist agenda. As the historian J. E. Cronin has remarked:

> the expansion of the state found considerable support in the upper reaches of society, and it makes little sense to attribute its progress to the gradual enfranchisement or the growing organisational strength of the working classes.[68]

The timing of the National Insurance Act, passed in December 1911, was largely in response to strikes by miners, dockers and railwaymen brought about by a rise in the cost of living, together with a reduction in wages of about 10% between 1900 and 1910.[69] The Act transferred the cost of the tubercular from local authority rates and working contributors to Friendly Societies, to workers' insurance contributions, employers and the Treasury. It thus reduced the burden on ratepayers, being initially financed by the 1909 "peoples' budget", which was eventually passed in 1911.

---

[66] *Final Report of the Departmental Committee on Tuberculosis*, Hansard, volume i, 1913, pp.7-8; N. McFarlane, Hospitals, Housing and Tuberculosis, 1988, p.67

[67] M. Pelling, V. Berridge, M. Harrison & P. Weindling, chapter 4, p.136, C. Webster, ed., *Caring for Health: History and Diversity,* Oxford University Press, 2001

[68] J. E. Cronin, The British State and the Structure of Political Opportunity, *Journal of British Studies*, volume 27, no.3, 1988, p.201

[69] D. J. Dutton, The Unionist Party and Social Policy 1906-1914*, The Historical Journal*, volume 24, no.4, December, 1981, p.874

It provided the state with more control, through an expanding and increasingly specialised health service, of the potentially infective working classes, thus assuaging middle class fears of contagion and the deterioration of the national stock. Moreover, the Act represented an unprecedented attempt, informed to a large extent by a social evolutionist ideology, to restore tens of thousands of consumptives to a condition of employability and to improve the health of future generations of workers, soldiers and mothers. The Labour movement's ambition of dissolving the Poor Law had, however, not been realised. Due to inadequate investment in sanatoria, a lack of employment following treatment and poor and short term disability pensions the majority of the working classes suffering from tuberculosis continued to be supported by the Poor Law into the 1930s.

CHAPTER ELEVEN

SANATORIUM TREATMENT FOR THE WORKING CLASSES: THE KENT TB SCHEME

Whilst the operation of the National Insurance Act from 1912 has been regarded by some historians as the manifestation of a new "social consciousness",[1] it has also been seen as largely unpopular and ineffectual.[2] This chapter considers how the new measures were received at a local level, how they were implemented, and to what extent they constituted a real transformation in approaches to public health.

From 1912 the responsibility for developing an integrated scheme for the treatment of tuberculosis shifted from local Town and Borough Councils to County Councils. Therefore, in addition to examining developments in public health at Folkestone, a broader perspective is adopted in this chapter, focusing on the early history of sanatoria in Kent.

The Sanatorium can be seen as fulfilling a number of different functions in the early twentieth century, and has been described as institutionally and ideologically "chameleonlike".[3] Theoretical approaches to the treatment of tuberculosis and the effectiveness of the sanatorium system until the 1930s are discussed through a study of Benenden, Grosvenor House and Preston Hall sanatoria in Kent. Were they therapeutic institutions for the cure of consumption, isolation units for the infectious, asylums for the incurable, work colonies for semi-invalids, places of social exclusion for the constitutionally defective, centres for the indoctrination of "hygienic" rituals and behaviour or

---

[1] J. Harris, *Private Lives and Public Spirit: Britain 1870-1914*, Penguin: London, 1993

[2] K. Laybourn, *Modern Britain Since 1906*, 1999, p.7; D. G. Green, *Working Class Patients and the Medical Establishment,* Aldershot: Gower Publishing Co. Ltd, 1985, p.178

[3] A. Bashford, Tuberculosis and Economy: Public Health and Labour in the Early Welfare State, *Health & History*, volume 4, no.2, 2002, p.24

experimental research establishments?

The Political Utility of the Sanatorium

Central to the question of whether the public treatment of tuberculosis can be seen as initiating a new era of socially oriented health reform lies an appreciation of how the disease was understood in the light of germ theory. As argued in chapter three, since the early 1890s the importance of a healthy diet and living conditions as the most effective means of preventing the active form of the disease had been repeatedly stressed by authorities on tuberculosis.[4] Ronald MacFie, for example, writing in *The Lancet* in 1905, saw improving the living conditions of the working classes as a more economic alternative to the construction of sanatoria:

> Consumption will be most speedily and economically abolished, not by means of sanatoriums but by hygienic improvements – better food, better housing, more open spaces, &c.[5]

Nevertheless, despite assurances from many public health officials and the staff of consumption hospitals that tuberculosis posed very little threat of infection, middle class anxieties over the moral and physical degeneration of urban inhabitants added to social pressure for the segregation of the tubercular poor.[6]

Sanatorium treatment provided an appealing solution to the problem of tuberculosis for a variety of reasons. Open-air therapy was already seen as a successful treatment for those who could afford it. Moreover it provided an option that, for one reason or another, satisfied the majority of public health officials. Not only was it generally accepted that the *bacillus* could not survive exposure to the light and air, these same conditions, it was believed, encouraged a strengthened resistance to the disease on the part of the host. In addition, the aggregation of consumptives in institutions created an opportunity to appraise them of the dangers of spreading infection by spitting and the benefits to their health of spending as much of

---

[4] For example, J. Niven, *Poverty and Disease*, Presidential Address to the Epidemiological Section of the Royal Society of Medicine, 22nd October, 1900, Proceedings of the Royal Society of Medicine, 3, part 2, 1910, pp.1-45; A. Ransome, Consumption, A Filth Disease, *The Lancet*, 1st January, 1898

[5] R. MacFie, Sanatoriums for the Poor and the Eradication of Consumption, *The Lancet*, 30th September, 1905, p.962; Sir W. Osler, The Prevention and Treatment of Tuberculosis, *The Lancet*, 18th July, 1914, p.167

[6] A. Hardy, *The Epidemic Streets*, Oxford University Press, 1993, p.258

their time as possible exposed to fresh air. It also, albeit for a short period of time, removed them from unhealthy environments and the risk of infecting their families and neighbours. As a medical historian has remarked in the case of AIDS:

> quarantine is a response not only to the actual mode of transmission, but also to a popular demand to establish a boundary between the "kind of person" so diseased and the "respectable people" who hope to remain healthy.[7]

The isolation of sections of society is generally a response to a complex of social concerns, and undoubtedly the legislation passed with the intention of providing for the compulsory sanatorium treatment of working class consumptives, Part II of the 1911 National Insurance Act, was influenced by social Darwinist ideology, albeit justified by appeal to germ theory.[8]

It has been suggested that the initial impact of germ theory in the late nineteenth century deflected attention away from the pressing need for environmental reforms, thus retarding improvements to the living conditions of many working class families and unnecessarily prolonging the prevalence of diseases such as tuberculosis.[9] If government investment in sanatorium treatment and health insurance was to some degree a tactical ploy intended to appease both the working classes and imperialist proponents of "national efficiency" at the expense of more fundamental social reforms such as housing then, arguably, this perception of the negative impact of germ theory on disease reduction may well be justified.

The 1909 budget had raised £25,000,000, largely through taxes on the affluent, and, although investment in the navy was seen as imperative,[10] by 1911 it would have been economically viable for the government to grant incentives to local authorities for a programme of housing reform. Although Lloyd George had committed himself in the 1909 budget to

---

[7] D. F. Musto, Quarantine and the Problem of AIDS, *AIDS – The Burdens of History*, eds., E. Fee & D. M. Fox, Berkeley, University of California Press, 1988, p.77

[8] J. Trostle, Early Work in Anthropology and Epidemiology: From Social Medicine to the Germ Theory, 1840-1920, *Anthropology & Epidemiology*, ed. Craig R. Janes, Dordrecht, Kluwer Academic Publishers, 1986

[9] F. B. Smith, *The Retreat of Tuberculosis, 1850-1950*, London: Croom Helm, 1988, p.168; J. Comaroff, Medicine: Symbol and Ideology, P. Wright & A. Treacher eds., *The Problem of Medical Knowledge*, Edinburgh University Press, 1982, p.61

[10] B. B. Gilbert, David Lloyd George, 1976, p.1063

"wage implacable war against poverty and squalidness",[11] it has been argued that the Chancellor had little interest in, or understanding of, urban social problems.[12] Nevertheless, he needed to compete with Chamberlain's promise of social reform to ensure the working class vote.

Despite the advice of many public health experts that consumptives would only benefit fully from sanatorium treatment if they were able to return to healthy homes,[13] expectations that tuberculosis would be swiftly vanquished by the new science of bacteriology and sanatorium treatment were high before the war. As an Irish health professional astutely observed in 1907:

> the essence of the discovery [of the *tubercle bacillus*] was that it proved that it was not an economic revolution that was needed but the destruction of the *bacillus*.[14]

The social reforms advocated by Lord Astor's report, particularly those relating to housing and environmental improvements, had been largely ignored by the Liberals in favour of a programme of health visiting, hygienic education and the confinement of the tubercular. This single-minded campaign against the *bacillus* was undoubtedly supported by elements of the medical establishment. From 1898 campaigns by the NAPC and pamphlets published by many local sanitary authorities, largely inspired by the pioneering work of Arthur Newsholme at Brighton publicising the dangers of personal infection, had encouraged a focus on the disinfection of houses and the testing and isolation of individuals.

On the other hand public health officials such as James Niven, MOH for Liverpool, and Arthur Ransome, MOH for Manchester, continued to emphasise the slum housing and poor diets of the working classes as large contributory factors to the spread of the disease. However, an entrenched attitude on the part of many politicians, doctors and social reformers of viewing sections of the poor as idle and dirty malingerers who posed a threat to the health and stability of the nation, together with a continuing adherence to the doctrine of "self-help", created resistance to any large

---

[11] D. J. Dutton, The Unionist Party and Social Policy 1906-14, *Historical Journal*, vol.24, no.4, December, 1981, p.876

[12] B. B. Gilbert, David Lloyd George, 1976, p.1060

[13] e.g. M. Quarry, Report of R.C.P.L., appendix volume II, 26th June 1906, Cd.21253,

[14] E. J. McWeeney, Popular Endeavours Against Tuberculosis (Paper read before the *Journal of Statistical and Social Enquiry Society of Ireland*, 19th April, 1907 published in pamphlet form), p.5 – quoted in Greta Jones, *Social Hygiene*, 1986

scale expenditure on the reform of slum areas.

Although the Housing Act of 1909 had encouraged local authorities to follow the innovatory policy of the newly created London County Council in making rehousing a part of slum clearance, this course of action was generally ignored and overcrowding became an increasing problem in the early twentieth century.[15] As one popular commentator on tuberculosis observed in 1910:

> improvements in housing, sanitation and food inspection have been made, but these have been so half-hearted that one despairs of anything tangible ever being accomplished.[16]

Lloyd George's reforms were to have little initial impact on the lives of the majority of working class consumptives. In the summer of 1913 Waldorf Astor, chairman of the Report on Tuberculosis of the previous year and MP for Plymouth, remarked on the "chaos and dissatisfaction" felt throughout the country regarding the treatment of tuberculosis. He blamed the obstruction of President of the LGB John Burns, whom he described as a "mid-Victorian reactionary",[17] for blocking the implementation of the Minority Report's proposals for social reform, remarking that "insured persons have been compelled to contribute for a benefit which is not worth the money they have been forced to pay".[18]

The Kent Tuberculosis Scheme 1908-1918

In Kent changes in the treatment of tuberculosis were more limited and gradual than generally portrayed. Local government was reluctant to intervene to ameliorate the hardships suffered by the poorest, leaving any assistance to private charity and the Poor Law. Local Councils were reluctant to implement any reformist legislation in the early twentieth century, and a County Medical Officer was not appointed until 1908. County Councillors, it has been argued, were concerned that a CMO would dictate policy to them and had declined to appoint one after the Local Government Act of 1888.[19]

---

[15] G. Sutherland, Social Policy in the Inter-War Years, 1973, p.430

[16] J. T. Nicholls, Can Consumption Be Cured?, *Health and Strength*, 19th March, 1910

[17] W. Astor, HC debate 12th June, 1913, volume 53, cc 1857-8

[18] Ibid, cc 1866

[19] P. Hastings & N. Yates, Health and Social Welfare, *Kent in the Twentieth Century,* ed. N. Yates, Woodbridge: Boydell & Brewer, 2001, pp.230-232

The Kent Insurance Committee managed to provide very few beds in sanatoria for the working classes until after the war. The county sanatorium at Lenham was not available for the civilian population until July 1919. Prior to this Kent County Council records reveal that the vast majority of cases notified to the County Medical Officer were either confined to what were, in effect, isolation homes for the dying, visited in their homes by charity workers or, from 1918 in Folkestone, visited by a female health visitor employed by the Sanitary Department.

Revolving shelters were also lent or rented by the Council. Arriving in sections they could be erected in gardens, yards or even on roofs. These open sided wooden huts isolated consumptives from their families whilst affording them a constant supply of therapeutic air. They could be revolved to protect the patient from strong winds, but were reportedly cold and lonely habitations,[20] and this therapeutic alternative to the sanatorium was generally unpopular:

> Do those who advocate domiciliary treatment on a large scale realise what it means to lie on one's back month in and month out in the same bed and in the same room with practically no distraction?[21]

Consumptives who lacked a garden or yard were directed to occupy a separate room if there was one. Otherwise they were likely to be isolated in any available institution. Thus, at least for Kent, the provision of sanatorium treatment in a sanatorium – the heart of the scheme originally advised upon under the Report of the Departmental Committee on Tuberculosis, 1912 – was almost entirely lacking until the 1920s.[22]

The circumstances of most destitute consumptives remained the same, although they were more likely to occupy segregated wards in Union infirmaries. Even following the National Insurance Act paupers suffering from consumption did not qualify for receipt of sanatorium benefit but either remained in workhouse infirmaries or were sent to other institutions for treatment or isolation under the administration of the Poor Law Guardians.[23]

Other than adapting their own workhouses for open air therapy, as at Sheppey where two balconies had been added, the only institutions

---

[20] M. Campbell, What Tuberculosis did for Modernism, 2005, pp.478-481

[21] Anonymous tuberculosis patient cited in E. Wittkower, *A Psychiatrist Looks at Tuberculosis,* London: NAPT, 1949, p.72

[22] Dr. A. S. MacNalty, Tuberculosis Work in England, 1924, p.165-169

[23] W. J. Howarth, MOH County of Kent, *Memorandum for Departmental Committee on Tuberculosis (Astor Report),* 1912, p.75

offering treatment for Kent's tuberculous paupers were the Sandgate sanatoria, offering 123 beds at one guinea per week, and St. Catherine's Hospital at Ramsgate, run by the Sisters of the Ordre-du-Croix, with 182 beds at fifteen shillings a week. Patients were sent to both institutions by the Guardians of Rochester, Chatham and Faversham, in north Kent, until at least 1914, demonstrating the dearth of resources for working class victims of tuberculosis in the county.[24]

As early as July, 1908 Dr. Heggs, Medical Officer for the Sittingbourne and Milton Joint Hospital Board, had criticised the County Council's inaction; "While we are waiting for a county sanatorium people are dying".[25] As a conviction of the infectiousness of tuberculosis grew amongst some local authorities, they became increasingly reluctant to accommodate pauper consumptives in workhouse infirmaries. In January 1909 Heggs described a situation common to most of the county at this time:

> There is no special accommodation for [consumptives] at our Union infirmary, and so, for the sake of the other inmates, these cases are preferably treated by out-relief. Thus these advanced cases, in the most infectious stage of the disease, are allowed and encouraged to stay at home where the risk of spreading the disease to those about them is very great indeed. Other members of the family become infected and they will ultimately become a charge on the rates. The house also becomes an infected area, and a danger to others who might inhabit it later.[26]

From 1st January, 1909 the notification of pulmonary tuberculosis amongst inmates of Poor Law institutions or those receiving outdoor relief came into operation under the Public Health (Tuberculosis) Regulations of 1908.[27] However, for most districts, including Kent, Poor Law infirmaries were not equipped to provide any specialised treatment for the tubercular. Although the government now provided half the cost of their treatment hardly any beds were available other than canvas pavilions or converted small-pox hospitals used for the isolation of advanced cases.[28]

Throughout the county there was a growing concern among local

---

[24] LGB correspondence relating to Kent TB Scheme, 1912-1917, NA MH 48/74

[25] Quoted from a meeting of the Sittingbourne Urban District Council, July, 1908, LGB correspondence Keycol Hill Tuberculosis Scheme, 1907-19, NA MH 48/75

[26] Sittingbourne UDC July, 1908, January, 1909, LGB correspondence Keycol Hill Tuberculosis Scheme, 1907-19, NA MH 48/75

[27] Folkestone Sanitary & Hospitals Committee, Minute Book March 1907-1910, Fo/AMc12/5

[28] A. Greenwood, KCC First Report upon Tuberculosis, 1914, p.117

authorities for the cost of continued inaction, both in terms of loss of life and of the financial burden borne by ratepayers. Heggs' report as MOH for Sittingbourne UDC in 1909 concluded that while "an enormous loss of life" was occurring in the district the local Council were doing nothing but waiting for the County to act and spending money on overcrowded institutions with enormous waiting lists, such as London's Brompton Hospital for Consumption.[29]

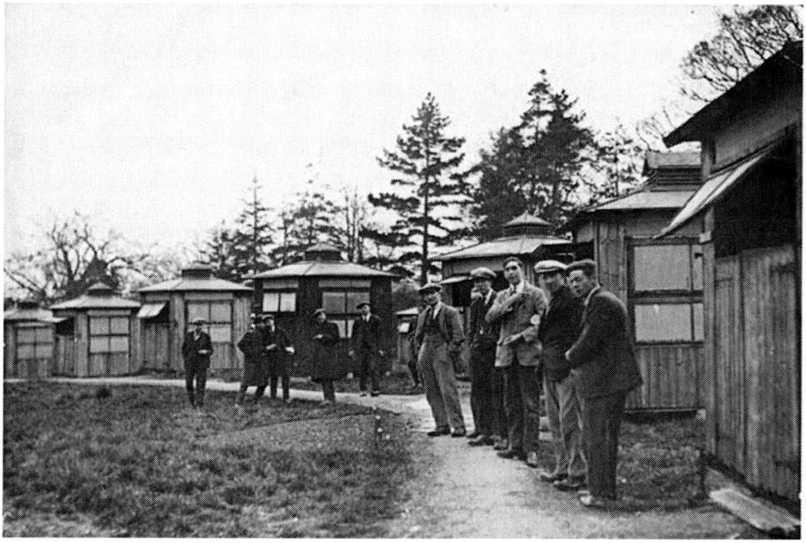

Illustration 11.1: Shelters at Papworth Tuberculosis Colony, Cambridgeshire, 1925-1930.

In May, 1909 the Medical Officer for Milton Regis UDC expressed the frustration felt by most health officials in the county:

> Can you tell me what place you can send an unlimited number [of consumptives] to, at two guineas a week? There is no place in Kent, and I do not know of any place in the country where you can depend on having all your cases accepted...With regard to the Maidstone sanatorium [Benenden], the Medical Superintendent there said that the kind of patients they had to deal with was the offspring of vicious and diseased parents, unhealthy and ill-fed, and drawn from their homes mostly in an advanced stage of the disease. These were the very worst sort of cases, and yet 50%

[29] Sittingbourne UDC meeting April 27th, 1909, MH 48/75

> were discharged as improved, and cured or ameliorated. In his opinion it would be difficult to find any beds at an existing sanatorium now…[there was] a case from the Guardians, they could not get it into a proper sanatorium, and it was sent to a quack institution with the result that it came back with no benefit. If they had to pay towards a county scheme they would be paying for the greater percentage of cases which would come from the slums of Chatham, Greenwich, Gillingham and other places.[30]

Apart from demonstrating the impersonal and dehumanising attitude adopted towards working class consumptives by many middle class professionals, the Medical Officer's report also illustrates the sense of optimism inspired by public sanatorium treatment. In addition it reveals local concern that provincial ratepayers would be subsidising the treatment of "vicious and diseased" urban "slum dwellers".

The problem of what to do with the tubercular was, to a certain extent, taken out of the hands of local authorities when from 1st January 1912 all cases of pulmonary tuberculosis were made compulsorily notifiable following the Public Health (Tuberculosis) Regulations of 1911. Individuals suspected of having contracted the disease were now referred to a public Tuberculosis Dispensary managed by the County Council, from where, in theory, they were directed to treatment in an institution. But as Waldorf Astor observed, few institutions had at this time been provided by County Councils. Many county authorities, it has been claimed, were in "open revolt" against government demands for the provision of sanatoria due to the difficulties of raising taxes locally.[31] Certainly, the provision of beds by Kent County Council was late and inadequate, the County sanatorium not being opened until after the war.

In Folkestone, Kent County Council proposals for the establishment of a Tuberculosis Dispensary in the town encountered resolute opposition from members of Folkestone Corporation and local traders who were concerned that fears of infection from working class consumptives would deter potential visitors. At a meeting in January 1914 Folkestone Council lodged an official protest against KCC's proposed dispensary in Dover Road. The County Council also received a petition from influential Folkestone residents, and the following month a spokesman for the East Folkestone Tradesmen's Association alleged that the dispensary would:

> directly and indirectly injure the town as a health resort…we think it is

[30] Milton Regis UDC meeting, May, 1909, MH 48/75

[31] C. Bellamy, *Administering Central-Local Relations,* 1988, p.66

> absolutely necessary that an isolated house on the border of the Borough be found immediately that would be as useful, and at the same time would not damage the town's reputation as a watering place.[32]

The selection of Folkestone as the embarkation port for hundreds of thousands of troops *en route* to France and Belgium was, however, shortly to have a greater impact on the town's image as a select health resort.

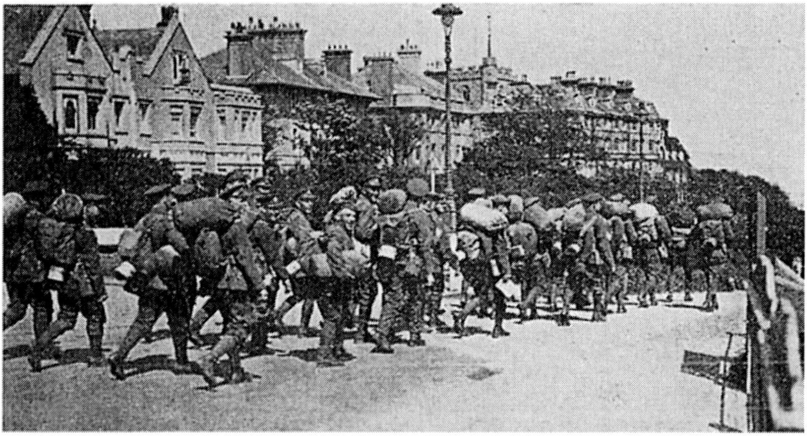

Illustration 11.2: Troops Marching through Folkestone prior to Embarkation c.1915.

The dispensary, one of eighteen in Kent, was eventually opened early in 1914 for one afternoon and one evening per week with Dr. Clark as Tuberculosis Officer. The County Council placated residents by agreeing to remove the brass plate and window notices bearing the words "County Tuberculosis Dispensary", and assured them there was no danger of infection and that there would be no publicity of any kind relating to the purpose for which the house was to be used. This attempt at concealment in a small town like Folkestone was, perhaps, more likely to have increased the alarm felt by residents as consumptives from a broad catchment area descended on the dispensary during the same afternoon and evening each week. The dispensary also served Cheriton, Hythe and Sandgate, a population of about 50,000. Both insured and uninsured

---

[32] Statement from meeting of East Folkestone Tradesmen's Association, 2nd February, 1914, Sanitary & Hospitals Committee Minute Books, 1913-1916, Fo-Amc12/8

workers (those ineligible for sanatorium benefit due to their income being in excess of £160 per year) were examined and treated, surgical operations were performed on non-pulmonary cases, and the vaccine *tuberculin* was administered to some cases.

Laboratory testing was now emerging as an important adjunct of public health. From February to April 1914 54 new cases were notified in Folkestone due to the tracing of contacts of known consumptives through the analysis of sputum samples performed by the county laboratory at Maidstone.[33] Although it is impossible to tell how common misdiagnosis was, these tests were not universally accepted as being reliable. In 1913 the journal *Public Health* claimed the sputum test did not distinguish between recent and healed pulmonary lesions, and that a positive reaction could be obtained from about 90% of healthy adults.[34] In any event, despite possessing the resources to identify individuals who had once been affected by tuberculosis, very few of these were to receive any form of sanatorium treatment at this time.

Although the National Insurance Act, as originally framed, had provided for "treatment in sanatoria or other institutions", subsequently the words "or otherwise" were appended to this statement. Thus "sanatorium benefit" did not refer solely to the provision of treatment in an institution, but was now extended to:

> treatment which can be given to the patient either at a dispensary, or at his home, or in shelters. In certain cases additional food, or a separate room or bed, may be provided as part of the treatment. Under proper conditions home treatment may constitute satisfactory sanatorium treatment.[35]

This amendment of the Act appears to have resulted from unexpected financial constraints. Although £1,500,000 had been provided by the Exchequer for the construction of sanatoria, dispensaries and other institutions for the tubercular, this sum proved inadequate and the remainder of the costs had to be provided by the rates, or from loans charged on the rates. In addition there were further burdens placed on

---

[33] Folkestone MOH Report, 1914, Folkestone Borough Council Sanitary & Hospitals Committee, Fo-Amc12/8

[34] *Public Health*, no.8, volume xxvi, May 1913, p.217; G. C. Bowker & S. L. Star, *Sorting Things Out: Classification and its Consequences*, Massachusetts Institute Of Technology, 1999

[35] A. Greenwood, KCC First Report upon Tuberculosis, 1914, p.134; W. J. Howarth, MOH County of Kent, *Memorandum for Departmental Committee on Tuberculosis (Astor Report),* 1912, p.75

ratepayers following a shortfall in contributions for tuberculosis treatment raised by the County Insurance Committees. As the scope of the revised Act was extended to apply to the uninsured, if they chose to contribute towards the cost of sanatorium treatment, half of these additional costs were met from the rates and, according to the Kent County Council Report on Tuberculosis, about half the costs for the treatment of insured cases were also to be met by local ratepayers.[36]

By 1913 KCC were proposing to construct a sanatorium of 100 beds for the county at an estimated cost of £15,000 and to provide a further 105 hospital beds for advanced cases in existing institutions. The provision of 100 sanatorium beds was recognised by the Council as being "far below the Astor standard", and their availability was long overdue. Following the guidelines of the Astor Committee the Insurance Committee calculated in 1913 that Kent required 136 beds but only had 45 available.[37] The County Sanatorium at Lenham was not constructed until 1917, and not opened for the treatment of tuberculosis until 1919.

For the years 1912 and 1913, out of a total of 1,762 cases of pulmonary tuberculosis notified in Kent, and 961 other tubercular cases – in all a small proportion of the actual number of people afflicted with the disease – the Kent Insurance Committee provided institutional treatment for 300 tuberculous patients, about three-quarters of whom were men. Of these 172 were sent either to the Bromley Sanatorium (a former smallpox hospital) or to Keycol Hill near Sittingbourne, both institutions for the segregation of advanced cases, eleven men went to the National Sanatorium at Benenden, and the rest to various institutions outside the county.

From the following table it can be seen that at this time most referrals were for the segregation of advanced cases at Keycol Hill and Bromley, the majority of other identified cases being visited at home by dispensary nurses or health visitors in order to be instructed how to minimise the risk of infection. In consequence of the shortage of beds locally the Committee was forced to look further afield. At the time it was felt appropriate to treat patients at a distance from their families in order to discourage visiting, which was said to compromise the patient's health, and in order to deter him from returning home before his disease had been arrested.

---

[36] A. Greenwood, KCC First Report upon Tuberculosis, 1914, p.134., pp.133-4

[37] A. Newsholme MOH report, LGB, 44, 1914-1915, xxiii, quoted in J. M. Eyler, *Sir Arthur Newsholme*, p.260

Table 11.1: Kent Patients Treated for Tuberculosis January 1912 - December 1913

Institution	male	female	total
Crooksbury Sanatorium		6	6
Bromley Sanatorium	86		86
Brompton Hospital	10	7	17
Dreadnought Hospital, Greenwich	2		2
Eversfield Chest Hospital, St Leonards-on-Sea		15	15
Fairlight Sanatorium	2		2
Keycol Hill	86		86
King Edward VII Sanatorium, Midhurst, Sussex	1	1	2
Maltings Farm Sanatorium, Nayland, Colchester	6	12	18
Mount Vernon Hospital		14	14
Pinewood Sanatorium, Wokingham, Berkshire	5		5
Royal National Sanatorium, Benenden	11		11
Royal National Sanatorium, Bournemouth	1	1	2
Royal National Sanatorium, Ventnor	5	1	6
Royal Sea Bathing Hospital, Margate	4	5	9
Whitmead Sanatorium, Telford, Surrey		16	16
Various	1	2	3
Grand Total	220	80	300

Source: KCC First Report on Tuberculosis and the Administration of Sanatorium Benefit, 1914

A major disincentive for consumptives accepting residential treatment was that their dependants were not guaranteed any financial assistance under the National Insurance Act of 1911.[38] In 1910 Charles Dowsing, an invalided soldier of Cheriton High Street was advised to enter hospital for his consumption to be treated but was unwilling to leave his wife. He received three shillings and sixpence from the Parish, a payment that would have stopped on his entering hospital, and Dowsing was concerned that his wife would have been evicted from their home:

> It's impossible for me to go and leave my wife at home starving and owing so much rent. I should simply die in hospital thinking about it so we may

[38] A. Greenwood, Kent County Council and Kent Insurance Committee, *First Report upon Tuberculosis and the Administration of Sanatorium Benefit,* Maidstone, 1914, p.134

as well be at home and starve as be separated.[39]

However, the Ministry of Health Act of 1919 devolved the provision of sanatorium treatment from Insurance Committees to local authorities, and subsequently both dependants and the uninsured were treated in Kent.[40]

Table 11.2: Kent Patients Treated for Tuberculosis Jan-March, 1914

Institution	male	female	total
Bromley Sanatorium	28		28
Brompton Hospital	2		2
Eversfield Chest Hospital, St Leonsards-on-Sea		4	4
Keycol Hill, Sittingbourne	17		17
King Edward VII Sanatorium, Midhurst, Sussex	1		1
Maltings Farm Sanatorium, Nayland, Colchester	5		5
Pinewood Sanatorium, Wokingham, Berkshire	1		1
Royal National Sanatorium, Benenden	3		3
Royal National Sanatorium, Bournemouth	1		1
Royal National Sanatorium, Ventnor	2		2
Royal Sea Bathing Hospital, Margate	3	2	5
Whitmead Sanatorium, Telford, Surrey		11	11
Grand Total	63	17	80

Source: KCC First Report on Tuberculosis and the Administration of Sanatorium Benefit, 1914

On 31st March 1914 the KIC had five adults being treated for non-pulmonary tuberculosis at the Royal Sea Bathing Hospital in Margate, whilst a further 75 consumptives were being treated at the above sanatoria, the majority of whom were advanced cases.[41] As can be seen in tables 11.1 and 11.2 after two years and three months of sanatorium treatment being available for insured working men and women in Kent only 92 out of 380 cases had been sent to sanatoria for treatment, most of these being described as advanced cases. The majority of patients, 217, were consigned to Bromley and Keycol Hill, institutions reserved for hopeless

[39] Letters from the Soldiers and Sailors Help Society, Fo/Z2/C4

[40] A. Salisbury MacNalty, MOH to Ministry of Health, Tuberculosis Work in England, *The Lancet*, 26th January, 1924, p. 166

[41] Local Government Board correspondence relating to Kent TB Scheme, 1912-1917, NA MH 48/74

cases who had no means of isolating themselves at home.[42]

In February 1914 25 beds were reserved by the Kent Insurance Committee at Benenden Sanatorium, which had opened near Ashford in 1907. Cases were also sent there by the King Edward VII Hospital Fund, the Insurance Committees of Middlesex, Nottinghamshire, Canterbury City Borough, Barrow in Furness, the Post Office Sanatorium Society, the Hearts of Oak Friendly Society, Manchester Unity and the Railwaymen's Union.

In 1915 Percy Jones, the proprietor of the Sandgate sanatorium business, opened the Grosvenor Sanatorium at Kennington, some fifteen miles away near Ashford, amidst alarmist headlines in the local press, such as "Consumption encampment disastrous for district" and "It spells ruin for Ashford".[43] The management of the Grosvenor had been so denigrated by local dignitaries for more than a decade that accommodation was unlikely to have been sought there at this time by the Kent Insurance Committee.

Following the 1911 National Insurance Act County and Borough Insurance Committees were keen to support any proposed sanatorium in order to fulfil their obligations under the Act by providing beds for local cases of tuberculosis. However, news of the proposed opening of the Grosvenor sanatorium at Kennington (named after the largest of the Sandgate sanatoria), was accompanied by fierce protest. Petitions were sent to local MPs, the LGB and the KCC. Kennington and Willesborough Parish Councils, East Ashford Rural District Council and Ashford Urban District Council objected that the sanatorium would reduce the value of local property, and that it was a threat to the health and prosperity of the neighbourhood.[44]

Kent County Council also protested to the Local Government Board claiming that the treatment of tuberculosis under the National Insurance Act ought to be dealt with by local authorities rather than "private speculators".[45] A sanatorium established for profit, it was argued, would not exercise the same regard for the interests of the patients and the locality. The necessary training, supervision and restraint of the patients would not be enforced and, in any event, the County Council was itself obliged to provide sufficient sanatorium accommodation for the County:

---

[42] A. Greenwood, *KCC First Report upon Tuberculosis and the Administration of Sanatorium Benefit*, 1914, p.33

[43] A. H. Joyce, Early Sanatoriums in Kent, *Bygone Kent,* volume 8, no.6

[44] Records of Grosvenor Sanatorium, 1912-1919, National Archives, MA 48/76

[45] Ibid.

> The Kent County Council have by their scheme undertaken the care and treatment of all tuberculous cases in the County, and they think it undesirable that a private venture of the character proposed should be allowed to be erected, and if the Board possess any power to veto such scheme the Council suggest that such power should be exercised.[46]

Laurence Hardy, M.P. for Hythe and Folkestone, sent a letter to John Burns, president of the Local Government Board, urging him not to license Jones' enterprise:

> Public bodies will put forward public grounds for enquiry, but I desire to approach you from another point of view. This sanatorium is promoted by a member of the Jones family, whose abuse of the sanatorium system has been before my eyes flagrantly during twenty years at Sandgate, and I most earnestly trust that a repetition of the same line of conduct at Ashford may be prevented. The records of your department fully show, I am sure, the evils which Sandgate has had to endure, and I need not detail them, but they are sufficiently well known to make you pause, before giving to this new venture the certification of your Board.[47]

The Local Government Board did not wish to lose the 200 beds provided by Jones' sanatoria, but in 1913 they considered his chances of establishing the new Grosvenor to be slight:

> In view of the local opposition it seems very unlikely that any local authority will be willing to include the proposed sanatorium in their scheme, but any further warning would be wasted upon Mr. Jones apparently.[48]

Although the LGB felt that it would be inconsistent to sanction the Sandgate Sanatoria on a permanent basis, it is clear from a memo of the time that they felt Jones' anticipated failure to secure an alternative site would result in the continuation of these Homes.[49] Apparently the LGB had no compunction in permitting Unions to continue sending tubercular patients to be treated in what were, largely, converted houses situated in the heart of a small town.

However, by July 1913 Jones had the support of about a dozen County

---

[46] W. B. Prosser, Clerk of KCC to LGB, 30th October, 1913, in Records of Grosvenor Sanatorium, 1912-19

[47] Ibid.

[48] Records of Grosvenor Sanatorium, 1912-19, LGB memo from Mr. Morse, 16th October, 1913

[49] LGB memo 23rd July, 1913, NA MA 48/76

and Borough Insurance Committees, including Warwickshire, Hampshire, Northamptonshire and London. As an integral part of the tuberculosis schemes of these bodies Jones was able to complete the purchase of Bockhanger estate, provide new buildings to accommodate 200 patients, and furnish it, for about £24,000 in March 1914. In March 1915 it was approved by the LGB under the 1911 National Insurance Act after the public furore had abated somewhat.

From 1916 there were many urgent applications for treatment from discharged soldiers. At the same time food was becoming increasingly expensive and difficult for Jones to obtain, and in July 1919 73 complaints about the quality and quantity of food were received by the Ministry of Pensions. Unnotified visits from the Medical Officers of various Insurance Committees and County Councils concluded that there were no grounds for complaint, as did a report conducted by Dr. MacNalty from the newly created Ministry of Health.

Jones was nevertheless becoming disillusioned with running the sanatorium:

> The difficulty of dealing with ex-servicemen makes the conduct of the Institution almost impossible, with the result that I have under serious consideration the question of using the sanatorium and estate for another purpose.[50]

The system of graduated labour employed to treat the tubercular in many sanatoria prior to the mid-1930s, when surgery increasingly came into vogue, was apparently difficult to enforce amongst ex-servicemen,[51] and by 1918 there were growing fears of social unrest due to shortages of food and housing. There were also concerns over the loyalty of soldiers and ex-servicemen.[52] Jones considered selling the estate, but the LGB saw no benefit in acquiring the sanatorium themselves:

> The sanatorium is practically always filled with patients sent by Local Authorities, Insurance Committees, and Boards of Guardians, and I do not think that the Chairman of the Board should be encouraged to purchase it…nothing would be gained by buying out the Limited Company. They would probably want a price considerably in excess of the original cost.[53]

[50] LGB, Grosvenor Sanatorium records, 1912-19, NA MH 48/76
[51] L. Bryder, *Below the Magic Mountain*, 1988, p.66
[52] G. Sutherland, Social Policy in the Inter-War Years, 1973, p.427
[53] Memo by A. B. Maclachen, 19th September, 1919, LGB correspondence relating to Grosvenor Sanatorium, NA MA 48/76

At the time both Preston Hall and Lenham sanatoria were being used as hospitals for injured servicemen, and throughout the country beds for consumptives were at a premium. By 1918 there would be 58,000 ex-servicemen judged to have contracted tuberculosis due to war service, and these were given priority when beds became available in sanatoria. A memorandum of 1919 from the records of the LGB reveals the importance of Jones' enterprise for the treatment of tuberculosis:

> The loss of this sanatorium for the treatment of tuberculosis would be serious and perhaps we might consider the question of extending the period for which it is approved.[54]

In summary, this episode in the development of open-air treatment for tuberculosis illustrates the pragmatic way in which the LGB mediated between local and national interests. It also demonstrates the increasing demand from County and Borough Councils and the Ministry of Pensions for beds for the treatment of tuberculosis after the war.

Over a period of about fourteen years perceptions of Jones' operations had shifted from his being denigrated for "trading in diseased paupers" to being considered an essential part of various County and Borough schemes for the treatment of tuberculosis. For an affordable fee (42 shillings per week in 1916) Jones provided treatment for poor consumptives at a time when few voluntary and charitable institutions could have survived financially, and Grosvenor House continued to operate as a sanatorium for the working classes until 1955. The aggregate treatment of those suffering from a chronic disease, which had not been attempted to any degree in England since the leprosaria of the middle ages, was gradually coming to be accepted, as were alternatives to charitably funded institutions, as the state increasingly extended control over the health and behaviour of the working classes.

Benenden and Grosvenor House Sanatoria 1910-1920

Patients of both sexes were also treated at Benenden, and the same charges and therapeutic regimes were in operation as at Grosvenor Sanatorium, however only 100 patients could be accommodated at the former in comparison to the 200 beds available at Jones' establishment. By 1916 Benenden was threatened with closure; support from the workers' organisations was poor, £30,000 had been spent on building and equipping

---

[54] Memo by A. B. Maclachen, 19th September, 1919, LGB correspondence relating to Grosvenor Sanatorium, NA MA 48/76

the sanatorium, and a debt of £7,325 remained. Charitable organisations were approached, and Princess Christina of Schleswig-Holstein, the president of the workers' organisation was appealed to for assistance. Even after the war financial pressures were not reduced; the cost of provisions was £2,100 more in 1919 than in 1918. Nevertheless, with the help of donations, and the economies achieved from the operation of a farm worked by patients, the sanatorium was to survive into the 1950s.[55]

Patients were originally admitted on a month long trial, and only early and treatable cases were retained. However, as the war progressed this rule was relaxed, and in 1915 Benenden was treating 40 "curative" cases, 40 "intermediate" and 17 "advanced". Their medical superintendent reported a rise in the death rate following the passing of the 1911 National Insurance Act which:

> gave rise in the public mind to an idea that all cases of pulmonary tuberculosis were more or less curable by sanatorium treatment, and the sanatorium of this country have, during the last twelve months, been flooded with unsuitable cases.[56]

At Grosvenor House at this time advanced cases were apparently "not objected to unless the patient is likely to die in the sanatorium",[57] but were treated separately from intermediate cases. Although the treatment records from 1915-1919 show that, on average, not more than about 5% of patients died at the sanatorium, this was due to patients being sent home or to isolation hospitals to die once it was considered that no further benefit would be obtained through treatment. Dr. A. N. Robertson, Medical Superintendent at Benenden between 1915-1919, considered the length of stay, on average 16 weeks, inadequate to complete the arrest of the disease, but this was the inevitable result of severe financial constraints; "in a large number of cases healing of the diseased lung is only starting when the patient leaves at the end of four months".[58]

The length of stay in a sanatorium was obviously critical to the success of the treatment. Doctors at private sanatoria in England at this time would generally recommend a stay of between six and twelve months in order to attempt a cure through open-air therapy. The average length of time

---

[55] B. McPate, *Benenden,* 2006, p.86

[56] W. J. Cox, Medical Superintendant, Annual Report, 1914, LGB records of Benenden Sanatorium, 1912-1918, NA MH 48/77

[57] From a Report of Special Inspection of the Grosvenor by the LGB, July, 1916.

[58] A. N. Robertson, LGB correspondence regarding Benenden Sanatorium, 1919, MH 48/77

working class patients were to be afforded was only three months, the minimum required by doctors and the maximum considered affordable by Insurance Committees.[59] If the length of treatment was, according to Benenden's Medical Superintendent, insufficient to realistically expect any long term improvement for the majority of cases, one is led to question the intended function of sanatorium treatment for the working classes.

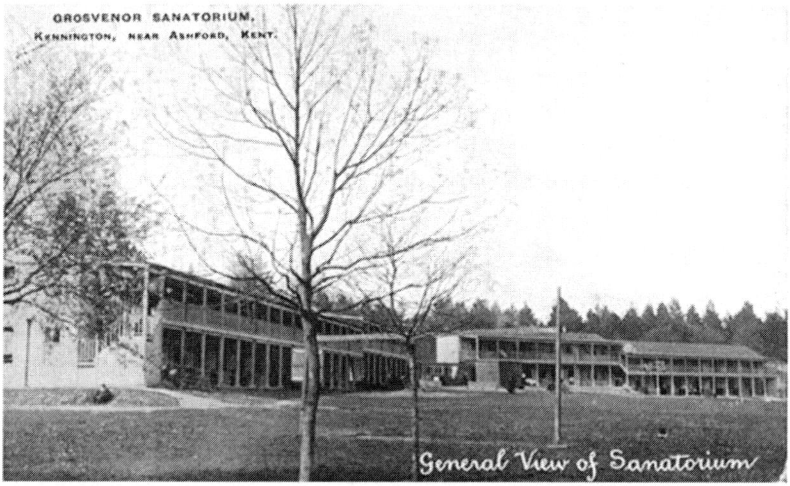
GROSVENOR SANATORIUM,
KENNINGTON, NEAR ASHFORD, KENT.
General View of Sanatorium

Illustration 11.3: Grosvenor Sanatorium near Ashford c.1921.

In 1911 Charles Garland, chairman of the Post Office branch of the National Sanatorium Association, and Thomas Lister, advisory physician to Benenden Sanatorium, saw the purpose of the institution as being primarily educational:

> The sanatorium is both hospital and convalescent home, in a sense, but it is also neither. It is really a training school of health, and to the indifferent or lazy patient is likely to be as useless as any other mode of treatment.[60]

The sanatorium may well have instructed the consumptive how to live with his disease, how to dispose of his sputum hygienically in a flask, not

[59] F. Condrau, The Social Structure of a Tuberculosis Sanatorium, *Journal of Interdisciplinary History*, volume 32, no.2, Autumn, 2001, p.247
[60] C. Garland & T. Lister, *Sanatoria for the People or the State Campaign Against Consumption,* London: Scientific Press, 1911, p.49

to share his cutlery or crockery, to live with open windows, to breathe through his nose, to avoid dust, to eat well, to avoid overexertion and to abstain from alcohol.[61] However, if the patient was not fit enough to secure employment after leaving the sanatorium he would only have an invalidity pension of five shillings a week to subsist on, and a relapse would have been the most probable outcome however much awareness of hygiene had been instilled in him.

LGB records for Benenden prior to 1914 include an annual follow-up of discharged cases that reveals a very high death rate over four years after leaving the sanatorium. Although deaths recorded in the sanatorium stood at about 5%, as at Grosvenor House, of 488 cases discharged between 1907 and 1911, 356 were dead by 1914. If this death rate subsequently rose in 1912, as claimed above, this suggests that at least 80% of patients died within four years of discharge between 1911 and the end of the war.

These figures are supported by the Australian tuberculosis expert Camac Wilkinson who, in 1912, subjected Englemann's results of open-air treatment in Germany, which had so impressed Lloyd George, to further scrutiny. The optimistic German statistics referred to many thousands of cases treated in 31 sanatoria, Wilkinson revealed that four fifths of patients were dead or invalids four years after being discharged.[62]

By 1920 there had, apparently, been little improvement; George Newman recorded that three quarters of cases treated in sanatoria in Germany and Britain were dead within five years.[63] It had been anticipated that the high percentage of advanced cases would decrease as time went on and patients were notified and treated at an earlier stage of the disease. Due to the lack of investment this did not happen. Some patients failed to respond to treatment and deteriorated, whilst others relapsed after returning home to overcrowded or insanitary conditions.[64]

The optimism felt by Charles Garland and Arthur Latham, the moving forces behind the Post Office Friendly Society and the Benenden Sanatorium, as well as by many other early campaigners against tuberculosis, was not justified. It had been hoped that the new dispensary system would facilitate the identification of early cases of tuberculosis and

---

[61] A. Greenwood, from pamphlet T.15, given to every patient in receipt of sanatorium benefit, *KCC First Report upon Tuberculosis and the Administration of Sanatorium Benefit*, 1914, p.16

[62] W. C. Wilkinson, *Tuberculin in the Diagnosis and Treatment of Tuberculosis,* London: J. Nisbet & Co., 1912, p.459, quoted in L. Bryder, *Below the Magic Mountain,* 1988, p.66

[63] G. Newman, letter to R.L. Morant, 1920, NA MH55/164

[64] LGB correspondence relating to Kent TB Scheme, 1912-1917, NA MH 48/74

that funding would be directed chiefly towards their cure. It had also been anticipated that tuberculosis could be cured within a generation once the "advanced cases" had naturally expired.[65] However, long waiting lists and long journeys to institutions meant that early cases, if they had been identified at tuberculosis dispensaries, would often have deteriorated by the time they arrived at their destination. Due to high unemployment, a lack of coordinated after care, and the unpredictable nature of the disease, all sanatoria in Kent were treating consumptives in all stages of the disease, whilst the Keycol Hill and Bromley institutions dealt largely with the bed-ridden.[66]

A lack of after-care for the working class tuberculosis sufferer was, as recognised by Kent's MOH, Alfred Greenwood, a major flaw of the system:

> the loss of employment while under treatment is only too common, and patients return to the difficulty of finding work. No work means no money, and no money means no food, which leads in time to a “relapse”. It is perhaps the most serious “vicious circle” in connection with the disease.[67]

Greenwood felt that public money spent on treatment would be wasted without the provision of adequate after-care, but no further funds were forthcoming from the Treasury at this time:

> At present I fear the question must be left to voluntary societies and private charity. It would, no doubt, be possible to have local after-care committees, which, in my opinion, might carry out valuable work; but such committees would need money, for without an income their scope for practical assistance would be limited.[68]

Training colonies, such as Preston Hall near Ashford, were eventually able to accommodate a certain number of discharged consumptives but the problem of employment remained largely intractable. In 1924 Dr. Thompson of Hastings observed at the annual conference of the NAPT that:

> in his area out of nine men...four were satisfactorily employed either at Preston Hall or Hastings Infirmary, whilst it has been impossible to find

---

[65] A. Latham & C.H. Garland, *The Conquest of Consumption*, 1911, p.14
[66] Sittingbourne and Milton Joint Hospital Board, 1907-09, NA MH 48/75
[67] A. Greenwood, *KCC First Report upon Tuberculosis and the Administration of Sanatorium Benefit*, 1914, p.125
[68] Ibid., p.125

employers of labour to take on the others.[69]

Nor was the identification of early cases for priority treatment a simple matter. Illustrating the difficulties associated with the diagnosis and prognosis of consumption, it is recorded in the minutes of the Benenden Sanatorium Committee of 1909 that consultant physician Arthur Latham disagreed with the medical referee in charge of admissions over whether cases were "early" or "advanced". This suggests that misdiagnosis was perhaps not uncommon.

As Robert Philip had indicated in the same year, diagnosis by *tuberculin* testing failed to discriminate between old quiescent tubercular lesions of the lung and fresh lesions of an aggressive nature indicating the rapid onset of consumption.[70] In 1920 H. H. Thomson, observed that: "tuberculin reactions have not proved of much practical value",[71] and that the experienced doctor must rely on his powers of observation for diagnosis:

> A fairly accurate estimate as to whether there exists an active or fibrotic pulmonary focus can frequently be made from the general and facial appearance of the patient.[72]

Even by 1936 the value of testing the contacts of tuberculous cases was felt by *The Lancet* to have produced "limited" results, particularly in the case of adolescents and children, and often even repeated x-ray examination proved inconclusive. In many cases "physical signs, even in the more chronic varieties of disease may be slight, negligible or absent".[73]

If the achievements of Grosvenor House and Benenden sanatoria were comparable to other institutions throughout the country before and during the war it seems probable that sanatorium treatment contributed little to the nation's economy, and indicates that their primary function would most likely have been perceived by staff and Insurance Committees as one of isolation rather than cure. Discipline was strict at both institutions and conditions whilst undergoing open-air treatment were often harsh. In 1915 Dr. Robertson decreed:

---

[69] NAPT Annual Conference, *The Lancet*, 12th July, 1924, pp. 80-81

[70] R. W. Philip, Progressive Medicine and the Outlook on Tuberculosis, *The Lancet*, 31st July, 1909, p. 283

[71] H. H. Thomson, *Tuberculosis and Public Health*, London: Longmans, 1920, p.64

[72] Ibid, pp.63-64

[73] Editorial, *The Lancet,* 25th July, 1936, pp. 196-7

> Patients are forbidden to close their front windows except in exceptionally stormy weather when it is sometimes necessary…The fresh air treatment increases the metabolism so that the appetite improves, night sweats are diminished and sleep is improved.[74]

However, although the staff generally relied on fresh air, diet and exercise to arrest the disease, one penny of each national insurance contribution had been set aside for medical research, eventually funding what was to become the Medical Research Council. In Kent all sanatoria were equipped with laboratories for the preparation of drugs and sputum analysis, and a certain amount of rather speculative chemotherapy and minor surgery was practised as sanatoria offered an ideal opportunity for research on patients who were generally perceived as being relatively expendable.

Tuberculin was being used therapeutically at Benenden in "a considerable amount of cases" from about 1911, but generally only in cases that were not responding to treatment, and whose constitution was considered strong enough to withstand it. The therapeutic use of *tuberculin* appears to have been particularly prevalent in Britain for three or four years from about 1911-1912, having been championed by Sir Robert Philip and Camac Wilkinson. However, whether due to the cost of the vaccine, or to the greater efficacy or benefits of *auto-inoculation*, the latter treatment prevailed and was a fundamental aspect of treatment in sanatoria in Kent and elsewhere in the country into the inter-war years.[75]

The system of graduated labour, originally devised by Dr. Marcus Paterson of Frimley sanatorium, was intended to *auto-inoculate*[76] patients with their own *tuberculin* – in effect to increase levels of the *bacillus* in the body in order to raise the body's resistance to it – through a system of carefully regulated exercise and work. This description of the process was given by Dr. Smyth, Benenden's Medical Superintendent, in 1912:

> When a patient is admitted he is kept at rest in bed for a probationary period, and when his pulse and temperature have shown that he is fit to move about he is allowed up for a short time. Next day he is sent for a short walk, and thus he is gradually brought along until he can walk eight or nine miles a day…he is gradually trained until he can do the heavy

---

[74] A. N. Robertson, Benenden Sanatorium 10th annual report, 1915

[75] C. T. Williams, Old & New Views on the Treatment of Consumption, *The Lancet*, 21st October, 1911, pp. 117-1124; R. W. Philip, Progressive Medicine and the Outlook on Tuberculosis, *The Lancet*, 31st July, 1909

[76] The concept of *auto-inoculation* was originally conceived by Sir Almoth Wright in the 1890s.

> navvy work of Grade D without fatigue, or undue rise of temperature.[77]

Work grades were assigned on Monday mornings, as at the Grosvenor, patients wore coloured badges to identify their status. Grade A patients were assigned jobs such as hoeing and weeding, whilst the attainment of Grade D entailed five hours of heavy work daily. W. J. Cox, Smyth's successor as Medical Superintendent, was convinced of the fundamental importance of *auto-inoculation* in the treatment of tuberculosis:

> If the patient is able to tolerate it, we may increase his dose of auto-inoculated *tuberculin* by giving him more exercise in proportion to his resistance and also to his physical powers. If he is showing signs of over-inoculation we must put on the brake and slow down his *tuberculin* production by giving more rest. If there is any secret of success in sanatorium treatment it is the observance of this simple rule.[78]

Exercise and work were regulated by the patient taking his temperature anally after work. Incautious over-exertion could result in fever and a relapse. In 1911 Smyth observed:

> After work the highest [temperature] was 102.4 Fahrenheit, after rest, in this case the temperature took two weeks to come down to its normal limits, and, therefore, presumably the patient was auto-inoculated too much'.[79]

At Grosvenor House between 1915-1919 half the patients were being treated solely by rest, graduated work and exercise, whilst the treatment of the other half was supplemented by drugs. The choice of treatment was decided by the resident Medical Superintendent employed at the time. For example Dr. Milne, arriving in 1919, discontinued the therapeutic use of *tuberculin* in particular cases, whilst he found the results of injection with *sanocrysin,* a preparation of gold, sodium and sulphur, to be encouraging in "bronchitic cases with copious sputum".[80] The side-effects of both these drugs were reported as being "traumatic".[81]

A range of other therapies were also constantly moving in and out of fashion. By 1914, although patients were still weighed regularly, less

---

[77] J. C. Smyth, Benenden records, 1912, LGB correspondence, NA MH 48/77
[78] W. J. Cox, Benenden records, 1912, LGB correspondence, December, 1914, NA MH 48/77
[79] J. C. Smyth, Ibid, 1914
[80] Grosvenor Sanatorium records, LGB correspondence, NA MH 48/76
[81] F. B. Smith, *The Retreat of Tuberculosis,* 1988

emphasis was placed on "kitchen physic":

> With regard to the diet, overfeeding has been avoided. In accordance with modern ideas, the administration of milk ad lib has long ago been abandoned at Benenden.[82]

At this time *heliotherapy* emerged as another therapeutic resource, and was to become prominent in the treatment of *lupus*, or tuberculosis of the skin, in ensuing decades:

> The beneficial influence of the sun's rays upon the skin should not be lost sight of. The "sunbath" is possibly quite as valuable to the body as the cold morning tub.[83]

In 1915 some Benenden patients were treated by *zomotherapy* whereby they were restricted to a diet of raw meat, apparently "with definite advantage".

In the same year two *artificial pneumothorax* operations were performed. This was a surgical technique employed from the late 1890s until the 1950s whereby air is injected into the chest cavity between the pleura and the lung in order to collapse the diseased lung and permit the organ to rest and its lesions to heal. Refills of air were required to be injected every three or four days. At Benenden the cases so treated were considered to be "distinctly improved, and the operation has given us a means of treating some otherwise hopeless cases".[84]

Carl Spengler's controversial IK serum was also employed but apparently failed to realise the promise claimed by its originator. The newly developed iodine therapy, however, reportedly achieved promising results in improving the general health of patients at Benenden. Surgery and laboratory medicine continued on an experimental level, each new treatment promising a spectacular breakthrough. However, from the late 1920s many doctors came to regard the main function of the sanatorium to be that of raising the resistance of the patient in order to counteract the *bacillus*.

The concept of *auto-inoculation* and the system of graduated labour has been elaborated at some length due to its neglect in recent accounts of sanatorium treatment, where it has either been ignored or treated as a

---

[82] W. J. Cox, Benenden records, 1914, NA MH 48/77

[83] Ibid.

[84] A. N. Robertson, Benenden records, 1915

medical justification for free labour.[85] Whilst the economic benefits derived from patient labour may have been a consideration for Medical Superintendents, it is evident from the records of all sanatoria operating in Kent that the therapeutic value of this treatment was not in doubt, and was in fact seen as central to building resistance to pulmonary tuberculosis.

The sanatorium routine at Benenden was rigidly structured. Patients rose at seven in the morning, took their temperature at least twice daily, were assigned graduated work, exercise or rest for an hour in the morning and afternoon, followed by a further hour of enforced rest and silence on the verandas. As may be imagined, in circumstances characterised by isolation and routine, where hope alternated with despair, the fundamental importance of strict discipline, and the inculcation of self-control, were central to the management of sanatoria.[86] Self control was the characteristic that distinguished the civilised from the bestial, and the compliant and redeemable consumptive from the expendable troublemaker.

Although a wilful contravention of the rules is often encountered in reports of sanatorium life, such behaviour was increasingly medicalised. Aberrant behaviour came to be seen as due to toxins from the *bacillus* affecting the central nervous system or, as the role of psychiatry in tuberculosis treatment became more pronounced, as part of a pattern of behaviour ultimately leading to resignation and acceptance of the patient's condition.[87] Nevertheless, failure to comply with the rules of the sanatorium could result in the patient's dismissal.

Autocratic management, loneliness and the lack of provision for dependants caused many patients to return home prematurely. Survivors were more likely to return to Poor Law relief than to find employment. Constantly inadequate funding, and often inadequate accommodation and diet, meant that many London Poor Law infirmaries were better equipped than sanatoria in Kent until the 1930s.[88] In addition the length of treatment was insufficient to achieve more than the beginnings of recovery and, consequently, and perhaps also as a result of food shortages, the mortality rate for tuberculosis rose during the war.

---

[85] cf. F. B. Smith, *The Retreat of Tuberculosis 1850-1950,* Beckenham, Kent: Croom Helm, 1988

[86] Dr. R. McFie, Medical Superintendent, Benenden, 1911, quoted in *Nursing Times*, 27th May, 1911; K. Figlio, Chlorosis and Chronic Disease in Nineteenth Century Britain, *Social History*, 3, No 2, 1978

[87] O. M. Holden, Mental Aspects of Tuberculosis, *The Practitioner*, 1922, p.109; E. Wittkower, *A Psychiatrist Looks at Tuberculosis,* London: NAPT, 1949, p.24

[88] I. Albery, MP for Gravesend, *Tuberculosis, Kent (Sanatorium Treatment),* House of Commons debate 12th November, 1930, Hansard, volume 244, cc1673-4

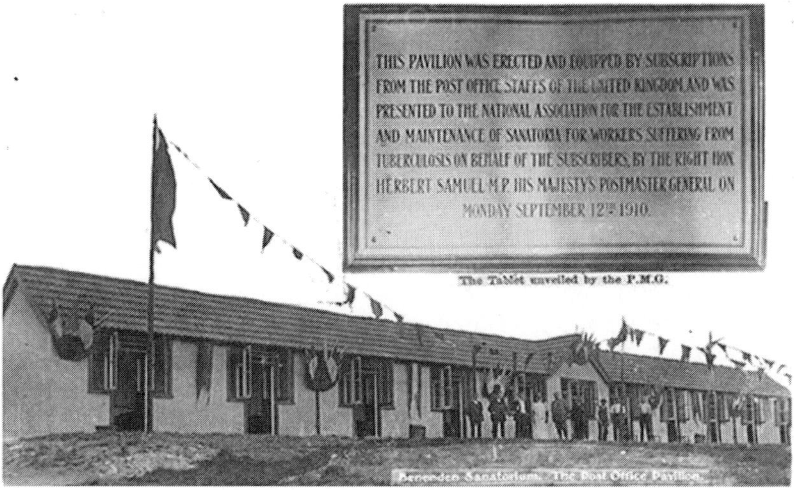
THIS PAVILION WAS ERECTED AND EQUIPPED BY SUBSCRIPTIONS FROM THE POST OFFICE STAFFS OF THE UNITED KINGDOM AND WAS PRESENTED TO THE NATIONAL ASSOCIATION FOR THE ESTABLISHMENT AND MAINTENANCE OF SANATORIA FOR WORKERS SUFFERING FROM TUBERCULOSIS ON BEHALF OF THE SUBSCRIBERS, BY THE RIGHT HON HERBERT SAMUEL M.P. HIS MAJESTY'S POSTMASTER GENERAL ON MONDAY SEPTEMBER 12TH 1910.
The Tablet unveiled by the P.M.G.
Benenden Sanatorium. The Post Office Pavilion.

Illustration 11.4: The Post Office Pavilion at Benenden Sanatorium, 1910.

Treatment of the tubercular was often harsh and patients were subjected to a range of experimental chemotherapies as well as daily maintenance and gardening work. Patients also appear to have been depersonalised and controlled in much the same manner as the destitute were treated under the Poor Law.[89]

Due largely to economic constraints, and the advent of the First World War, but also to the persistence of deeply entrenched evolutionist attitudes towards the poor and tubercular, both workhouse infirmaries and the harsh disciplinary ethos inherent in the Poor Law remained integral to the national struggle against tuberculosis until the dissolution of Boards of Guardians in 1929 and beyond. Although the rational and scientific administration of the sanatorium held the promise of a more egalitarian and socially progressive future for the working classes their chances of survival if diagnosed with tuberculosis had not improved significantly by the mid-1920s.

Public sanatorium treatment exemplified a programme of liberal health reform that was ostensibly humanitarian but led to an expansion of state control that reached into the subjective life of individuals. Bureaucratic and scientific structures dominated every aspect of the lives of patients, instilling into them an ethic of social responsibility and conformity.

---

[89] A. Bashford, Cultures of Confinement, p.139

The regimentation and control of the errant and infected body of the consumptive by the rational, scientific techniques of the expert occurred in a space that was moral as well as medical. Tuberculosis was viewed by many in the medical profession as a symptom of a more general moral and physical malaise,[90] often being associated with alcoholism and syphilis,[91] and treatment was supplemented with lectures and sermons that reinforced moral strictures relating to alcohol and sex.

The regulation of sanatorium life into a strict daily routine facilitated the inculcation of rigid values of social duty and personal hygiene; "things were rubbed into him there and became part of his existence, and when he went home he thoroughly realised what he had to do".[92]

Compliance in patients and ex-patients was achieved more through self-regulation than coercion. The sanatorium experience increased their awareness of the possibility of relapse and death and, at least at Beneneden, patients were instructed that they could not consider their disease arrested until they had been free of symptoms for two years, and that they should always refrain from visiting public places such as theatres and music halls.[93]

The public campaign against tuberculosis also contributed greatly to the hygienic self-regulation of the population as a whole. The delineation and standardisation of "healthy behaviour" and the creation of hygienically conscious citizens served to construct a medicalised norm that was reinforced by repeated precepts in workplaces, schools, churches and by health visitors. Families seen to deviate from this norm were increasingly liable to be labelled as anti-social, "dirty" and morally and hygienically suspect.

---

[90] G. Chatterton-Hill, *Heredity and Selection in Sociology*, London: Adam & Charles Black, 1907; R. A. Nye, Sociology: The Irony of Progress, *Degeneration*, eds. J. E Chamberlin & S. Gilman, New York: ColumbiaUniversity Press, 1985

[91] This was a common assumption amongst the medical profession at the time, see D. S. Barnes, *The Making of a Social Disease: Tuberculosis in Nineteenth Century France*, Berkeley, 1995; Dr J. Edward Squire, Senior Physician, Mount Vernon Hospital, quoted in *The Hospital*, 2nd December, 1911

[92] *East Kent Gazette*, 23rd July, 1910, reporting on the cost effectiveness of monthly educational stays in sanatoria, as opposed to 'curative therapy'.

[93] Anonymous Benenden patient, *Hospital Saturday Fund Journal*, 30th December, 1914

CHAPTER TWELVE

THE MEDICALISATION OF WORKING CLASS LIFE, 1912-1926

Medicalisation, the appropriation of previously personal and domestic space by the expert, together with the institutionalisation of individuals who failed to conform to the expert's standard of fitness, were the dual strategies employed in promoting the Edwardian middle-class ethos of hygiene, self-control and social responsibility. The hygienic mission of sanitary officers and health visitors to the poorly housed and malnourished in the early twentieth century disseminated a medicalised version of middle class mores and values.

From the 1920s the medicalisation of exercise and diet reflected a concern with strengthening the resistance of working class city dwellers to disease through the ministrations of organisations such as the League of Health. Self-sufficiency, physical exercise, cleanliness, sport, order, moderation and self-control were seen as essential to the cultivation of the English ideal of *mens sano corpore sano*.

Conformity to these principles was inculcated in schools, youth movements, factories, the church, the military and by government and charitable agencies and health visitors in order to establish the hygienic self-regulation of the population. The medicalisation of previously private aspects of family and community life, such as nutrition, the rearing of children and domestic and personal hygiene, meant in practice that, increasingly, all areas of working class life were becoming subject to state control and public health intervention.[1]

For example, reflecting the new concern with the health and welfare of mothers and children, particularly following the Report on Physical Deterioration of 1904, legislation designed to detect tuberculosis and other diseases in schools and factories was introduced at this time. The 1911

[1] J. Harris, *Private Lives,* 1993, p.231; A. Bashford, Cultures of Confinement, in *Isolation: Places and Practices of Exclusion*, eds. Caroline Strange & A. Bashford, London: Routledge, 2003, p. 135

National Insurance Act provided a framework, together with related legislation, such as the 1907 School Medical Services and the Maternal and Child Welfare Act of 1918, for the systematic supervision and treatment of sections of the population whose increased fitness or segregation from society, the government considered, would be of benefit to the future health and economic competitiveness of the nation.[2]

In 1912 tuberculosis specialist Robert Philip claimed that 30% of schoolchildren examined by him bore "tuberculosis stigmata", and cited the work of continental researchers showing that most working-class city children had been affected by tuberculosis by the age of fifteen.[3] The instilling of good sanitary habits into this urban youth who harboured the "seedlings of tuberculosis", was, he claimed, key to the reinvigoration of the nation. At an NAPT conference in 1914 Philip maintained that the alleviation of the tuberculosis problem lay in "projecting a searchlight into the home", and that "the object lesson of the sanatorium must be enforced in the home".[4]

Philip's metaphor implies a constant surveillance of working class homes in order to detect behaviour considered to be deviant or dangerous to the public health, rather than any intervention designed to improve the well-being or domestic conditions of working class families. The lesson of the sanatorium was complete deference and obedience to the professional classes and a perpetual struggle against dirt, often a vain pursuit for a large family living in old housing stock with a limited water supply and precarious income.

Early in the twentieth century the health visitor emerged as an employee of the local authority, albeit initially poorly trained and paid, and working class families became subject to increasing scrutiny from various health and welfare officials. Whilst the value to the nation of what was perceived as an aspect of preventive medicine was enthusiastically welcomed by the middle classes, these intrusions into the life of the poor were often resented. This was quaintly acknowledged in the presidential address to health visitors at the Folkestone Health Congress of 1921:

> People don't like to have numbers of visitors enquiring into their health and happiness. You and I, when we are tired, find it rather a bore, when some of our own acquaintances call for purely social reasons. Picture what we

---

[2] A. Hardy, *Health and Medicine in Britain since 1860*, Basingstoke: Palgrave, 2001

[3] L. Bryder, 'Wonderlands of buttercup, clover and daisies', 1992

[4] Sir R. Philip, Conference of NAPT, Leeds, 7th & 8th July , 1914, *The Lancet*, 18th July, 1914

should feel like if we had to interview instead all the different official visitors, to which the unfortunate working-class home is laid open'.[5]

The concerted action of the tuberculosis dispensary, school medical inspections and the various home visitors did apparently have a noticeable effect on the fitness of the working-classes in Folkestone after the War. In 1921 the Mayoress of Folkestone observed:

> It was a pleasure on a recent Empire Day to see in the March Past the improved physique of the boys and girls compared with those of the past decade.[6]

Although levels of nutrition for the working family had probably improved by this time the diet of the working classes was not prioritised by medical authorities. Rather, the health propaganda disseminated to the poor was essentially the moral and sanitary message of vigilance against dirt:

> it ought not to be difficult to ensure that a clean body should provide the healthy mind, and yet we find in the poorer homes there is a great lack of personal cleanliness. This is, no doubt, due to the bringing up of the Mother...[7]

Condemnation of the insanitary and immoral behaviour of elements of the working classes was at this time an invariable part of the campaign against tuberculosis. The NAPT contributed greatly to the stigmatisation of the disease, associating it with other social problems that were understood as being caused by inherited dispositions. In 1911 Dr. A. Maxwell Williamson, MOH for Edinburgh, speaking at the Annual Conference of the NAPT, saw the decline in the incidence of tuberculosis as being related to a reduction in venereal disease together with a decrease in *per capita* expenditure on alcohol. Alcoholism was, he asserted, "the most potent factor in propagating tuberculosis".[8] This perception of

---

5 G. Tuckwell, Presidential Address to Health Visitors at Folkestone Health Congress, 1921, *Journal of the Royal Sanitary Institute*, volume xlii, no.5, March 1922

6 Mrs. R. G. Wood, Address on Personal and Domestic Hygiene, Folkestone Health Congress, 1921, *Journal of the Royal Sanitary Institute*, volume xlii no.3, November, 1921

7 Ibid.

8 Dr. A. Maxwell Williamson, Transactions of the NAPT, Annual Conference, Caxton Hall, Westminster, July 19-21, 1911, London: Adlard & Son, p.24

alcoholism, syphilis and tuberculosis as related "social scourges" was not uncommon amongst the middle classes in the early twentieth century.[9]

What has been perceived by historians as the enlightened implementation of public health measures for the benefit of the masses was, in general, unpopular with the working classes, as was the National Insurance Act, partly due to the compulsory deductions imposed on workers.[10] The social stigmatisation and alienation experienced by the families of the tuberculous poor, whose homes had become the site of public inspection, and who were themselves the object of sanitary education with its associated moral implications, must have persuaded many sufferers to avoid tuberculosis dispensaries and health visitors and trust to the efficacy of patent medicines. The aversion of landladies to letting accommodation to consumptives and the fear of loss of employment has also been cited as a common reason for the tubercular adopting a life of secrecy concerning their disease.[11]

Although the emergence of what can be seen as "social medicine" potentially threatened the liberty of the individual, medical officials appear, in general, to have been mindful of England's tradition of individuality. Powers for the compulsory removal of advanced cases of tuberculosis from their homes to special isolation hospitals had been granted to local authorities, but there is little evidence of their being called into use.

Alfred Greenwood, Medical Officer of Health for Kent County Council, expressed his reservations on the question of the compulsory removal of consumptives shortly after notification was introduced:

> However important a measure this may be, I am not sure public opinion is ready for the general enforcement of such a step at the present time, whatever may happen in the future. At all events, I am of opinion that persuasion by the general medical practitioners, the Tuberculosis Officer and the Tuberculosis Nurse should be tried first. It is also obviously undesirable that any of these institutions should gain the reputation of being homes for the dying, if such can be avoided. It is a most difficult problem to solve.[12]

---

[9] H. de Carle Woodcock, *The Doctor and the People,* 1912, p.184

[10] G. R. Searle, *The Liberal Party: Triumph and Disintegration,* London: MacMillan, 1992, p.112

[11] E. Wittkower, *A Psychiatrist Looks at Tuberculosis*, 1949, p.82

[12] A. Greenwood, *KCC First Report upon Tuberculosis and the Administration of Sanatorium Benefit*, 1914, p.117

The apparent compliance of the working classes seems remarkable when one considers that thousands of people judged to be in an advanced stage of consumption were taken to isolation hospitals from which there was very little chance of returning. Both official and social pressure to seek treatment would, however, have been strong, and sometimes even family members were reluctant to continue living with a consumptive.

There is little evidence that medical treatment for the working classes improved before the First World War. Dr. F. J. Smith, a consultant doctor representing the Royal College of Physicians on the Departmental Committee on Sickness Benefit Claims under the National Insurance Act of 1914-16, declared in April, 1914 that medical provision for the working classes, including sufferers from tuberculosis, was "distinctly and emphatically" no better than in previous years. Furthermore, he claimed that doctors on local insurance panels were overburdened with patients, sometimes being responsible for more than 3,000 cases, and that the Poor Law culture of suspecting patients of malingering remained evident.[13]

The Report also confirmed that initially hardly any sanatorium treatment was available nationally, and that pressure was sometimes put on tuberculosis patients by sick visitors to cancel their claim for sanatorium benefit.[14] Mr. H. Dyer, General Secretary of the Royal Oak Benefit Society, remarked that there was a heavy drain on approved insurance societies due to there being no sanatorium treatment, and often no sanatorium benefit available for patients.[15]

This would have provided a further argument for transferring the responsibility for treating tuberculosis from Insurance Committees to County Councils. The Report noted an initial increase in sickness claims, especially by women, and particularly for chronic complaints which had often been neglected when the necessity of working had precluded treatment. It would appear that chronic illness amongst the civilian working classes was still largely untreated during the war. In 1916 the Chief Tuberculosis Officer for Birmingham warned that individuals diagnosed with tuberculosis should not stop work due to long waiting lists for sanatorium treatment and the consequent risk of increased poverty and malnutrition.[16]

Between 1915 and 1918 mortality and morbidity due to consumption increased substantially at both a national and a local level, despite the

---

[13] F. J. Smith, Report of the Departmental Committee on Sickness Benefit Claims under the National Insurance Act, 1914-16, Hansard, p.1143, Cd 7688

[14] Ibid., p.947, Hansard, Cd 7691

[15] H. Dyer, *Ibid.*, p.725, Hansard, Cd 7676

[16] H. Dyer, Hansard, Cd 7691, p.647; Hansard, Cd 7688-89

incidence of death from disease falling in general. Deaths from consumption had risen by 25% between 1913 and 1918, and by as much as 35% for women. It has been argued that this was as a consequence of deteriorating housing conditions due to a nationwide postponement of housing reform, reduced food supplies leading to malnutrition, in addition to large movements of workers, particularly women, from the country to urban munitions factories.[17] However, the fall in the death rate in 1920 to 9% below the rate in 1913 suggests that nutrition was a major factor.[18] The availability of food had increased in the immediate post-war period whilst overcrowding generally remained a problem until the 1930s.

In Folkestone notifications of tuberculosis rose from 43 in 1919 to 83 in 1920 following the influenza epidemic of the previous year, adding weight to the argument that infectious diseases can weaken resistance to tuberculosis, or reactivate old tubercular lesions. However it should be noted that, due to the stigma associated with tuberculosis as well as the pressure applied by local authorities for the tubercular to enter institutions, perhaps the majority of consumptive cases were not notified. As late as 1927 Dr. Rose Jordan, Tuberculosis Officer for Lewisham, recorded that 47% of deaths diagnosed as being due to tuberculosis in London were either not notified or notified only within three months of their death.[19]

Yunge-Bateman records that influenza spread most rapidly in families occupying small houses. Apparently the military were initially the most affected, probably spreading the disease through travelling in poorly ventilated trams between Sandgate and Folkestone. The epidemic struck in October 1918 and was over by 20th January, 1919, disproportionately affecting residents of the poorest districts.[20] Many of the 84 residents notified with pulmonary tuberculosis in 1920 had previously been affected by the influenza virus, the incidence being most common among domestic servants and servicemen. In the same year there were also 121 notifications of scarlet fever and 665 notifications of measles and german measles which may also have had an effect on the continuing high number of notifications for tuberculosis during 1922 and 1923.[21]

---

[17] L. Bryder, The First World War: Healthy or Hungry?, *History Workshop*, 24, 1987, pp.141-157.
[18] Ibid., pp.146-7
[19] *BMJ*, 21st April, 1928, p.692
[20] Yunge-Bateman, Folkestone MOH report, 1918
[21] Ibid., 1920

Table 12.1: Deaths from Influenza in Folkestone 1918-1919

	male	female	total
west ward	9	3	12
north ward	10	15	25
east ward	11	10	21

Source: Folkestone MOH report, 1918

A further cause of increased morbidity and mortality from tuberculosis during the war may well have been the virtual suspension not only of sanatorium treatment for civilians, but also of their isolation in Poor Law institutions as priority on waiting lists was given to ex-servicemen. Despite their being prioritised, the fact that tubercular ex-servicemen were still on waiting lists for treatment, and still being accommodated in Poor Law infirmaries themselves, remained a concern in the House of Commons as late as 1928.[22]

From August 1916 until June 1919 Elham workhouse and infirmary were used as a military hospital for Canadian soldiers[23] and, as happened at many Union infirmaries, the destitute sick were sent home to their families or housed in other institutions.[24] The Poor Law system survived the advent of compulsory insurance and, following the recommendations of the Majority Report of the Royal Commission on the Poor Laws, workhouse infirmaries were retained for the *residuum* and the "undeserving".[25] And, whilst County Councils managed their own tuberculosis schemes in the inter-war period, workhouse infirmaries continued to accommodate advanced consumptive patients.[26]

Some infirmaries appeared to function as both isolation units and clearing houses. According to a Ministry of Health report on the treatment

---

[22] J. Hayes, MP for Liverpool, House of Commons debate, November 12th, 1928, Hansard, cc 610-11

[23] *Elham Poor Law Union,* pamphlet produced by Kent Archives Service, p.2

[24] M. A. Crowther, *The Workhouse System,* London, Routledge, 1983, p.93; Marcus Paterson, superintendant of Frimley sanatorium claimed that cases of advanced consumption were housed in lunatic asylums during the First World War (Paterson, 1921)

[25] M. A. Crowther, Paupers or Patients? Obstacles to Professsionalisation in the Poor Law Medical Service Before 1914, *Journal of the History of Medicine and Allied Sciences*, 39:1, 1984, p.46;

[26] M. A. Crowther, 1983, p.96; Hansard, House of Commons debate 13th July, 1926, volume 198, cc303

of tuberculosis in Poor Law hospitals of 1922-23, infirmaries tended to be used for "chronic cases and as waiting places for early patients", who apparently received "very little treatment". Many of these had already undergone treatment at sanatoria. For instance, Miss Wyborne, a 49 year old single dressmaker was admitted to Islington infirmary in 1922. Described as a chronic case, she had previously been at the County Sanatorium in Lenham and attended the tuberculosis dispensary at Dover. She had been admitted to the infirmary through the workhouse and was waiting to be transferred to an institution at Eastry.[27]

In 1923 questions were raised in Parliament demanding to know what action was being taken to provide accommodation for the tubercular other than in Poor Law institutions, as had been the intention of the 1911 Act.[28] In that year 3,000 cases of tuberculosis were reportedly still being treated in London Poor Law infirmaries and charged on London rates.[29] In 1919 Lord Henry Cavendish-Bentinck, MP for Nottingham South, summarised the impact of the tuberculosis scheme:

> We know perfectly well that the sanatorium benefit by itself is perfectly useless. It is all very well for persons well-to-do, but to the poor man who has to go back to crowded surroundings and insanitary homes it is of very little use.[30]

Despite the shortcomings of the National Insurance scheme, the notification of pulmonary tuberculosis from 1912 and the inauguration of the dispensary system can be seen as providing an early model for the development not only of a nationwide system of public health, but for a wider form of state intervention into the moral life of the nation, and into working class culture in particular. It also heralded an unprecedented move towards professionalisation and specialisation in the field of medicine, even though coordinated administration was initially lacking. The diagnosis and treatment of consumption was gradually becoming standardised and, following this model, subsequent medical and educational structures, such as the health clinic, were elaborated in order to examine, categorise, regulate and educate larger sections of the population.

---

[27] Ministry of Health report on *Poor Law Hospitals, The Treatment of Tubercular Persons,* 1922-23, NA MH 55/145

[28] Mr. Briant to representative of Ministry of Health, Hansard, House of Commons debate, 7th March, 1923, volume 161, cc498-9

[29] Mr.Touche, Ibid.

[30] Lord H. Cavendish-Bentinck, House of Commons debate, 30th June, 1919, Hansard, volume 117, c 686

The compulsory notification of tuberculosis, like the earlier notification of acute infectious diseases, was accepted by the working classes and welcomed by the better off, who generally regarded it as the responsibility of the state to protect the population from infection. Changes in the treatment of tuberculosis signalled not merely an expansion of social medicine in order to improve the health of the poor and vulnerable, but the introduction of a system designed to protect the middle classes from possibly degenerate, and now potentially infectious, elements of the increasingly disaffected poor. In addition the dispensary system, already established in France, Germany and Scotland,[31] provided a new model for the surveillance and control of sources of infection, now perceived by many health officials as emanating from human rather than environmental sources.

[31] A. Latham & C. H. Garland, *The Conquest of Consumption*, 1911, p.31

CHAPTER THIRTEEN

TUBERCULOSIS AND HOUSING

Despite continued warnings by prominent public health professionals from the 1880s of the threat to the health of working class communities from poor housing and overcrowding these problems remained evident in many towns and cities well into the twentieth century. This is borne out in the case of Folkestone, where housing conditions in many working class districts did not improve until the mid-1930s.

In 1910 the Council's Hospital and Sanitary Committee again acknowledged the dilapidated condition of working class housing, but felt unable to implement orders to condemn properties under the Housing of the Working Classes Acts due to an acute shortage of housing and problems of overcrowding. A letter from the Local Government Board of 1913 reiterated the concerns of the previous decade, noting that the housing shortage resulted in the sub-letting of rooms and overcrowding due to insufficient building and the closing and demolition of houses. It recommended that the Council should act quickly to avoid liability under the Excess Sickness clause of the National Insurance Act:

> the Authority should accelerate their procedure so as to close the houses in the Borough which are unfit for human habitation more promptly, having regard to the provision of the National Insurance Act, whereby approved societies [insurance companies] can claim compensation from a local authority where the sickness experience is more than 10% above that expected when the Act was framed, and where such excess sickness can be proved to be caused by neglect of the Authority to enforce sanitary and housing provisions.[1]

However, the Council would have been aware that neither the LGB nor approved societies possessed any real power to enforce penalties.[2]

---

[1] Letter from LGB to Folkestone Borough Council, August, 1913, Folkestone Sanitary and Hospitals Committee Minute Book 1910-1913

[2] C. Bellamy, *Administering Central-Local Relations*, 1988, p. 245

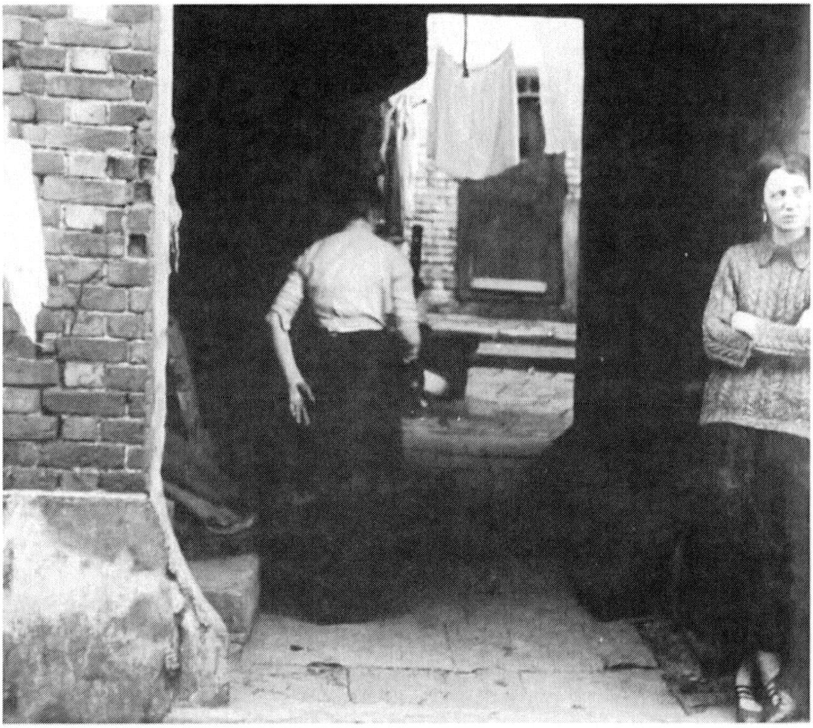

Illustration 13.1: Entrance to Dunns Alley, Folkestone, 1928.[3]

In May, 1917 Folkestone's Sanitary Inspector, John Pearson, wrote on behalf of the Borough Council's Sanitary and Hospital's Committee to the LGB requesting that the Board sanction the purchase and erection of temporary huts to house working class residents who were occupying various properties classified as unfit for human habitation.

In September the LGB replied that they were not in favour of the erection of huts for the displaced working classes of the town, and conditions appear to have remained the same in 1918. The health visitor, who was responsible for the supervision of cases of tuberculosis in the town, reported dozens of consumptives living in dirty and overcrowded homes such as the following:

Another case of tuberculosis reported – the patient and four children are

[3] Folkestone East Ward, 25th January 1928, EKAC Fo-S1/96/1

living and sleeping in one room. The kitchen is in a very bad state, there is no ventilation and practically no light. When the patient was asked why the family occupied one room she stated there was vermin in the bedrooms.

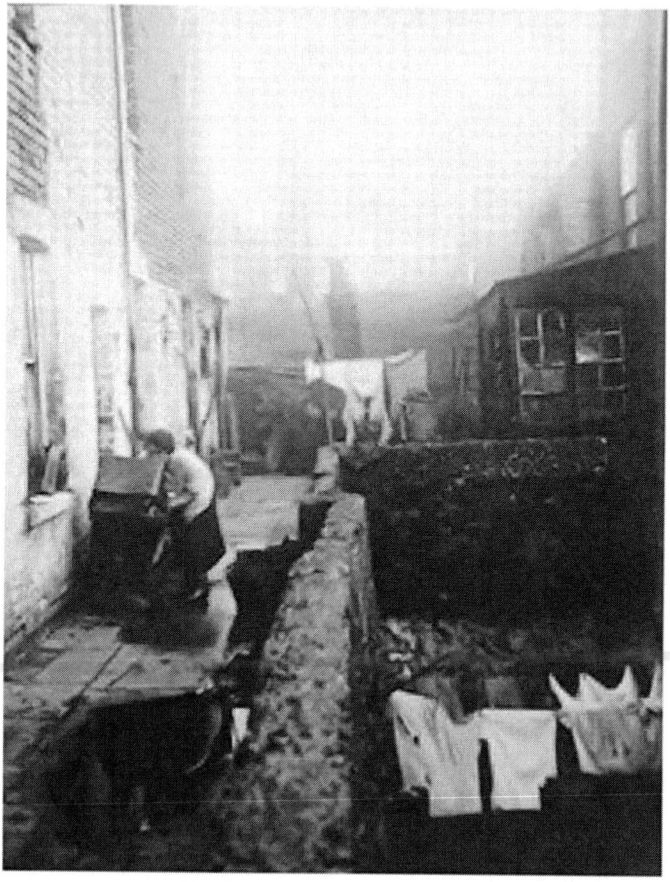

Illustration 13.2: Bates Alley, Folkestone, 1928[4]

After the war the shortage of housing for returning soldiers, overburdened welfare facilities and the task of reconstructing the dilapidated town exacerbated the existing class divisions in Folkestone. The renown and prosperity the town had enjoyed as an exclusive health

[4] Folkestone East Ward, 25th January 1928, EKAC Fo-S1/96/1

resort in the later nineteenth century was never to be recaptured. The relationships between social classes had also subtly but irrevocably altered.[5]

Workers were less ready to accept work that involved long hours in return for low pay. The wealthy found it cheaper to visit Mediterranean resorts, and Folkestone Councillors were forced to appeal to the upper middle classes to resort to the west of the town, while the east of the town began to be frequented by trippers from London's east end and elsewhere.[6]

The medical profession continued to lobby for housing reform, particularly in connection with the spread of tuberculosis. In 1920 H. H. Thomson, the MOH for Hertfordshire, citing the discovery of Dr. Tatham of the General Register Office that the death rate for tuberculosis in back-to-back housing in Salford was 5.2 per thousand compared to 2.8 where no such housing existed, asserted:

> It is no exaggeration to state that the solution of the problem of tuberculosis, more especially the pulmonary form of the disease, resolves itself into a solution of the housing problem with the abolition of those insanitary conditions of life of which tuberculosis is the most insistent and tragic expression.[7]

By 1918 there was a shortage of 600,000 houses in Britain which, in addition to food shortages, was the cause of widespread discontent leading to the threat of rent strikes.[8] The Folkestone and District Trades and Labour Council sent a letter to the Borough Council in December, 1918 expressing their serious concerns over the housing shortage for the working classes and anticipating:

> the dangerous social unrest that will inevitably ensue when the thousands of men that have been on His Majesty's Service return to civil life and find that no homes are available for many of them, and that no adequate provision has been made to remedy the shocking housing conditions that prevailed even before the war.[9]

---

[5] P. Donaldson, *Ritual and Remembrance: The Memorialisation of the Great War in East Kent,* Cambridge Scholars Publishing, 2006, p.19

[6] C. H. Bishop, *Folkestone: The Story of a Town,* 1973, pp.134-135

[7] H. H. Thomson, *Tuberculosis and Public Health*, pp.28-30

[8] G. Sutherland, Social Policy in the Inter-War Years, 1973, p.430

[9] Letter from Folkestone & District Trades & Labour Council, 26th December, 19 18, Folkestone Sanitary and Hospitals Committee Minute Book 1916-1919

They appealed against rising rents and threatened "uncompromising opposition, and in all probability a RENT STRIKE".[10] The Folkestone Express also reported that on 3rd January 1919 10,000 men had marched to the centre of Folkestone to voice their frustration with the slow process of demobilisation and the shortage of housing.[11]

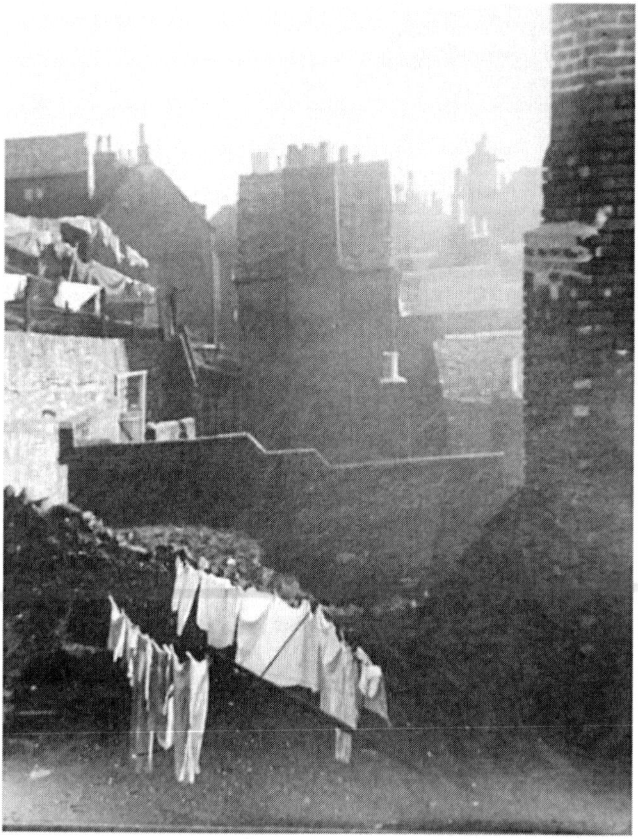

Illustration 13.3: Clouts Alley, Folkestone, 1928[12]

---

[10] Ibid.

[11] *Folkestone Express,* 15th May, 1920,

[12] Folkestone East Ward, 25th January 1928, EKAC Fo-S1/96/1

Although the working classes were more politically organised after the War, working class Councillors posed no significant challenge to the political establishment in Kent during the first half of the twentieth century. The Conservatives' dominated politics in East Kent throughout the 1920s with their share of the vote remaining above 65%.[13] One historian claims that "even committed activists" adopted a non-party approach when elected to local Councils, and that the local model does not, in this instance, necessarily conform to national trends.[14]

Folkestone's housing problems were exacerbated by the military occupying "nearly 100 of the largest houses in the town" whilst dozens more large houses remained empty. In 1919 the LGB suggested that these properties could be turned into flats for the working classes. But despite continued pressure from Yunge-Bateman, the Local Government Board, the Ministry of Health and the District Housing Commissioner the Borough Council continued to resist the accommodation of working class residents in formerly select areas of the town. They subsequently rejected the LGB's recommendations on the grounds that the houses were unsuitable for working class dwellings and converted them into high rent apartments.[15]

In order to deter mounting unrest the government introduced housing subsidies between 1919 and 1921. And, although not all local authorities responded, 170,000 houses were constructed in 1919.[16] In 1920 Sir Philip Sassoon's Model Housing Society eventually built sixteen cottages and eight flats for the working classes on Folkestone's East Cliff, taking advantage of subsidies provided under the Housing Act. However, the Ministry of Health was forced to intervene to prevent the local Council building the houses, mostly intended for fishing families, two miles from the harbour on a site that had previously been condemned as unsuitable due to poor drainage.[17]

---

[13] Sir Philip Sassoon was Conservative MP for Hythe (the constituency incorporating Folkestone) between 1912 and 1939.

[14] B. Atkinson, Politics, *Kent in the Twentieth Century*, ed. N. Yates, Woodbridge: Boydell & Brewer, 2001, p.184

[15] Folkestone Borough Council, Sanitary & Hospitals Committee, Minute Book November 1919-October 1921

[16] G. Sutherland, Social Policy in the Inter-War Years, 1973, p.430

[17] Folkestone Borough Council, Sanitary & Hospitals Committee Minute Book November 1919-October 1921. Following pressure from the Ministry only half of the development was situated on the Walton Farm site proposed by the Borough Council.

Yunge-Bateman's report of 1925 reveals no improvement. The expenditure on Poor Law relief had increased by about 60% from £3,084 in 1921 to £4,801 in 1925, and at least 270 houses were needed "immediately" for the town. He again observed that there existed a serious degree of overcrowding with "entire families inhabiting one or two small rooms" and sub-letting by tenants being a common practice. No houses had been constructed in the town since 1914 apart from the sixteen cottages and eight flats built on the East Cliff under Sir Philip Sassoon's Model Housing Scheme in 1920.[18] The overcrowded and insanitary area close to the fish market was not demolished until 1935, at which time the death rate for the district was still two and a half times greater than for the rest of the town.[19]

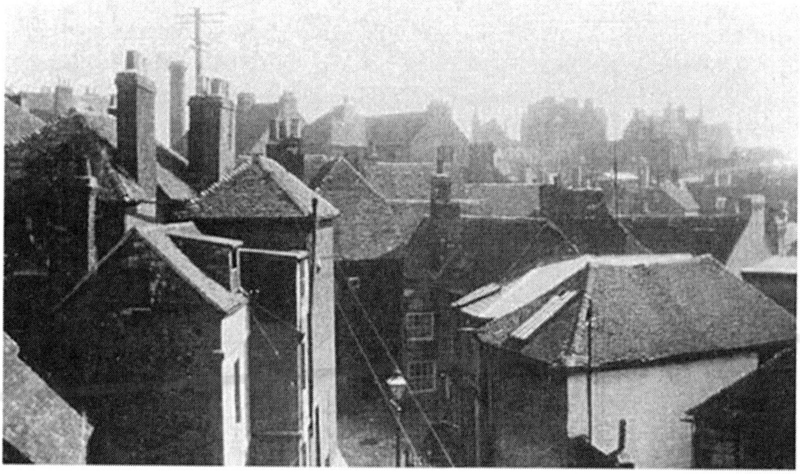

Illustration 13.4: Castle's Yard in Folkestone's crowded east ward c.1930. In the distance is St. Andrew's Convalescent Home on the East Cliff.

Lord Radnors' reluctance to improve working class housing in Folkestone typifies the widespread resistance to slum demolition and rehousing that still existed at the turn of the twentieth century.[20] This

[18] M. Yunge-Bateman, MOH report 1925, p.8, p.30

[19] *The Times*, 6th April, 1933; 16th February, 1934; 11th October, 1934

[20] D. Byrne and J. Keithley, *Housing and the Health of the Community,Unhealthy Housing: Research, Remedies and Reform*, London, Routledge, eds. R. Burridge & D. Ormandy,1993, p.57; N. McFarlane, Hospitals, Housing and Tuberculosis, 1988, p.75

suggests that housing reform was both ideologically and economically unacceptable to many at this time. It seems probable that deeply entrenched beliefs in the values of individualism and self-help, and concerns that granting material assistance to the poor would undermine their work ethic, contributed to the low priority attached to housing reform by many local authorities. In Folkestone, for example, slum housing continued to have a damaging effect on the health of working families until at least the mid-1930s.

CHAPTER FOURTEEN

PRESTON HALL SANATORIUM AND TUBERCULOSIS COLONY, 1919-1930

The early years of Preston Hall tuberculosis colony provide an example of the disregard and abuse that virtually powerless victims of tuberculosis could be exposed to in sanatoria. Between 1920 and 1924 the tuberculosis settlement apparently operated as little more than a corruptly managed and poorly disciplined dumping ground for tubercular ex-servicemen.

Preston Hall, at Aylesford near Maidstone, began as a private philanthropic enterprise. Originally opened in 1919 as a sanatorium and settlement for tubercular soldiers and sailors, the management sought to maintain it through creating a self-sufficient colony for ex-patients. The sanatorium was approved by the Ministry of Health in March, 1920 under the management of Chief Medical Officer Dr. T. L. Bonar, and by the following year the Exchequer had sanctioned grants to provide accommodation for 50 ex-patients in addition to a total of £43,560 being invested to fund the 242 bed sanatorium.

The management of the sanatorium was problematic from its inception. Bonar's "dictatorial manner" and his tendency to summarily discharge men he considered unsuitable was reminiscent of the workhouse and led to criticism from the British Legion. According to Ministry of Health records Bonar had no compunction in dismissing patients in order to benefit from their tuberculosis pensions and training bonuses, which were paid to the colony by the Ministry of Pensions but forfeited by patients on their dismissal.

Patients and colonists, who expected to remain for life, were reportedly intimidated by Bonar's dictatorial power and his dog. Their vulnerability was underlined when their welfare committee was disbanded by Bonar after requesting him to reconsider two such dismissals.[1] Although it would

[1] Ministry of Health records of Preston Hall,NA MH52/73 LGB correspondence, NA MH 52/66

have involved the loss of benefits and possible destitution for their families about half the 1921 admissions had left or wanted to leave.[2]

By 1923 another £10,000 had been granted by the government for the construction of a further 25 cottages. 1,119 men had been treated and trained since the sanatorium opened, in 1924 there were 555 men, women and children in the colony, rising to 654 in 1928, 122 of whom were settlers and 131 under treatment in the sanatorium.

Colonists and their families originally reared poultry, pigs and bees and, from 1928, printing and fibre and leather case making and angora rabbit breeding were added to the colony's enterprises. As their payment from the Ministry of Pensions stopped when they ceased to be patients, they were paid fifteen shillings per week by the enterprise, less two shillings and sixpence for heating and lighting, for working a 44 hour week.

Despite complaints by colonists of inadequate wages and training and poor conditions the Chief Medical Officer was supported by Preston Hall's executive committee, whose chairman described the colony as "happy and contented", and Bonar as:

> a man of outstanding ability, and one of the best administrators; his whole interest in life is in the welfare of the Colony, which without him would not have reached its present stage of development.[3]

The committee found no evidence of any need for an enquiry, and the complainants were characterised as agitators suffering from "that irritability of manner to which tubercular patients are particularly prone".[4]

Eventually, in 1924, an enquiry was initiated by the Ministry of Health, and complaints were compiled by the British Legion, 103 men being interviewed over three days. It was found that patients and trainees had been exploited as labourers, the commercial development of the colony taking precedence over the training, and that supervision and procedures for complaints were poor. In addition the hygiene, food and accommodation were found to be inadequate and, as a consequence, the health of the patients had not improved. The inside of huts were covered in snow in winter, blankets were never fumigated and spitting was said to be

---

[2] F. B. Smith, *The Retreat of Tuberculosis*, p.83

[3] Letter to Ministry of Health from G. Reeves Smith, chairman of Preston Hall Executive Committee, December, 1923, LGB correspondence, MH 52/66-70

[4] Letter to Ministry of Health from G. Reeves Smith, chairman of Preston Hall Executive Committee, December, 1923, LGB correspondence

promiscuous and not discouraged.[5]

Poor morale had resulted in financial scandals involving the organisation of boxing tournaments for which public donations had been solicited. In addition, Dr. Chapman of the Ministry concluded that there existed:

> a universal want of confidence shown in him (Bonar) as in the institution generally by the men here...[and that] gambling, drunkenness and immorality have gone on very little checked.

No action was taken against Bonar, who by this time was in an advanced stage of consumption, and it appears he lived out his days amongst the colonists.[6]

In 1925 the colony was placed under the management of the British Legion and the ultimate control of Pendrill Varrier Jones, Chief Medical Officer of the celebrated Papworth Hall Tuberculosis Colony in Cambridgeshire, for reorganisation. By 1927 a new Chief Medical Officer, Dr. McDougal, had introduced a more co-operative spirit to the colony, placing more emphasis on therapy than had previously been the case.

Despite a Ministry of Health directive of 1922 that advanced cases, particularly those living with children, needed to be isolated for the remainder of their lives in tuberculosis hospitals or "in suitable wards of other residential institutions",[7] and that sanatorium treatment of intermediate cases be "limited to that necessary to restore their general health and working capacity,"[8] McDougal's patients included "a considerable number" with advanced tuberculosis, many intermediate and few early cases. As at Papworth Hall consumptives in all conditions were now accepted and treated, sometimes for years. Varrier Jones believed that even cases that were generally considered hopeless could be effectively treated by *auto-inoculation*.[9]

A constant supply of patients was also necessary in order to support the colony as no further funding from the Ministry of Pensions was available

---

[5] Enquiry on Preston Hall by Dr. Chapman, Ministry of Health, 28th July, 1924, MOH records, NA MH 52/66-73

[6] Ibid.

[7] LGB records of Tuberculosis Treatment Schemes, MH55/130, circular 280, January, 1922. Marcus Paterson, 1921, claimed that cases of advanced consumption were housed in lunatic asylums during the war.

[8] Ministry of Health Treatment Schemes, LGB correspondence, National Archives, MH 55/130

[9] Marcus Paterson, *The Shibboleths of Tuberculosis*, London: John Murray, 1920

for settlement and training from 1928, and the Ministry of Health refused to encourage local health authorities to send patients to Preston Hall at the expense of the County Sanatorium at Lenham.[10] Dr. Chapman, visiting on behalf of the Ministry in January, 1928 was, however, reassured to find "no indication that patients are retained to keep the beds occupied or to afford cheap labour to the industries".[11]

Table 14.1: The expansion of Preston Hall Tuberculosis Settlement

	1925-6	1926-7	1927-8	1928-9
Average number of settlers	49	82	117	134
Average sanatorium patients	70	107	140	150
Profit or loss	£1,563.00	£875.00	-£2,328.00	-£4,420.00
Profit or loss per settler	£31.00	£11.00	-£20.00	-£33.00

Source: Ministry of Health records of Preston Hall, National Archives

That year there were 111 settlers and 147 ex-servicemen in the sanatorium but fewer received a pension, which was only awarded in the case of tuberculosis being contracted during war service. Whilst it was anticipated that civilian patients would eventually have to be accepted, the British Legion urged that colonists be limited to the relatives of ex-servicemen.

McDougal felt that the colony was inadequately supported by the health authorities, partly due to its being perceived as primarily a settlement rather than a sanatorium. In 1929 he persuaded his executive Council of the importance of Preston Hall's sanatorium, and initiated interviews with representatives of local authorities in order to attract patients. By October 1929 the sanatorium's 180 beds were constantly filled and the population of the village was 539 with an average age of 37. Settlers' wages were about one shilling per hour for a 40 hour week and rents were between four and nine shillings per week [12]

The losses for 1927-29 were due to a fire and to the bankruptcy of a supplier, however, notwithstanding this setback the experiment was largely

---

[10] Ministry of Health, Correspondence relating to Preston Hall Tuberculosis Settlement 1928-1931, NA MH52/73

[11] Ibid.

[12] Ibid.

seen as a success. As well as isolating notoriously difficult consumptive ex-servicemen at an estimated total cost of £525 per settler in 1930 it provided some purpose in the lives of men who had often repeatedly undergone the tedium of sanatorium treatment.[13]

Recommendations for the expansion of tuberculosis village settlements had been published by the Inter-departmental Committee on Tuberculosis of 1919, however the proposals were rescinded during the post-war economic slump in the cost-cutting Geddes Report of 1922. By 1930 the Ministry of Health:

> more and more realised that substantial economy could be achieved by maintaining patients in settlements instead of throwing them on the Poor Law.

Consequently, in 1930, the Ministry of Health proposed the establishment of "five or six" new tuberculosis settlements.[14]

The combination of moral and medical instruction characteristic of sanatorium life provided an early template for later institutions and social strategies intended not merely to categorise the socially defective, but to foster compliance with the state and indoctrinate moral and hygienic values through, for example, the development of physical exercise and sport in schools, industry and the armed forces, and the introduction of health centres and psychiatric hospitals.

The provision of sanatorium treatment following the National Insurance Act of 1911 was probably the first instance of state intervention into the "minutiae of social life",[15] the mores, habits and beliefs of the working population of Britain.

By the late 1920s a different emphasis was placed on the function of sanatoria, brought about largely due to the experimental work of sanatorium doctors, and a shift away from a primary focus on the *bacillus* becomes evident. In accordance with the views of Varrier-Jones at Papworth and Paterson at Frimley, Dr. James Watt, Medical Superintendant of the King George V sanatorium at Godalming, articulated this change of approach in 1932, claiming that the development of immunity through the open-air regime, a healthy diet, rest and exercise was more effective than a focus on the *bacillus*:

---

[13] Memo by Dr. Coutts, Ministry of Health, Correspondence relating to Preston Hall, 28th June, 1928, National Archives, MH52/73

[14] MoH memo, Ibid.

[15] D. Armstrong, *The Political Anatomy of the Body*, Cambridge University Press, 1983

> while Medical Officers of Health and bacteriologists tended to concentrate their efforts in fighting tuberculosis on avoidance of infection, clinicians – particularly those working in sanatoriums – were far more impressed with the state of the patients' defences. The facts that no child living in the tuberculosis village settlements at Papworth and Preston Hall had developed tuberculosis, that members of the staffs of sanatoriums living among open cases showed no greater incidence than the general population, and the relative infrequency of conjugal tuberculosis, led to the conclusion that even repeated or continuous dosage [of the bacillus] was not the cause of the disease.[16]

An initial focus on the dangers of infection posed by tuberculosis had, despite reassurances to the contrary by many experts in the disease, intrinsically informed measures contained in the 1911 Act and subsequent government legislation relating to the disease. This emphasis on isolation and hygienic training had sidelined recommendations by pioneering sanatorium administrators and public health experts, contained in the report of the 1912-13 Committee on Tuberculosis, that social reforms would provide the most effective means to counter the disease.

These proposed reforms to improve housing and ameliorate the appalling conditions of many working families had largely been ignored by Asquith's government. However, the experience of public sanatorium treatment persuaded many doctors that tuberculosis would be more effectively controlled through improvements to the general health and living conditions of the working classes.

---

[16] Dr. J. Watt, Annual Conference of NAPT, London, *The Lancet*, 30th July, p. 241, 1932

CHAPTER FIFTEEN

PUBLIC HEALTH AND SOCIAL REFORM, 1922-1930

The view that the active onset of tuberculosis was triggered when the immune system was somehow compromised due to poverty, sickness or anxiety was not uncommon in the English medical profession throughout the first half of the twentieth century. This perspective, sometimes linked to theories of constitutional predisposition to the disease, was supported by the researches in Switzerland of Nägeli in 1898 and Reinhart in 1917, which revealed the almost universal presence of tubercular lesions in post-mortem studies of urban inhabitants.[1]

Increasingly, as the twentieth century progressed, influential public health workers and physicians emphasised the improved resistance to the disease to be gained through the provision of better housing and nutrition for the poorest and most vulnerable members of society.[2] And by the inter-war period tuberculosis came to be perceived by the English medical profession more as an endemic disease that was occasionally rendered active due to adverse environmental and genetic factors than as a simple consequence of inhaling the *bacilli*.[3]

Thus an exclusive concern with the eradication of the *bacillus* was by no means a monolithic response in public health discourses relating to tuberculosis. As one historian of medicine has observed:

> Twentieth century opponents of the pasteurisation of milk...argued that

---

[1] M. Morris, The Past & Future of the Crusade Against Tuberculosis, *BMJ*, 16th November, 1918, p.539

[2] F. B. Smith, *The Retreat of Tuberculosis*, 1988, p.224

[3] Dr. C. H. Browning, Glasgow University, 12th Annual NAPT conference, *BMJ*, v.2 (3418), 10th July, 1926, p.67. The researches of Reinhart of Berne in 1917, claiming that 96% of children tested there gave a positive response to the tuberculin test, also helped to consolidate this perspective, quoted in M. Morris, The Past & Future of the Crusade Against Tuberculosis, *BMJ* 16th November, 1918, p.539

> some exposure to tubercle bacillus was necessary. In their view a tubercularised body was a healthy body, resistant to the onset of disease.[4]

Indeed, in the 1930s the medical profession remained undecided as to whether an early infection conferred immunity or contributed to the onset of later disease.[5]

Exposure to the sun and fresh air, it was widely believed, improved immunological resistance to tuberculosis and was seen as hugely beneficial for the urban inhabitants of dark and ill-ventilated homes. In 1916 George Newman, then Chief Medical Officer to the Board of Education, saw the introduction of the open-air school, which had been pioneered in Germany, as potentially revolutionary for the future health of the nation:

> No one can measure the national gain that will accrue from their increased well-being, even as no-one can estimate the loss in defective and devitalised man-power which the nation has sustained for many years, due to the lack of appreciation, and even systematic neglect, of the value to the body of fresh air and sunlight. The open-air school is a simple and economical way of applying a method of national education to the susceptible mind and body of the child.'[6]

For Newman, who was appointed Chief Medical Officer to the Ministry of Health in 1919, the benefits of sunlight and fresh air on urban slum dwellers appeared to offer more hope for preventing disease than the development of laboratory medicine. Indeed the aim of the new ministry was to consolidate the idea and practice of preventive medicine which was tied to a vision of broader social and behavioural reform, and for the first time a department solely responsible for combating tuberculosis was established under Dr. F. J. H. Coutts.[7]

Although the Ministry of Health has generally been seen as a continuation of the LGB in all but name,[8] a more reformist approach can

---

[4] D. Cantor, The Diseased Body, *Medicine in the 20th Century*, ed. R. Cooter & J. V. Pickstone, Harwood Academic Publishers, 2000, p.351

[5] F. J. H Coutts, ex-Senior Medical Officer of Health to the Ministry of Health and head of department responsible for tuberculosis, espoused the former view. NAPT Annual Conference, *The Lancet*, 30th July, 1932, p. 241.

[6] G. Newman, Report of CMO to Board of Education, 1916, quoted in L. Bryder, 'Wonderlands of Buttercup, Clover and Daisies', 1992, p.77

[7] A. S. MacNalty, Tuberculosis Work in England, *The Lancet*, 26th January, 1924, p.167

[8] G. Sutherland, Social Policy in the Inter-War Years, 1973, p.425

be detected, and for the inter-war period, it has been argued, the attention of the medical profession was focused on the "soil", the constitution, general fitness and environment of the individual, at least as much as on the "seed" or germ.[9]

This shift in approach towards prevention of the disease is apparent in the attitude of medical professionals confronting the problem of tubercular infection from milk. The eradication of the disease in cows was one aspect of the campaign against tuberculosis that had made little headway, due largely to obstruction from agricultural interests. The increasing focus on the health of the child was, however, eventually to result in a more systematic regulation of the milk supply. In September, 1918 a London conference of Sanitary Inspectors declared themselves:

> of the opinion that, in view of the prevalence of tuberculosis in Great Britain, and of the suffering, pauperism, and death resulting therefrom, the sale and consumption of tuberculous milk and meat should, in the interest of public health, be made impossible,

and urged the government to enact legislation to abolish private slaughterhouses and to secure the health of the national herd.[10] Possibly due to the government's attention being directed towards the global influenza pandemic at this time no measures were enacted.[11]

By 1921 the work of local sanitary authorities had effected little or no improvement in dairy herds, and it was claimed that from 6-10% of milk supplied to the public contained *tubercle bacilli*, and that 42% of the nation's herds were infected with tuberculosis.[12] Fears of a loss of milk production and the expense of systematically *tuberculin* testing cattle had resulted in lengthy government procrastination, despite the recommendations of two commissions on tuberculosis. Eventually, during the 1930s, the Peoples' League of Health initiated a campaign for *tuberculin* tested milk, but it was not until the Milk Act of 1949 that all milk was ordered to be pasteurised or tested.[13] As the Director-General of the Army Veterinary

---

[9] S. Sturdy, Hippocrates and State Medicine, 1998, p.16

[10] Quoted in Folkestone Hospitals and Sanitary Committee minute book, Nov. 1916-Oct. 1918

[11] In an outbreak from October-December 1918 58 people died from influenza in Folkestone and many more in Shorncliffe Barracks.

[12] S. G. Moore (MOH Huddersfield), Milk and Disease, paper read at Folkestone Health Congress, *Journal of the Royal Sanitary Institute,* volume xlii, no.4, January 1922

[13] L. Bryder, *Below the Magic Mountain*, 1988, p.247; G. Jones, *Social Hygiene*, 1986, pp.76-77

Service commented in 1922:

> one is inclined to the opinion that too much consideration is being given to vested interests, and not enough to the welfare of our nation's greatest asset, our children'.[14]

From an analysis of post-war medical journals it becomes evident that neither medical or veterinary experts were in agreement on the causes or means of eradicating the disease. In 1920 a letter from the Research Institute in Dairying at Reading to the *British Medical Journal* drew attention to the recent tendency of farmers' trade journals to report expert opinion downplaying the effects of infection and suggesting that the virulence of the *bacillus* was over-estimated. Quoting a medical opinion previously published in the same journal stating that:

> the tendency of modern thought is to challenge the whole germ theory of tuberculosis and to shift the angle of vision from specific to social causes of the disease,

the correspondent requested that a sufficiently prestigious body representing the medical profession be asked to advise whether or not it was a worthwhile endeavour to attempt to eradicate *tubercle bacillus* from the nations milk supply.[15]

This gradual shift of focus amongst many health professionals from the germ to the social and economic conditions of the working classes was significant in that it precipitated a move away from measures of isolation and disinfection towards a more holistic concern with nutrition, exercise, improved housing and the relief of poverty. In the same issue of the *BMJ* Dr. C. Muthu, a physician from the Mendip Hills Sanatorium and the author of a recent book on the treatment of pulmonary tuberculosis,[16] questioned the emphasis on the dangers of infection from tuberculous milk and *bacilli* in general at the expense of focusing on social conditions:

> Not till England comes to see, as America has done, that tubercle bacillus is no longer tuberculosis can any progress be made in solving the problems of tuberculosis. The theory that "stamp out bacteria and you will stamp out disease" is becoming more and more untenable at the present day...Here

---

[14] Major-General Sir Layton Blenkinsop, Presidential address at Folkestone Health Congress, *Journal of Royal Sanitary Institute*, volume xlii, no.5, March 1922

[15] R. Stenhouse Williams, letter to *BMJ* 4th December, 1920, p.873

[16] C. Muthu, *Pulmonary Tuberculosis and Sanatorium Treatment*, London: Baillière, Tindall and Cox, 1910

> lies the beginning of the tragedy of the tuberculous child. Improve the social and economic and moral conditions of the people, so that the country may rear strong and healthy mothers who would feed their children with their own milk, then tuberculosis among children will become as rare as in so-called savage countries.[17]

This change of emphasis during the 1920s, from a concern with infection towards an understanding of active tuberculosis as invariably being due to low immunological resistance caused by poor living conditions, did not, however, result in any change in health policy.[18] Too much had been invested in sanatorium treatment by this time, and there was also the moral improvement (as recognised by Dr. Muthu above) of the working classes to consider. The NAPT, who included many owners of private sanatoria,[19] certainly continued to stress the importance of alcohol and sexual promiscuity in the spread of the disease.[20]

The form of treatment for pulmonary tuberculosis offered in sanatoria during the 1920s had altered little from that practised in the 1850s. In fact the shift of focus adopted by much of the medical profession from the identification and disinfection of the germ to a broader environmental approach can be seen in general as a reversion to the pre-germ theory approach of developing the body's resistance to tuberculosis. Diet, rest, fresh air and regulated exercise under the strict supervision of an experienced physician remained central to sanatorium treatment.

This utilisation of the healing powers of nature to effect a cure was at the heart of the form of preventive medicine which came to the fore in the early twentieth century, and particularly in the inter-war years when it was championed by George Newman, the first Chief Medical Officer of the Ministry of Health.

Newman encouraged an understanding of the body as a responsive, organic whole, capable of defending itself against disease if provided with sufficient nourishment and fresh air. Following the example of Hippocrates, the good physician, he advised, should work with and not against nature;[21] the martial metaphors derived from a tradition of Enlightenment inspired science advocating the mastery and control of

---

[17] C. Muthu, *BMJ*, 4th December, 1920, pp. 872-3

[18] N. McFarlane, Hospitals, Housing and Tuberculosis, 1988, p.75

[19] Ibid, p.84

[20] A. M. Williamson, Transactions of the NAPT, Annual Conference, Caxton Hall Westminster, July 19-21, 1911, London: Adlard & Son, p.24

[21] G. Newman, *An Outline of the Practice of Preventive Medicine: A Memorandum Addressed to the Minister of Health,* London: HMSO, 1919, p.39 quoted in S. Sturdy, Hippocrates and State Medicine, 1998, p.16

nature were giving way to a new appreciation of the efficacy of natural therapeutics:

> it is this *vis medicatrix naturae*, no longer an abstraction but an ordered sequence of actions and reactions, which the wise physician and surgeon will seek not to destroy or pervert but to release and supplement at the bedside.[22]

This movement away from a reductionist focus on germs to a more holistic approach becomes increasingly apparent after about 1925. As the influential Dr. F. R. Walters stated in 1927:

> It is a mistake to regard the disease as mainly due to infection. Lack of resistance, temporary or permanent, together with the conditions of life, have much more to do with it. In proportion as a community becomes immunised against *tubercle*, so does the relative importance of causes other than infection increase.[23]

And, in the same year, this view of the disease was supported by John Robertson, MOH for Birmingham, who contended that healthy people would not contract tuberculosis.[24]

This shift from associating the spread of tuberculosis with the *bacillus* to a greater focus on environmental conditions was pioneered to a great extent by the staff of sanatoria and Medical Officers of Health and reflects a growing awareness that tuberculosis was a disease of poverty. Dr. D. P. Marais, visiting from South Africa in 1932, remarked that English perceptions of consumption had:

> gone from the extreme of frightening people by talking of the universality of infection by tuberculosis to the opposite extreme of suggesting that infection was of very little importance.[25]

This shift of perspective, propagated mainly by public health officials, eventually led to wider social reforms as a focus on developing the natural resistance of individuals to tuberculosis was consolidated in the later 1920s and 1930s. For example, reflecting a greater acceptance of the

---

[22] G. Newman, *An Outline,* 1919, p.21

[23] F. R. Walters, On Estimating the Value of Remedies in Pulmonary Tuberculosis', *The Lancet*, 11th June, 1927, p.1272

[24] Sir J. Robertson, NAPT 13th Annual Conference, *The Lancet*, 9th July, 1927, p.69

[25] Dr. D. P. Marais, NAPT 18th Annual Conference, *The Lancet*, 30th July, 1932, p. 242

effects of poor housing on health, mortality and morbidity statistics for tuberculosis were consistently employed during the inter-war period in attempts to promote slum clearance.[26]

This broader approach to public health is also evident at a local level for the inter-war period. In October 1921 Austin Priestman was employed by Folkestone Borough Council as Assistant MOH, School Medical Inspector, Medical Inspector of Aliens and Maternity and Child Welfare Officer.[27] He was to serve as Folkestone MOH from 1925 to 1936, and his perspective on infection provides a further example of this more holistic approach to disease, and a contrast to his predecessor Yunge-Bateman's emphasis on the isolation and destruction of the bacillus. Writing in the *Medical Officer* in 1935 Priestman argued that nature can provide a more effective resistance to the onset of disease than a vaccine as long as the individual is healthy, well-nourished and fulfilled:

> It is safer to help man and his resistance through the healing channels of work and food and recreation, and to leave to Nature an immunisation which she will give, perhaps more slowly than we wish, but more efficiently and with a more true economy.[28]

Here preventive medicine is directed towards strengthening the immune system and general health of the individual rather than adhering to a bacteriological model focusing on isolation and vaccination. In an article entitled "Epidemic Diphtheria" in the *Medical World* of 1931, Priestman typified the attitude of many medical professionals in the inter-war period in advocating the therapeutic effects of fresh air, sunlight and nutrition rather than artificial immunisation:

> Rather than attempt wholesale immunisation by artificial means we should adopt the same plan of campaign against *bacillus diphtheriae* as we adopted against the bacillus of tuberculosis—namely, provide better ventilated, better lighted and better equipped schools, and feed all children who need feeding.[29]

Priestman's approach to countering tuberculosis in his capacity of School Medical Officer was to emphasise that improvements in nutrition and living conditions for the poorest, both at home and at school, would develop their resistance to disease. He blamed the incidence of

---

[26] D. Byrne & J. Keithley, Housing and the Health of the Community, 1993, p.61

[27] Report of Folkestone Health Committee, 1921-23, Fo/AmC12/11

[28] A. Priestman, *Medical Officer,* 9th March, 1935, p.99

[29] A. Priestman, *Medical World*, 6th February' 1931, p.627

tuberculosis on overcrowding, density of population, "bad home conditions" and poverty. In a paper on tuberculosis amongst schoolchildren in Folkestone published in 1925 he concluded that the efforts of the medical profession were largely negated due to the persistence of poverty and poor housing. His research, he claimed, demonstrated:

> the righteousness and urgency of the lamentation of medical officers of health, which says "all efforts made by the medical profession to alleviate and abolish the incidence of tuberculosis and other diseases, some of which, especially measles and whooping cough, act either as predisposing agents or as wind for a smouldering fire, are frustrated by economic and housing considerations".[30]

Priestman was also convinced, as were many of his contemporaries, of the existence of an hereditary predisposition to tuberculosis. His understanding of tuberculosis reflects the tradition of statistical research into the disease pioneered by Francis Galton and continued by Karl Pearson, Leonard Darwin, Major Greenwood and others of a eugenic persuasion in the inter-war period. It also provides evidence of the persistence of evolutionist ideas. Priestman's School Medical Officer's report of 1929, for example, records that 14.2% of tuberculosis cases examined were the result of an inherited predisposition.[31]

This concern with heredity reflects the emergence of a more socially oriented approach to medicine that incorporated elements of sociology and biology. During the inter-war years the marriage and reproduction of the tubercular, for example, was actively discouraged by the medical profession, abortion occurred "on a considerable scale", and the sterilisation of tubercular women was commonly recommended by doctors in order to avoid the generation of children possessed of a tubercular *diathesis* or predisposition.[32]

The new political landscape following the war, the ardent struggles for reconstruction, the impact of the Russian revolution and the antagonism felt by many younger professionals and intellectuals towards the unregulated capitalism of the previous generation all contributed to a more egalitarian vision of social progress for many young doctors.

---

[30] A. Priestman, Hygienic and Economic Factors in the Incidence of Tuberculosis Amongst School-children, *British Journal of Tuberculosis,* volume 19, pt.3, 1925, p.150

[31] Ibid.

[32] *BMJ*, 5th December, 1931, p.1059; *The Lancet*, 4th November, 1933, p.1056; F. B. Smith, *The Retreat of Tuberculosis*, p.230

For some, preventive medicine and social reform were linked with evolutionary inspired theories of social planning. One manifestation of this tendency was a socialist ideal of public health, informed by eugenics, and pioneered by, amongst others, Julian Huxley and John Ryle.[33] The perception of tuberculosis as an hereditary affliction also reinforced the social stigma associated with the disease. The identification of tuberculosis in a family could result in the loss of employment through fears of contagion, but equally a sense of shame in being marked out as having "tainted blood" was often very real. As late as 1949 a nursing sister confessed "when I first knew I had TB I was horrified. I felt as if I had a slur on my character".[34]

Priestman's synthesis of natural therapeutics, heredity and bacteriology exemplifies a return to a more holistic approach to medicine, characterised by open-air schools, a focus on health as well as disease, and a greater willingness to question the advances of science following the disjunctures of war. This move away from an over-reliance on bacteriology, also contributed to by the Lübeck tragedy of 1921, when 249 babies were mistakenly injected with massive doses of *tubercle bacillus,* also led to the introduction of the BCG vaccine for tuberculosis being deferred in Britain until the 1960s, whereas on the continent it was widely adopted in the 1920s and 1930s.[35]

The positivist and newly standardised perception of both the *tubercle bacillus* and the infected body, that had been employed in the national fight against tuberculosis from the late 1890s was, to a large extent, superseded in the inter-war years by an understanding of the disease as a more protean and dynamic process, and the body as an interactive part of a larger environment.

---

[33] D. Porter, John Ryle: Doctor of Revolution?, D.&R. Porter eds., *Doctors, Politics and Society: Historical Essays,* Amsterdam, Atlanta, 1993, p. 257

[34] Miss M. C., quoted in E. Wittkower, *A Psychiatrist Looks at Tuberculosis,* London, 1949, p.21

[35] R. & J. Dubos, *The White Plague: Tuberculosis, Man and Society,* Rutgers University Press, [1952], 1987, p.123

CONCLUSION

In conclusion this study of Folkestone and Sandgate can be summarised in three interconnected points. Firstly, it demonstrates that the causes of tuberculosis, as well as the choice of medical responses, remained contested by the English medical profession throughout the early twentieth century, and contradicts accounts of a paradigmatic shift in medical attitudes following Koch's work on tuberculosis in the 1880s.[1]

This examination of responses to the disease highlights how scientific knowledge was framed in accordance with specific political perspectives. These divergent interpretations of medical theory can only be understood with reference to early twentieth century culture and ideology and reflect conflicting attitudes to the related problems of chronic disease and poverty.

Secondly, Part III shows that historians have both overestimated the impact and misinterpreted the significance of the introduction of sanatorium treatment for the working classes. Very few civilians were treated in sanatoria in Kent before 1930, improvements to public health were minimal, and the main effect of the 1911 National Insurance Act was to undermine the power of workers' Friendly Societies.

Thirdly, this account of cultural change in Folkestone and Sandgate, highlighting disparities in social class, is essentially the story of resistance by a local elite to external pressures for reform. This research demonstrates the extent to which local power structures, seeking to maintain traditional social values and protect economic interests, can deflect forces for change. In this instance Folkestone Borough Council resisting pressure to improve local housing and enforce the inspection of milk. It considers the relationship between the MOH, the Borough Council and other local institutions, and underlines the distinctiveness of the local and its particular interrelation with outside forces. For example, the Local Government Board's intervention to prevent closure of the Sandgate sanatoria, and how this controversy contributed to the debate on infection and precipitated calls for the compulsorary notification of tuberculosis

[1] e.g. K. C. Carter, The Development of Pasteur's Concept of Disease Causation and the Emergence of Specific Causes in Nineteenth Century Medicine, *Bulletin of the History of Medicine*, 65, 1991, p.548

nationally.

The expert testimony provided at the reading of the Sandgate Bill by a succession of experienced and prestigious medical professionals demonstrates that Arthur Newsholme's conviction of the importance of isolating consumptives in an early or intermediate stage of the disease was a minority view by 1905. In the following year the LGB inspector, Timbrell Bulstrode, in his Report on Sanatoria, concluded that:

> the presence of the *bacillus* may not be such an overwhelming factor in the causation of the malady as was once supposed; ... the resistance of the body to the *bacillus* is the major factor.[2]

In Bulstrode's opinion consumption was mostly caused by a weakened constitution which was often hereditary but could also be due to malnutrition, overwork, poor housing and the debilitating effects of other diseases. He believed that the decline in the tuberculosis death rate from the 1870s was the result of improvements in sanitation, cheaper food and improved housing and was unconnected with the discovery of the *tubercle bacillus*.[3]

On the other hand this study shows that a concern with the infectiousness of tuberculosis was evident in Folkestone particularly in 1898 and 1899. As recounted in chapters six and seven both Charles Fitzgerald in 1898, and Marcus Yunge-Bateman in 1899, strongly advocated measures to counter the infectiousness of tuberculosis which, Yunge-Bateman claimed, had been established through research "during the last few years".[4] 1899 was also the year in which Arthur Newsholme initiated a scheme for the isolation of consumptives at Brighton, and in which the NAPC was founded with the express intention of alerting the public to the infectious nature of tuberculosis.[5]

This research identifies the influence of economic, social and political interests at both a local and a national level on the interpretation and application of medical theory. A focus on the infectiousness of tuberculosis both facilitated arguments for the institutionalisation of poor consumptives

---

[2] H. Timbrell Bulstrode, *Report on Sanatoria for Consumption,* 1905-1906, p.117

[3] H. Timbrell Bulstrode, On the Causes, Prevalence and Control of Pulmonary Tuberculosis, *The Lancet*, ii, 1903, pp. 76, 206, 304-5

[4] C. E. Fitzgerald, The Prevention of Tuberculosis, *The Lancet*, 8th October, 1898, pp.932-933; Folkestone MOH Report on Consumption, Folkestone Sanitary & Hospitals Committee Minute Book, 1899, Fo-Amc12/1

[5] A. Newsholme, Public Health in Relation to the Struggle Against Tuberculosis, *Journal of Hygiene*, iii, 1903

and sidelined demands for social reform. The Liberal government's intervention in public health was not merely due to the failure of traditional philanthropic structures to cope with problems related to destitution and chronic disease.[6] Reformist legislation also demonstrated that concerns over the health of the nation were being addressed, and managed to deflect attention away from the wretched conditions in which the industrial classes lived and worked.[7]

Government responses to the problem of tuberculosis were primarily motivated by political ideology and expediency. The recommendations of a majority of Medical Officers of Health and sanatorium administrators that addressing social and economic factors such as housing, employment and nutrition were paramount in combating tuberculosis were ignored in favour of more short term solutions such as the notification, isolation and supervision of working class consumptives. Bacteriological explanations for the spread of tuberculosis were employed selectively by politicians, social reformers and some in the medical profession. They were employed to reinforce a well established and apparently successful sanitarian approach to the prevention of tuberculosis that emphasised the dangers associated with an unclean home and immoderate behaviour.

This incorporation of bacteriology within an essentially sanitarian perspective provided the necessary scientific justification for the comprehensive indoctrination of the working classes into the rituals of *bourgeois* cleanliness, sobriety and industry.[8] Much of this social propaganda, particularly the promotion of breastfeeding, and the growing ability of MOHs to apply pressure to local authorities to improve water resources, was beneficial to the health of the working classes.

However, the benefits to health of ritualised domestic hygiene, essentially a confused moral and sanitarian antipathy to "dirt" – in a Chadwickian sense - were limited whilst slum housing and chronic poverty remained unaffected. It was not until the re-emergence of a more holistic approach to health during the inter-war years when some of these social and economic factors, such as poor housing and tuberculous milk, were addressed that the problem of tuberculosis was more successfully contained. The campaign against tuberculosis demonstrates how, throughout

---

[6] K. Laybourn, *Modern Britain Since 1906*, London: Tauris and Co., 1999

[7] F. B. Smith, 1988, p.168; N. McFarlane, Hospitals, Housing and Tuberculosis, 1988, p. 85

[8] Whilst the accommodation of germ theory within older medical models has been acknowledged few aspects relating to the import of this phenomenon have been elaborated, with the exception of M. Worboys, *Spreading Germs*, Cambridge University Press, 2000

the 50 year period under study, medical knowledge can be variously formulated to highlight infection, immoral and insanitary behaviour, inherited predisposition or poverty as the primary cause of the disease.

The introduction of the 1911 National Insurance Act was designed chiefly to appease middle class fears of social degeneration and to undermine politically and ideologically inspired initiatives aiming at more far reaching social reforms. It served to overshadow the political challenges of both the SMOHs campaign against destitution, and that of "municipal socialism", whereby local Acts of Parliament to initiate health reforms had been passed, mostly by London boroughs and northern industrial towns.[9] The Liberal Party largely rejected the advice of public health experts to improve the living standards of the urban poor, acting mainly on the recommendation of Timbrell Bulstrode's more eugenically influenced report on sanatoria for the LGB.

This extension of state health control was then chiefly motivated by economic and political concerns relating to the control and regulation of manpower. In particular, the expansion of medical and welfare structures can be seen as directly related to a burgeoning "eugenic consciousness" at the beginning of the twentieth century whereby more social planning was seen to be required by government in order to avert what was widely perceived as the threat of a "biological crisis".[10]

At a time when rational economics and notions of national efficiency were mobilised in the service of a failing empire, and particularly in the inter-war years, conceptions of the hereditary nature of consumption served, for many of the middle classes, as an explanation for the perceived deterioration of the health of the nation. This view of tuberculosis as indicative of a degenerate hereditary strain led to calls for the permanent isolation of consumptives in colonies, and even their sterilisation as a means to the scientific promotion of a healthier stock.[11]

At Folkestone these social Darwinist attitudes towards the chronically sick and destitute were institutionalised in the local Charity Organisation Society and the Elham workhouse. The individualist principles of the Folkestone COS continued to hold sway at least until the war. Poverty and sickness were also largely viewed by the sanitary department and the local establishment as being due to the working classes' own ignorance and neglect. Consequently legislation that permitted the Council to implement

---

[9] D. Watkins, The English Revolution in Scientific Medicine, 1984, p.440

[10] *BMJ*, 1929, p.114; R. Overy, The Morbid Age, Britain Between the Wars, London: Allen Lane, 2009, pp.100-105

[11] G. Jones, *Social Hygiene in Twentieth Century Britain*, Beckenham: Croom Helm, 1986, p.22

improvements to the housing or diet of the poor was resisted as long as possible.

In Kent the implementation of Part II of the National Insurance Act from 1912, originally intended to provide sanatorium treatment nationally, can hardly be seen as constituting a watershed in state health care. This research demonstrates that most men and women suffering from tuberculosis were still treated at home or in Poor Law institutions well into the 1920s.[12] This account of tuberculosis treatment in Kent largely continuing to be managed by mutual aid societies, independent entrepreneurs, charitable agencies and the Poor Law is at odds with the assumption of many historians of medicine[13] that Koch's discovery of the *tubercle bacillus* prompted a revolution in attitudes towards the disease that led to universal sanatorium treatment.

Chapters eleven and twelve show that few real improvements to the health of the working classes were achieved in the two decades after the National Insurance Act of 1911, with little if any more treatment for the tubercular than had been provided by Friendly Societies, religious charities and some workhouse infirmaries. A significant effect of the introduction of state sanatorium treatment was an erosion of the power of workers' Friendly Societies as providers of health insurance and treatment for consumptive workers which, in turn, strengthened the financial independence of the medical profession.[14] The consolidation of doctors opposed to the dominance of Friendly Societies and medical clubs is exemplified in Folkestone by their boycotting of the Provident Societies Medical Association and the establishment of a doctors' Medical Association.[15]

The stated intention of Asquith's 1908-1916 government was to separate the treatment of tuberculosis from the Poor Law and to restore thousands of tuberculous workers to a condition of employability.

---

[12] LGB correspondence relating to Sanatoria in Kent, NA MH 48/74-78

[13] S. L. Cummins, *Tuberculosis in History*, London: Baillière-Tindall, Cox, 1949; R.Y. Keers, *Pulmonary Tuberculosis: A Journey Down the Centuries*, London, Baillière-Tindall, 1978; H. Williams, *Requiem for a Great Killer: The Story of Tuberculosis,* London: Health Horizon, 1973; W. Spink, *Infectious Diseases: Prevention and Treatment in the Nineteenth and Twentieth Centuries*, Folkestone: Dawson, 1978; K. C. Carter, The Development of Pasteur's Concept of Disease Causation and the Emergence of Specific Causes in Nineteenth Century Medicine, *Bulletin of the History of Medicine,* 65, 1991; F. Ryan, *The Forgotten Plague,* New York: Little, Brown, 1993

[14] D. G. Green, *Working Class Patients*, 1985, p.149

[15] *The Lancet*, 22nd December, 1894, p.1498; 29th December, 1894, p.1574, 18th March, 1905, p. 378; *Folkestone Up-to-Date*, 14th December, 1895, p.6

However, this restructuring of the management of tuberculosis generally failed to diagnose and treat cases before the onset of advanced disease, and contributed little to the improved health or productivity of the nation. Although the incidence of tuberculosis continued to fall, apart from a resurgence of the disease between 1915 and 1918, the evidence from sanatoria in Kent strongly suggests that although sanatorium treatment may have been effective in treating tuberculosis, the insurance system lacked the necessary funding and after-care needed to sustain the health of patients. Where records for the survival of sanatorium patients in the county exist they show that few survived more than five years after being discharged.[16]

In contrast to criticism of tuberculosis experts for pusuing sanatorium treatment when survival rates were so poor, this research finds that superintendents of sanatoria and MOHs were largely unequivocal in stressing that poor living conditions and unemployment were the cause of relapses in ex-patients.[17] There was a general belief in the benefits of open-air therapy. The failings of the system can rather be seen as due to a lack of political investment or intent.

After the war the effectiveness of the sanatorium experiment was increasingly criticised, chiefly on the grounds of inadequate investment which dictated that treatment rarely exceeded three or four months, and a general lack of after-care often leading to a reactivation of the disease. Subsequently more stress came to be placed on environmental considerations in regard to the treatment of the working classes, such as nutrition, housing and employment, and the development of more self-sufficient colonies for the tubercular were planned.

The advantage of a local study is that it offers a more nuanced picture than emerges from national studies. Public health problems and solutions in England varied regionally as well as over time.[18] Previously neglected details and factors specific to particular localities can illuminate the impact of wider social, economic and ideological currents on the lives of individuals and communities. And more general and abstract debates, such as that focusing on reasons for the decline of tuberculosis during the

[16] W. J. Cox, Medical Superintendant, Annual Report, 1914, LGB correspondence, Benenden Sanatorium, 1912-1918, NA MH 48/77

[17] F. B. Smith, *The Retreat of Tuberculosis*, 1988, pp.244-245

[18] C. Hamlin, *State Medicine in Great Britain,* D. Porter, ed., *The History of Public Health and the Modern State*, Amsterdam, Rodopi, 1994

twentieth century, can be more readily contextualised.[19]

This examination of tuberculosis in Folkestone and Sandgate illustrates how contrasting meanings were assigned to the disease along lines of social class. It compares the promotion and practice of open-air therapy as a cure for tuberculosis amongst the affluent with the extension of this treatment to the working classes. Whilst various studies of seaside resorts have charted their economic and demographic expansion,[20] very little research has focused on the influence of climatology in general, or open-air therapy in particular, in the growth of the coastal resort.

This relatively neglected chapter in medical history is important for an analysis of disparities in medical treatment and living conditions between social classes. It provides an example of how a privileged ideal - in this instance the quasi-symbolic purification of lungs perceived to be infected with the corrupt breath of a degenerate underclass - is translated into a harsh regimen of discipline, social isolation and exposure to the elements.

This study also reveals these towns' history of social polarisation and their dual aspects as both exclusive health resorts and as centres of poverty and disease. Folkestone's rapid success led to overcrowding in the cramped, overbuilt and increasingly neglected working class districts of the town. Epidemics of infectious disease in the poorest districts particularly affected the health of children. Whilst the de Bouverie family's investment in the creation of a well-located, spaciously planned and exclusive health resort had provided employment for thousands of working people, consideration of their health and welfare remained secondary to the promotion of the town's reputation as a socially exclusive health resort.

The Lord of the manor and much of the local establishment with financially vested interests in the resort were not deeply connected to the area, many having retired there or moved to Folkestone for their health. This enterprise designed to attract affluent health seekers was run entirely through private investment and lacked any ethos of social cohesion or co-operation that had characterised the original community of boatmen and fishermen.

The refusal of the Borough Council to implement the majority of Yunge-Bateman's proposed preventive measures against tuberculosis and

---

[19] T. McKeown, *The Modern Rise of Population*, 1976; J. M. Winter, Public Health and the Political Economy of War, 1988, pp.163-173; L. Bryder, The First World War: Healthy or Hungry?, 1987, pp.141-157

[20] S. Farrant, London By The Sea, 1987; J. Hassan, *The Seaside, Health and the Environment*, 2002; D. Cannadine, *Lords and Landlords,* 1980; J. K. Walton, *The British Seaside*, 2000

their reluctance to invest in their sanitary department reflects the predominantly *laissez faire* approach to local government and public health held by Folkestone Councillors and Poor Law Guardians at the beginning of the twentieth century. Similarly, Lord Radnor's attempts to prevent disclosure of inadequate and overcrowded housing in Folkestone underlines how the short term social and economic interests of power elites were able to obstruct public health interventions.

The ground landlord, supported by the Borough Council, most of whose members had financial interests in Folkestone's reputation for exclusivity, was largely responsible for ensuring that house construction for the working class population continued to be restricted in order to maintain the town's "social tone". Before 1918 the middle and lower middle classes predominated in the electorate, the raising of local rates for reform was unpopular, and very few members of the Borough Council represented the interests of the working man (women of course still having no rights to representation).

Apart from their exploitation as a source of labour, the Sunday sermon and the appeals to sobriety and morality of churchmen and women and pious local charities, intervention in the lives of the working classes had traditionally been minimal. This relative unconcern for the health, living conditions and habits of the working classes in Folkestone was not altered significantly until the appointment of Marcus Yunge-Bateman and John Pearson to Folkestone Council's Sanitary Department in the 1890s.[21]

Yunge-Bateman's training in bacteriology undoubtedly inspired his initiation of a variety of preventive public health interventions in the lives of Folkestone's working classes. But although the MOH slowly acquired more authority and influence over the implementation of health measures following the Liberal reforms of the early twentieth century, his powers remained subordinate to the interests of the privileged until the late-1920s. Despite his successful intervention in effecting improvements to the quality and supply of water, sanitation, childcare and domestic hygiene, successive MOHs lacked authority to address the problems of infected milk and overcrowding until the 1930s.

Another original contribution to medical history provided by this study is the part played by seaside convalescent homes in the treatment of tuberculosis. The tubercular were usually only admitted to general hospitals for the relief of acute symptoms and, before the availability of sanatoria for the working classes after the First World War, there were few specialised institutions, such as the Brompton Hospital, for consumptives.

---

[21] EKAC-Fo/A/M/c/12/1-7

This presented a critical problem particularly for Friendly Societies and Boards of Guardians in industrial towns and cities where destitution and tuberculosis were inter-related problems.[22] Seaside convalescent homes at this time not only relieved overcrowding in urban workhouse infirmaries, but provided a form of open-air therapy that was already established as an effective treatment for the more affluent, and probably extended the working lives of consumptive members of Friendly Societies and Trade Unions.

From the mid-1880s a combination of workers' mutual aid societies, private enterprise and charitable institutions run by religious organisations had provided treatment for poor consumptives sent by some local authorities, Boards of Guardians and Friendly Societies. Convalescent homes within these sectors often provided the only respectable means of relief from a cycle of overwork and chronic disease for working men and women who had contracted tuberculosis. Although patients generally received only a minimum of attention from doctors, and nurses often lacked any formal training, convalescent homes, many of which were to be found on the south coast of England, played an important role in the care of the tubercular from about 1880 until the 1920s which has been almost entirely overlooked.

Highlighting local differences that diverge from other accounts of the history of tuberculosis, this study shows that the National Association for the Prevention of Tuberculosis had a limited role in Folkestone. Religious charities and Friendly Societies played a more important part in the care of the tubercular.[23] The local COS and Board of Guardians were largely composed of Borough Councillors, churchmen and retired military officers, and constituted a form of civil power that shared many of the values and interests of the governing elite. Both organisations operated a system of granting relief for the chronically ill that was morally selective and bitterly resented and feared by the working classes.

---

[22] Evidence of Dr. M. Quarry, M.O. Lambeth Union, Minutes of proceedings before the Select Committee of the House of Lords on the SUDC Bill, 22nd March, 1905, pp.236, 245; Report of RCPL, appendix volume ii, 26th June 1906, Cd.21253, 21271-3, 21290, 4499, pp.993, 1004, 1013; RCPL, volume xlii, p.92; J. S. Davy, Report for the Local Government Board on the Sandgate Homes, 23rd December, 1898; J. S. Davy, Head of Poor Law Division, Royal Commission on the Poor Laws, 1909, appendix volume i, 19th February, 1906, Cd. 4625, 3808; The Renewal of the Sandgate Sanatoriums Scandal, *The Lancet*, 18th June, 1904

[23] F. B. Smith, *The Retreat of Tuberculosis*, 1988; L. Bryder, *Below the Magic Mountain,* 1988

These paternalist structures served to distinguish the respectable and industrious from the undeserving poor. The function of the local Board of Guardians and the Charity Organisation Society was to deter pauperism, reliance on the state and charity and to encourage self-reliance. This individualist ethic conflicted with a more centralised vision of social health modelled on preventive medicine.

By only being available when consumption became so advanced as to render the sufferer incapable of work, Poor Law and charitable relief was inimical to the introduction of public health measures designed to prevent infection. The attitudes and concerns of members of both organisations indicate that they were influenced by a social evolutionist perspective that viewed pauperism as a mark of biological deficiency.

The changes to approaches in public health during the period under study in Folkestone can be characterised according to the attitudes of the towns three successive Medical Officers of Health. William Bateman's term of office pre-dated the concern with preventive medicine adopted by his nephew Marcus in the wake of the growing acceptance of the infectious nature of tuberculosis. William's joint role as Poor Law Officer would have involved aggregation of the sick in the workhouse infirmary at a time when tuberculosis was a fact of life amongst the working classes, and a fatalistic attitude to the spread of the disease amongst the destitute was common.[24] No provision either for its treatment or for financial assistance would have been available other than outdoor relief or, possibly, a sponsored visit to the Brompton Hospital for Consumption in the rare case of a benefactor being found.

Marcus Yunge-Bateman's interventionist approach to disease and his focus on the prevention of infection, particularly in 1898 and 1899, reflected a new optimism in public health and the treatment of disease involving laboratory testing, the identification of carriers and the disinfection, education and isolation of infected individuals.

After the war and the influenza pandemic Austin Priestman was more concerned with the body's immunological resistance to disease and maintaining the economic and social support that ensured individual and social health:

> There can be little doubt that, as with the great bulk of diseases in elementary school children, the cause is primarily weakened resistance to disease brought about by insufficient or unsuitable feeding, or both,

---

[24] Miss M. Loane, a district nurse writing in 1909, comments on the fatalistic attitude held by many of the older generation with regard to the outcome of disease in general, Outlines of Routine in District Nursing, London, 1909, p.146

> combined with parental ignorance of the simplest rules of domestic hygiene.[25]

Whilst, like his predecessors, condemning parental ignorance, if not neglect, Priestman was convinced that poverty was the prime cause of disease, particularly tuberculosis, and he argued for improvements in diet, housing and better conditions in workplaces and schools in order to reduce the spread of the disease. This evidence of a movement away from a focus on infection in the 1920s, together with the research on Preston Hall industrial colony, supports the contention that a more holistic and environmental approach emerged in medical practice at this time.[26]

Doctors, politicians, social reformers, international development agencies and historians have all tended to frame the issue of tuberculosis according to their political sensibilities and values. The response of individuals and institutions with a vested interest in maintaining the political and economic *status quo* in a global society characterised by great economic disparities remains in essence the same as that adopted by the Liberal government in 1911. The testing of target populations and medium term treatment of the tubercular, often including isolation. This approach to community health, supported by powerful multi-national pharmaceutical corporations, still largely predominates in national and international health programmes.

Conversely, echoing the appeals of MOHs such as Arthur Ransome and Austin Priestman, other academics and commentators on public health and global politics continue to emphasise that treatment that ignores the social and economic conditions of the tubercular is ineffectual and that only a determination to ensure adequate housing, diet and sanitation can effect a sustainable reduction in deaths from tuberculosis.[27]

---

[25] A. Priestman, Work of the School Medical Officer, London: Oxford University Press, 1915

[26] S. Sturdy, Hippocrates and State Medicine, 1998, p.16; N. McFarlane, Hospitals, Housing and Tuberculosis, 1988, p.75

[27] P. D. van Helden, The Economic Divide and Tuberculosis, *EMBO Reports*, volume 4 (supplement), June, 2003

BIBLIOGRAPHY

Primary Sources: Manuscripts

East Kent Archive Centre

G/EL/3/1-20, Elham Union Application and Report Books, September 1902-March 1930

G/EL/4/4/5, Elham Union Ladies Visiting Committee Books, 1894-1952

G/EL/4/3/4/2, Elham Union Register of Deaths, 1898-1914

Fo/A/M/c/1-5, Folkestone Borough Council Minutes of Committes, 1836-1898

Fo/A/M/c/5/17, Folkestone Borough Council General Purposes & Miscellaneous Committees Minute Book, November 1894-June 1895

Fo/A/M/c/12/1-14, Folkestone Borough Council Sanitary & Hospitals Committee (Health Committee from 1921) Minute Books, January 1898- October 1931

Fo/A/M/c/23, Folkestone Borough Council Special Committees, October 1912-July 1918

Fo/Z/1/A/D/1-10, Folkestone COS Diary & Committee Report Books, 1886-1920

Fo/Z/1/A/M/1-4, Folkestone COS Minutes of monthly meetings, January 1886-September 1913

Fo/Z/1/F/2-3, Folkestone COS Journals for Relief, February 1908-July 1923

FoZ/1/C, Folkestone COS, correspondence, 1907-1940

Fo/Z/2/C, Folkestone Soldiers and Sailors Help Society, correspondence, 1905-1912

Fo/A/Z/6, Folkestone Health Congress, 1904, papers and memoranda

Fo/A/Z/7, Folkestone Health Congress, 1921, papers and memoranda

F/1987/8, Manuscripts of Samuel Pilcher, 1839-c.1912

Fo/A/Z/6/4, Pearson, J. *Milk Supplies and their Dangers, with Local Experiences*, paper delivered at Folkestone Health Congress, 1904

Fo/L/5/9, Report on the Sanitary Condition of Folkestone, 1893

Fo/L/5/17, Report on the Sanitary Condition of Folkestone, 1894

Fo/L/6/7, Report on the Sanitary Condition of Folkestone, 1918

Fo/L/7/1, Report to the General Board of Health on the Sanitary Condition of Sandgate, 1849-1850

UD/Sg/A/M/1/6-16, Sandgate LBH & UDC minutes, 1881-1921
UD/Sg/A/M/4/1-2, Sandgate UDC Special Purposes Committee, 1900-1906
F/1954/3/Q2, Sandgate Dispensary minute book, 1875-1946,
UD/Sg/A/M2/2-3, Sandgate UDC minutes of committees, 1908-18

Victoria Hospital annual reports, 1893-1904
MH/SEK6/1/1/4, Victoria Hospital committee minutes, April 1897-October 1909

Benenden Chest Hospital
Annual Reports
Scrapbooks

Berkshire Record Office
D/EX1675/1/12/21/1, records of Community of Saint John the Baptist, St. Saviour's Mission, Folkestone, 1887-1955
D/EX 1675/14/2/1-6, records of the Community of St. John the Baptist, St. Andrews, Folkestone, 1875-1919
D/EX1675/14/1/1, Minutes of Transactions at Council meetings & building committee meetings, St. Andrews Home, Folkestone, 1881-1935

British Library
Jones, J. J. *Advantages of the Dominion of Canada*, December, 1883, rare books section

Canterbury Cathedral Archives
CCA-DCb-F/F/Fo/1, Sister Miriam, Letter to Archbishop of Canterbury, March 8th, 1896

Centre for Kentish Studies
Do/C/A/11/7/1, Grosvenor House Convalescent Home, 1900
Do/C/D/H/2, Tuberculosis Report by Medical Officer of Health, 1901
K610, 362.196995, A. Greenwood, First Report upon Tuberculosis and the Administration of Sanatorium Benefit, Centre for Kentish Studies

National Archives
Local Government Board correspondence:
MH 48/77 Benenden sanatorium, 1912-1919
MA 48/76 Grosvenor sanatorium, 1912-1919

MH 48/70 East Kent No.3 Combined District, 1905-1920
MH 12/5040 Elham Board of Guardians, 1897-1898
MH 12/5041 Elham Board of Guardians, 1899-1900
MH 12/5053 Elham Correspondence
MH 12/5045 Folkestone Sanitary Papers 1893
MH12/5046-49 Folkestone Sanitary Papers 1894-1896
MH 12/5052 Folkestone Sanitary Papers 1897-1898
MH 12/5053 Folkestone Sanitary Papers 1899-1900
MH 48/74 Kent Tuberculosis Scheme, 1912-1917
MH 48/75 Kent Tuberculosis Scheme, 1907-1919
MH 48/75 Keycol Hill Tuberculosis Scheme, 1907-19
MH 48/78 Lenham Sanatorium, 1913-1919
MH 113/42 LGB Medical Department Memos & Reports, 1905
MH 52/66-73 Ministry of Health, correspondence relating to Preston Hall Tuberculosis Settlement 1919-1935
MH 55/145 Ministry of Health, Report on Poor Law hospitals, The Treatment of Tubercular Persons, 1922-23
MH 55/164 Newman, G. letter to R.L. Morant, 1920
MH 12/5050 Sandgate Sanitary Papers, 1893-1896
MH 12/5051 Sandgate Sanitary Papers, 1897-1900
MH 55/130 Kent Tuberculosis Treatment Schemes, 1907-1919

Parliamentary Archives

HL/PO/PB/5/71/23, minutes of proceedings before the Select Committee of the House of Lords on the SUDC Bill, 1905

HC/CL/PB/10/3, minutes of proceedings before the Select Committee of the House of Commons on the SUDC Bill, 1905,

Primary Sources: Printed

British Library

Black, G. *Family Health Book*, London: Ward, Lock & Co., 1892

—. *Health for the Household: Based on a knowledge of air, water, food, clothing, drink and the Training of the Mind'*, London, 1858

Davos Guide Book, Illustrated Europe Series, London: C. Smith & Son, 1882, 000881362

Folkestone Library

Blackwell, T. E. *Report to the General Board of Health on the Drainage and Water Supply of Sandgate, in connexion with the late Outbreak of Cholera in that Town,* 21st February, 1855, 614.514

Chadwick, E. *Report to the General Board of Health on the town of Sandgate*, 1849, 614.514

Fitzgerald, C. E. Folkestone as a Health Resort, paper delivered at a meeting of the Association of Public Sanitary Inspectors at Folkestone in 1889, 614 folk

Fynmore, R. J. *Fynmore Collection*, Scrapbook of Press Cuttings relating to Folkestone, Sandgate & Hythe 942.23 folk

Rammell, T. W. *Report to the General Board of Health on a Preliminary Inquiry into...Sandgate*, HMSO, 1849, 628.2

Cooper, G. H. *Notes on Street Names of St. Saviour's Parish Compiled by G. H. Thompson,* St Saviours Parish Magazine, 1969, 929.3

Kelly's Directory of Folkestone, 1898-1899, 1903-1904, 1927-1930 microform, 942.23 folk

Kelly's Handbook to the Titled, Landed & Official Classes for 1913, 1929, London, Kelly's Directories Ltd, 920.042

Parliamentary Papers

Addison, Dr. C. House of Commons debate 12th July, 1911, volume 28, cc396-7

Albery, I. MP for Gravesend, *Tuberculosis, Kent (Sanatorium Treatment),* House of Commons debate 12th November, 1930, volume 244, cc1673-4

Astor, Lord W. House of Commons debate 12th June, 1913, volume 53, cc1857-8, 1866

Briant, Mr. to representative of Ministry of Health, House of Commons debate, 7th March, 1923, volume161, cc498-9

Bulstrode, H. T. *Report on Sanatoria for Consumption and certain other aspects of the Tuberculosis Question*, Supplement to the 35th Annual Report of the Local Government Board 1905-6, Cd. 3657

Burns, J. Debate on Poor Law Administration, House of Commons debate, 27th April, 1911, volume 24 cc2029-30

Cavendish-Bentinck, Lord Henry, House of Commons debate, 30th June, 1919, volume 117, c 686

Chapple, Dr. W. House of Commons debate, 27th April, 1911, volume 24, cc2046

Davy, J. S. Royal Commission on the Poor Laws, 1909, appendix volume I, 19th February, 1906, Cd. 4625, 3808

Dyer, H. Report of the Departmental Committee on Sickness Benefit Claims under the National Insurance Act, 1914-16, p.725, Cd 7676, Cd 7691, p.647, Cd 7688-89

Final Report of the Departmental Committee on Tuberculosis, 1913, Cd.6641

Hayes, J. MP for Liverpool, House of Commons debate, November 12th, 1928, cc 610-11

Interdepartmental Committee on Tuberculosis, 1919, HMSO, pp.139-184, cmd. 317

Lloyd George, D. *Memorandum Explanatory of National Insurance Bill,* London: HMSO, May 1911, Memorandum 147, p.15

Newman, G. *An Outline of the Practice of Preventive Medicine: A Memorandum Addressed to the Minister of Health,* London: HMSO, 1919

Newsholme, A. 39th Annual Report of LGB 1909-10. *Supplement to Report of Board Medical Officer containing a report on Infant and Child Mortality,* PP 1910/xxix, Cd.5263

Report of the Departmental Committee on Sickness Benefit Claims under the National Insurance Act, 1914-16, Cd 7688

Report of the Inter-Departmental Committee on Physical Deterioration, 1904, Cd.2175

Report of the Royal Commission on the Poor Laws, 1905-1909, Cd.4499

Smith, F. J. Report of the Departmental Committee on Sickness Benefit Claims under the National Insurance Act, 1914-16, p.1143, Cd 7688

Wilson, H. J. Parliamentary Debates House of Commons, Returns of Commons, 1905, p.51, Hansard, 4th series: volume 1-199, 1886-1908, UKC library

Sandgate Society

London Samaritan Society and Homerton Mission, *Particulars of Beach Rocks Convalescent Home, Sandgate,* London Samaritan Society, 1894

Wellcome Library for the History and Understanding of Medicine

The Abolition of Poor Law Guardians, Fabian Tract no.126, 1906

British Spas & Health Resorts, Official Publication of British Federation of Spas, London: Ed. J. Burrow & Co., 1920

Burns, J. *Transactions of the NAPT*, Annual Conference, Caxton Hall, Westminster, London: Adlard & Son, July 19-21, 1911,

Clunn, H. *Famous south coast pleasure resorts past and present*, London: T. Whittingham & Co., 1929

Dickens, A.L. *Report to the General Board of Health on an Inquiry with respect to the proceedings of the Local Board of Health, the state of the public works of water supply and drainage &c. of Sandgate*, May 30th, 1856

Howarth, W. J. MOH County of Kent, *Memorandum for Departmental Committee on Tuberculosis,* 1912

Folkestone MOH report, 1898, b13562514

Views and Reviews – Special Edition, Brighton: W. T. Pike & Co., 1896

Williamson, Dr. A. M. *Transactions of the NAPT*, Annual Conference, Caxton Hall, Westminster, London: Adlard & Son, July 19-21, 1911,

Yunge-Bateman, M. G. MOH Reports, 1894, 1896-1898, 1903-1911, 1913-1915, 1919-1920, b13562514

An Account of the Infirmary for Asthma, Consumption and Other Diseases of the Lungs, Union St., Bishopsgate, established 1814, Annual Report, 1827

Primary Sources: Popular Literature

Austen, J. Sanditon, *Minor Works Volume VI*, ed. R.W. Chapman: Oxford University Press, 1963

Bronte, C. *Jane Eyre*, Harmondsworth: Penguin, 1966

Dickens, C. *Nicholas Nickleby*, Harmondsworth: Penguin, 1994

—. *Dombey and Son,* Harmondsworth: Penguin, 1986

—. *Our Mutual Friend,* London: The New Illustrated Dickens, 1947-58

Eliot, G. *Daniel Deronda,* London: Cox & Wyman, 1970

—. Janet's Repentance, *Scenes of Clerical Life,* Edinburgh: W. Blackwood, 1878

James, H. *The Wings of the Dove*, New York: Charles Scribner's Sons, 1909

Kingsley, C. *Alton Locke*, London: MacMillan & Co., 1862

Maugham, W. S. *The Sanatorium*, in *Creatures of Circumstance,* 1947

Shaw, G. B. *The Doctor's Dilemma,* London: Penguin, 2004

Shelley, P. B. *'Essay on the vegetable system of diet',* in *'Shelley's Prose, or The Trumpet of a Prophecy*', ed. David Lee Clark, Albuquerque: University of New Mexico Press, 1966, p.93 (date unknown)

Smollett, T. *Travels Through France and Italy,* Oxford University Press, ed. Frank Felsenstein, 1979

Sterne, L. A *Sentimental Journey & Other Writings,* [1768] Oxford University Press, 2008

Wells, H. G. *Anticipations of the Reaction of Mechanical and Scientific Progress upon Human Life and Thought,* London: Chapman & Hall, 1901

—. *An Experiment in Autobiography,* volume 1, London: Faber & Faber, 1934

Primary Sources: Medical/ Medico-Popular and Sociological Books

Anonymous, (Probably T. Hawkesley) *Engineers and Officials; an Historical Sketch of the Progress of 'Health of Towns Works' (between 1838 and 1856) in London and the Provinces,* London: E. Stanford, 1856

Anonymous, *Health for the Household: Based on a knowledge of air, water, food, clothing, drink and the Training of the Mind,* London: Jarrold & Sons, 1858

Anonymous, *The Family Physician, A Manual of Domestic Medicine by Physicians and Surgeons of the Principal London Hospitals,* London: Cassell & Co., 1894

Beddoes, T. *Essay on the Causes, Early Signs and Prevention of Pulmonary Consumption for the Use of Parents and Preceptors,* Bristol: Biggs & Castle, 1799

—. *Hygiea,* Bristol: Phillips, 1802

Beevor, Sir H. *An Oration on the Declension of Phthisis*, London, n.p., 1899

Bennet, J. H. *On the Treatment of Pulmonary Consumption by Hygiene, Climate and Medicine*, London: John Churchill, 1866

Beveridge, W. H. *Unemployment: A Problem of Industry,* London: Longmans, Green & Co, 1909

Black, G. *Family Health Book*, London: Ward, Lock, Bowden & Co., 1892

Booth, C. *The Life and Labour of the People in London*, 9 volumes, London: Macmillan & Co, 1901

Booth, General, *Darkest England and the Way Out*, London: Charles Knight & Co. Ltd, 1890

Braun, J. *The Curative Effects of Baths and Waters*, London: Smith, Elder & Co., 1875

Churchill, J. F. *Consumption and Tuberculosis,* London: Longman, Green & Co., 1875

Chatterton-Hill, G. *Heredity and Selection in Sociology*, London: Adam & Charles Black, 1907

Clouston, T. S. *Clinical Lectures on Mental Diseases,* London: J.A. Churchill, 1883

Clark, J. *Medical Notes on Climates, Diseases, Hospitals and Medical Schools in France, Italy and Switzerland,* London: T&G Underwood et al., 1820

Copland, J. *The Forms, Complications, Causes, Prevention and Treatment of Consumption and Bronchitis*, London: Longmans, 1861

Culpepper, N. *The English Physician; Enlarged with 369 Medicines made of English Herbs,* Crosby Oxford University, 1814 (originally published 1653)

Epps, J. *Consumption, Its Nature and Treatment*, London: Sanderson, 1859

Ewart, W. *Marine Climates in the Treatment of Tuberculosis,* London: Bailliere, Tindall & Cox, 1907

Garland C. & Lister, T. *Sanatoria for the People or the State Campaign Against Consumption,*
London: Scientific Press, 1911

Galton, F. *Inquiries into Human Faculty and its Development*, London: MacMillan, 1883

Garland, C. & Lister, T. *Sanatoria for the People or the State Campaign Against Consumption,* London: Scientific Press, 1911

Hill, H. W. *The New Public Health*, London: MacMillan, 1916

Huber, J. B. *Consumption: Its Relation to Man and his Civilisation. Its Prevention and Cure,* London: J.B. Lippincott, 1906

Larking, A. E. *Notes on Folkestone Historical, Climatological and Medical*, London: J&A Churchill, 1889

Latham, A & Garland, C. *The Conquest of Consumption,* London: T. Fisher Unwin, (1910), 2nd ed., 1911

London, J. *The People of the Abyss*, [1903] London: Pluto, 1998

Luke, T. D. *Spas and Health Resorts of the British Isles*, London: A.&C. Black, 1919

Mackie, S. J. *A Handbook of Folkestone for* Visitors, London: J. English, Simpkin & Marshall, 1856

—. *A Descriptive and Historical Account of Folkestone and its Neighbourhood with Gleanings from the Municipal Records*, [1856], Reprinted from the "Folkestone Express". 2nd edition. Folkestone: J. English, 1883

Macleod-Munro, D. G. *The Psycho-Pathology of Tuberculosis*, Oxford University Press, 1926

Maudsley, H. *Body and Mind: An Inquiry Into Their Connection and Mutual Influence, Specially In Reference To Moral Disorders,* London: MacMillan & Co., 1870

Morris, M. *The Book of Health,* London: Cassell, 1883

Moseley, G. *Sandgate as a Residence for Invalids*, London: John Churchill, 1853

Muthu, C. *Pulmonary Tuberculosis and Sanatorium Treatment*, London: Bailliere, Tindall & Cox, 1910

Newman, G. *Infant Mortality. A Social Problem*, London: Methuen, 1906

Newsholme, A. *The Prevention of Tuberculosis*, London: Methuen, 1908

Osler, W. *The Principles and Practice of Medicine*, New York: Appleton, 1904

Paterson, M. *The Shibboleths of Tuberculosis*, London: John Murray, 1920

Pearson, K. *A First Study of the Statistics of Pulmonary Tuberculosis* , London: Dulao & Co., 1907

—. *A Second Study of the Statistics of Pulmonary Tuberculosis: Marital Infection,* London: Dulau & Co., 1908

—. *The Problem of Practical Eugenics,* London: Dulao & Co., 1909

Priestman, A. *Work of the School Medical Officer,* London: Oxford University Press, 1915

Richardson, B. W. *The Hygienic Treatment of Pulmonary Consumption*, London: John Churchill, 1857, pp.336-344

Rogers, J. *Reminiscences of a Workhouse Medical Officer,* London: Fisher, 1889

Rowntree, B. S. *A Study of Town Life*, London: Macmillan & Co, 1901

Sims, G. How the Poor Live, London: Chatto & Windus, 1883

Thomson, H. H. *Tuberculosis and Public Health*, London: Longmans, 1920

Thomson, S. *Health Resorts of Britain; and how to profit by them*, London: Ward & Lock, 1860

Tressell, *The Ragged Trousered Philanthropists,* London: Lawrence & Wishart, 1914

Tyndall, J. *New Fragments*, London: Longmans, 1892

Walters, F. R. *Sanatoria for Consumptives*, 3rd edition, London: Swan Sonnesnschien, 1905

Webb, S. & B. eds., *The Break-Up of the Poor Law: Being Part One of the Minority Report of the Poor Law Commission,* London: Longmans, Green & Co, 1909

Webb, B. & S. *The State and the Doctor,* London: Longmans, 1910

Wells, H. G. *Anticipations of the Reaction of Mechanical and Scientific Progress upon Human Life and Thought,* London: Chapman & Hall, 1901

White, A. *Efficiency and Empire*, 1901, Brighton: Harvester Press, 1973

Wilkinson, W. C. *Tuberculin in the Diagnosis and Treatment of Tuberculosis,* London: J. Nisbet & Co.,1912

Wittkower, E. *A Psychiatrist Looks at Tuberculosis,* London: National Association for the Prevention of Tuberculosis, 1949

Wood, N. *Health Resorts of the British Isles,* University of London Press, 1919

Woodcock, H. de C. *The Doctor and the People*, London: Methuen, 1912

Yeo, J. B. *Climate and Health Resorts*, London: Chapman & Hall, 1885

Young, T. *A Practical and Historical Treatise on Consumptive Diseases*, London: Thomas Underwood, 1815

Primary Sources: Medical Journals and Newspapers

Anonymous Benenden patient, *Hospital Saturday Fund Journal*, 30th December, 1914
Anonymous speaker, NAPT 13th Annual Conference, *The Lancet*, 9th July, 1927
Barr, Sir J. *BMJ*, 30th December, 1911
—. Doctors' Ultimatum to Ministers, *The Times*, 24th July, 7, 1912
—. *BMJ,* 27th July 1912
Beale, L. S. The open-air treatment of tuberculosis, *The Lancet*, 10th December, 1898
The Black Hole of Etchinghill, *The Star,* 22nd August, 8th & 11th September, 1893
Blenkinsop, Major-General Sir Layton, Presidential address at Folkestone Health Congress, *Journal of Royal Sanitary Institute*, volume xlii, no.5, March 1922
Blundell, N. *The Great diurnal of Nicholas Blundell of Little Crosby, Lancashire,* Transcribed and annotated by F. Tyrer, ed. J. J. Bagley. 3 vols. Manchester: Record Society of Lancashire & Cheshire, volume I, 1968-72
BMA Medico-Political Committee, *An Investigation into the Economic Conditions of Contract Medical Practice in the United Kingdom,* BMJ Supplement, 22nd July, 1905
Brabazon, Lord, R. State Directed Colonisation; Its Necessity, *Nineteenth Century*, volume xxxi, April 1887
Browning, Dr. C. H. 12th Annual NAPT Conference, Glasgow University, *B.M.J.*, v.2 (3418), 10th July, 1926
Bulstrode, H. T. On the Causes, Prevalence and Control of Pulmonary Tuberculosis, *The Lancet*, ii, 1903
Burton-Fanning, F. W. The Open-Air Treatment of Phthisis in England, *The Lancet*, 26th March, 1898
Chubb, W. L. *B.M.J.*, 3rd May, 1890, p.1055
Clark, J. Tubercular Phthisis, or Consumption, Phthisis Tuberculosa, Phthisis Pulmonalis, J. Forbes, A. Tweedie & J. Conolly (eds.), *The Cyclopaedia of Practical Medicine,* volume iv, London, Gilbert & Piper, 1832-35
de Terrason, E. The Open-Air Treatment of Consumption, *Chambers's Journal,* Sixth Series, ii, December 1898-November 1899, pp.134-138

Dixon, G. B. The Domiciliary Treatment of Tuberculous Patients, *British Journal of Tuberculosis*, volume 9, pp.19-22

Doctor Koch's Discovery, *The Spectator*, 65, 22nd November, 1890, pp. 726-727

Edelston, B. G. The Ostracism of the Tubercular, *The Lancet*, 16th July, 1949

Ellis, H. Eugenics and St. Valentine, *Nineteenth Century*, 59, 1906

Emmanuel, J. G. Tuberculosis and Insurance, *Journal of the Federated Insurance Institute,* 11, 1908

Eugenics: Its Definition, Scope and Aims, *The American Journal of Sociology,* volume 10, no. 1, 1904

Fitzgerald, C. E. The Prevention of Tuberculosis, *The Lancet*, 8th October, 1898

Folkestone Slums, *The Star*, 6th October, 1894

Galton, F. & Mahomed, F. A. An Inquiry into the Physiognomy of Phthisis by the method of Composite Portraiture, eds. H. G. Howse & F. Taylor, *Guy's Hospital Reports,* 3rd Series, volume xxv, London, J&A Churchill, 1881, pp.475-493

Hillier, A., Tuberculosis and Public Action, *Fortnightly Review,* 71, 424, April, 1902, pp.700-712

Holden, O. M. Mental Aspects of Tuberculosis, *The Practitioner,* 1922

Howells, W. D. In Folkestone out of Season, *Harper's Monthly Magazine*, November 1904

Local Misgovernment, *Public Health,* 1899-1900, volume xii

Lindsay, J. A. Inaugural Address on the Problem of the Consumptive Poor to the Ulster Medical Society, November 4th, 1897, *The Lancet*, 4th December, 1897

McFie, R. Sanatoriums for the Poor and the Eradication of Consumption, *The Lancet*, 30th September, 1905

—. *Nursing Times,* 27th May, 1911

MacNalty, A. S. Tuberculosis Work in England, *The Lancet,* 26th January, 1924

Mackenzie, Sir L. The Production of Fitness, paper delivered at Folkestone Health Congress, 1921, *Royal Society of Health Journal,* volume xlii, no.4, January, 1922

Marais, D. P. NAPT 18th Annual Conference, *The Lancet,* 30th July, 1932

Moore, S. G. Milk and Disease, paper read at Folkestone Health Congress, *Journal of the Royal Sanitary Institute*, volume xlii, no.4, January 1922

Morris, M. The Past and Future of the Crusade Against Tuberculosis, *B.M.J.*, 16th November, 1918

Muthu, C. *B.M.J.*, 4th December, 1920

NAPT Annual Conference, *The Lancet*, 12th July, 1924

Newsholme, A. The Notification of Phthisis Pulmonaris, *Practitioner*, 67, 1901

—. Public Health Authorities in Relation to the Struggle against Tuberculosis in England, *Journal of Hygiene*, 3, 1903, pp.446-467

—. The Relative Importance of the Constituent Factors involved in the Control of Pulmonary Tuberculosis, *Transactions of the Epidemiological Society*, 25, 1905-6, pp.31-140

—. An Inquiry into the Principal Causes of the Reduction in the Death Rate from Phthisis during the last 40 years with special reference to the Segregation of Phthisical Patients in General Institutions, *Journal of Hygiene*, 6, 1906, pp.304-384

—. Some Conditions of Social Efficiency in Relation to Local Public Administration, *Public Health* 22, 1908-9

—. National Changes in Health and Longevity, *Quarterly Publications of the American Statistical Association*, volume 17, no.134, June, 1921

Niven, J. *Poverty and Disease*, Presidential Address to the Epidemiological Section of the Royal Society of Medicine, 22nd October, 1900, Proceedings of the Royal Society of Medicine, 3, part 2, 1910, pp.1-45

Osler, Sir W. The Prevention and Treatment of Tuberculosis, *The Lancet*, July 18th, 1914

Pearson, J. Milk Supplies and their Dangers, *Journal of State Medicine,* volume xii, no.9, September 1904

—. Thirty Years Sanitary Experience in Folkestone with Local Experiences, *Journal of the Royal Sanitary Institute*, volume xlii, no.1, July 1921, pp.293-297

—. Thirty Years Sanitary Progress in Folkestone, *Journal of the Royal Sanitary Institute*, volume xlii, no.5, March 1922

Philip, R. W. Progressive Medicine and the Outlook on Tuberculosis, *The Lancet*, 31st July, 1909

—. Conference of NAPT, Leeds, 7th & 8th July, 1914, *The Lancet,* 18th July, 1914

—. The Outlook on Tuberculosis, *B.M.J.*, 10th January, 1931

Poore, G. V. Climate in its Relation to Health, *Journal of Society of Arts*, 33, 21st November 1884 – 13th November 1885, pp.908-922

Powers of Inspection by Sanitary Authorities (The Folkestone Case), *The Lancet*, 6th May, 1893

The Preventive Provisions of the Insurance Bill, *Public Health*, volume 25, 1911-12

Priestman, A. Hygienic and Economic Factors in the Incidence of Tuberculosis Amongst School-children, *British Journal of Tuberculosis*,

volume 19, pt.3, 1925
—. *Medical World*, 6th February, 1931
—. *Medical Officer*, 9th March, 1935
Public Health, no.8, volume xxvi, May 1913
Ransome, A. Consumption, A Filth Disease, *The Lancet*, 1st January, 1898
Report on the Paris Commission on Consumption, *Science,* volume xiv, no.345, September 1899
—. Phthisis rates: their significance and their teaching, *Transactions of the Epidemiological Society*, 1904-5
Raw, N. Sanatoria for Consumption, *Folkestone Chronicle & Observer and Canterbury Register*, 30th July, 1904
The Renewal of the Sandgate Sanatoria Scandal, *The Lancet*, 29th June, 1907
Report on the Paris Commission on Consumption, *Science,* volume xiv, no.345, September, 1899
Report on the Sanitary Condition of Folkestone, *The Lancet,* 17th April, 1875
Rivers, W. C. The Atavistic-Degenerative Diathesis of Tuberculosis, *The Lancet*, 20th January, 1923
Robertson, J. *Journal of the Royal Sanitary Institute*, volume xli, no.4, March, 1921
Robertson, Sir J. NAPT 13th Annual Conference, *The Lancet*, 9th July, 1927
Smith, H. G. *Journal of the Royal Sanitary Institute*, volume xli, no 4, March 1921
Squire, Dr J. E. *The Hospital*, 2nd December, 1911
The Coastal Health Resort, *The Lancet,* 12th March, 1932
The Infectiousness of Phthisis, *The Lancet*, 18th March, 1899
The Work of the NAPC, *B.M.J.*, 29th July, 1916
Tuberculosis and the Poor Law, *British Journal of Tuberculosis*, 1908
Tuckwell, G. Presidential Address to Health Visitors at Folkestone Health Congress, 1921, *Journal of the Royal Sanitary Institute,* volume xlii, no.5, March 1922
Tyson, W. J. Presidential Address to the Preventive Medicine Section, Folkestone Health Congress, *Journal of State Medicine*, volume xii, no.9, September 1904
Unidentified author, The Fight Against Consumption, *The Practitioner*, July, 1901
Walters, F. R. On Estimating the Value of Remedies in Pulmonary Tuberculosis', *The Lancet,* 11th June, 1927
Watt, Dr. J. Annual Conference of NAPT, London, *The Lancet*, 30th July,

1932

Weber, F. P. *B.M.J.*, 20th December, 1919

—. A Change of Air in young adult life and early middle age, *The Practitioner,* no. 481, volume 81, no.1, July, 1908

Weber, H. The Croonian Lectures on The Hygienic and Climatic Treatment of Chronic Pulmonary Phthisis, *BMJ*, 14th March, 21st March, 28th March, 4th March & 11th April,1885, pp.517-522, 575-576, 641-643, 688-690, 725-727

Wells, H. G. A Touchstone for Mr. Kidd's Prognostic, *Pall Mall Gazette,* 24th May, 1895

White, A. The Nomad Poor of London*, Contemporary Review*, May 1855, volume xlvii

Williams, C. T. Old & New Views on the Treatment of Consumption, *The Lancet*, 21st October, 1911

Williams, R. S. Letter to *B.M.J.,* 4th December, 1920

Wood, Mrs. R.G. (Mayoress of Folkestone), Address on Personal and Domestic Hygiene, Folkestone Health Congress, 1921, *Journal of the Royal Sanitary Institute,* volume xlii, no.3, November 1921

Wood, Alderman R.G. Presidential Address to Folkestone Health Congress, 1921, *Journal of the Royal Sanitary Institute*, volume xlii, no. 4, January 1922

Young, Dr. R.A. & Findlay, Dr. L., The Coastal Health Resort, *The Lancet,* 12th March, 1932

Secondary Sources: Books

Abel-Smith, B. *Hospitals 1800-1948*, Heinemann: London, 1964

Aries, P. *The hour of our death*, Harmondsworth: Penguin, 1983

Armstrong, D. *The Political Anatomy of the Body,* Cambridge University Press, 1983

Arthur, M. *Lost Voices of the Edwardians,* London: Harper Collins, 2006

Bagley, J. J. & A. J. *The English Poor Law*, London: Macmillan, 1966

Banfield, M. A. *Health Biographies of Alexander Leeper, R. L. Stevenson and Fanny Street*, Modbury, S. Australia, 2001

Barnes, D. S. *The Making of a Social Disease. Tuberculosis in Nineteenth Century France*, Berkeley: University of California, 1995

Bates, B. *Bargaining for Life: A Social History of Tuberculosis, 1876-1938,* Philadelphia: University of Pennsylvania Press, 1992

Bellamy, C. *Administering Central-Local Relations 1871-1919*, Manchester University Press, 1988

Berridge, V. *Opium and the People: Opiate Use and Policy in 19th Century and Early 20th Century Britain*, London: Free Association Books, 1998

Bishop, C. H. *Folkestone: The Story of a Town,* London: Headley Brothers, 1973

Bonham, V. *A Joyous Service*, V. Bonham/CSJB, 1989

Bourdieu, P. *Outline of a Theory of Practice,* Cambridge University Press, 1977

Bowker, G. C. & Star, S. L. *Sorting Things Out: Classification and its Consequences*, Massachussets Institute of Technology, 1999

Brand, J. *Doctors and the State*, Baltimorre: Johns Hopkins Press, 1965

Braithwaite, W. J. *Lloyd George's Ambulance Wagon,* London: Methuen & Co., 1957

Bryder, L. *Below the Magic Mountain, A Social History of Tuberculosis in Twentieth Century Britain,* Oxford University Press, 1988

Bynum, W. F. and Porter, R. eds., *Brunonianism in Britain and Europe*, London: Wellcome Institute, 1988

Byrne, K. *Tuberculosis and the Victorian Literary Imagination,* Cambridge University Press, 2011

Cannadine, D. *Lords and Landlords: The Aristocracy and the Towns 1774-1967,* Leicester University Press, 1980

Clarke, P. *Lancashire and the New Liberalism,* Cambridge University Press, 1971

Cordery, S. *British Friendly Societies 1750-1914,* Houndmills, Basingstoke: Palgrave MacMillan, 2003

Crowther, M. A. *The Workhouse System,* London, Routledge, 1983

Cummins, S. L. *Tuberculosis in History*, London: Bailliere, Tindall, Cox, 1949

Cunningham, A. & Jardine, N. eds., *Romanticism and the Sciences,* Cambridge University Press, 1990

De Almeida, H. *Romantic Medicine and John Keats,* Oxford University Press, 1991

Digby, A. *The Evolution of British General Practice, 1850-1948*, Oxford University Press, 1999

Donaldson, P. *Ritual and Remembrance: The Memorialisation of the Great War in East Kent,* Cambridge Scholars Publishing, 2006

Dormandy, T. *The White Death: A History of Tuberculosis*, London, The Hambledon Press, 1999

Dubos, R. *Mirage of Health*, [1952] New York: Harper & Row, 1959

Dubos, R. & J. *The White Plague: Tuberculosis, Man and Society,* Rutgers University Press, 1987

Dwork, D. *War is Good for Babies and Other Young Children: A History of the Infant and Child Welfare Movement in England 1898-1918,*

London, Routledge, 1987
Eyler, J. M. *Sir Arthur Newsholme and State Medicine, 1885-1935*, Cambridge University Press, 1997
Fee, E. & Fox, D. M. eds., *Aids: The Burden of Histor,y* Berkeley: University of California Press, 1988
Frawley, M. H. *Invalidism and Identity in Nineteenth Century Britain,* University of Chicago Press, 2004
Galdston, I. *Social and Historic Foundations of Modern Medicine*, New York: Brunner/Mazel, 1981
Gaudillière, J. P. & Löwy, I. eds. *Heredity and Infection* Routledge: London, 2001
Geertz, C. *The Interpretation of Cultures: Selected Essays,* New York: Basic Books, 1973, pp.3-30
Gilman, S. *Franz Kafka, The Jewish Patient*, London, Routledge, 1995
Green, D. G. *Working Class Patients and the Medical Establishment,* Gower Publishing Co. Ltd, Aldershot, 1985
Haley, B. *The Healthy Body and Victorian Culture,* Cambridge, Massachusetts, Harvard University Press, 1978
Hardy, A. *The Epidemic Streets*, Oxford University Press, 1993
—. *Health and Medicine in Britain since 1860*, Basingstoke: Palgrave, 2001
Harker, D. *Tressell: The Real Story of the Ragged Trousered Philanthropists,* London, Zed Books, 2003
Harris, J. *Private Lives and Public Spirit: Britain 1870-1914*, Penguin, London, 1993
Hassan, J. *The Seaside, Health and the Environment in England and Wales since 1800,* Aldershot: Ashgate Publishing Ltd, 2002
Herzlich & Pierret, *Illness and self in society,* Baltimore: Johns Hopkins University Press, 1987
Himmelfarb, G. *The Idea of Poverty: England in the Early Industrial Age*, New York: Random House, 1985
Hobsbawm, E. *The Age of Revolution,* New York: World Publishing, 1962
Jones, G. *Social Darwinism and English Thought*, Brighton: Harvester Press, 1980
Jones, G. *Social Hygiene in Twentieth Century Britain*, Beckenham: Croom Helm, 1986
Keers, *R. Y. Pulmonary Tuberculosis: A Journey Down the Centuries*, London: Baillière-Tindall, 1978
Kemp, W. *The Desire of my Eyes,* New York: Farrar, Strauss & Giroux, 1990

Lawlor, C. *Consumption and Literature,* Basingstoke: Palgrave, MacMillan, 2006

Laybourn, K. *Modern Britain Since 1906,* London: Tauris & Co., 1999

Marland, H. *Medicine and Society in Wakefield and Huddersfield, 1780-1870,* Cambridge University Press, 1987

Marwick, A. The Deluge: British Society and the Great War, London: Bodley Head, 1965

Matthews, W. ed., *The diary of Dudley Ryder, 1715-1716,* London: Methuen, 1939

Mazumdar, P. M. H. *Species ad Specificty*, Cambridge University Press, 1995

—. *Eugenics, Human Genetics and Human Failings: The Eugenic Society, its Sources and its Critics in Britain,* London: Routledge, 1992

McKeown, T. *The Modern Rise of Population*, London: E. Arnold, 1976

—. *The Role of Medicine: Dream, Mirage, or Nemesis?*, Princeton University Press, 1979

—. *The Origins of Human Disease*, Oxford: B. Blackwell, 1988

McLeod, H. *European Religion in the Age of the Great Cities 1830-1930,* London: Routledge, 1995

McPate, B. *Benenden, The History of the Benenden Healthcare Society 1905-2005*, York: William Sessions Ltd, 2006

Nevill, A. *Dickens in Folkestone*, Folkestone and District Local History Society, 2002

—. *The Story of Folkestone*, Eastbourne: A. Rowe, 2009

Overy, R. *The Morbid Age, Britain Between the Wars*, London: Allen Lane, 2009

Pedlar, F. J. *The Maitland Story,* Maitland Trust, ca. 1968

Pick, D. *Faces of Degeneration, a European Disorder, c.1848-1918,* Cambridge University Press, 1989

Pike, E. R. *Human Documents of the Lloyd George Era*, London: George Allen & Unwin, 1972

Porter, J. D. & McAdam, K. P. (eds) *Tuberculosis: Back to the Future,* Chichester: J. Wiley & Sons, 1994

Porter, R. *George Cheyne: The English Malady,* London: Routledge, 1991

Richardson, A. *Love and Eugenics in the Late Nineteenth Century*, Oxford University Press, 2003

Rothman, S. *Living in the Shadow of Death: Tuberculosis and the Social Experience of Illness in American History*, New York: Basic Books, 1994;

Rousseau, G. S. *Nervous Acts: Essays on Literature, Culture and Sensibility*, Basingstoke: Palgrave, MacMillan, 2004

Searle, G. R. *The Liberal Party: Triumph and Disintegration,* London: MacMillan, 1992

Shaw, A. & Reeves, C. *The Children of Craig-y-nos: Life in a Welsh Tuberculosis Sanatorium, 1922–1959,* London: Wellcome Trust Centre for the History of Medicine, UCL, 2009

Slater, G. *Poverty and the State,* London: Constable & Co., 1930

Smith, D. C. ed., *Correspondence of H.G. Wells, volume 1,* London: Pickering & Chatto, 1998

Smith, F. B. *The Retreat of Tuberculosis*, Beckenham: Croom Helm, 1988

Spink, W. *Infectious Diseases: Prevention and Treatment in the Nineteenth and Twentieth Centuries*, Folkestone: Dawson, 1978

Stedman Jones, G. *Outcast London*, Oxford University Press, 1971

Stedman, G. *Stemming the Torrent*, Aldershot: Ashgate Publishing, 2002

Walton, J. K. *The English Seaside Resort: a social history 1750-1914*, Leicester University Press, 1983

Wilkinson, E. *The Town that was Murdered, The Life Story of Jarrow,* London: Gollancz, 1939

Williams, H. *Requiem for a Great Killer: The Story of Tuberculosis,* London: Health Horizon, 1973

Williams, R. *The Country and the City,* Oxford University Press, 1975

Winter, J. M. *The Great War and the British People*, London: MacMillan, 1986

Wohl, A. S. *The Eternal Slum: Housing and Social Policy in Victorian London,* New Brunswick: Transaction Publishers, [1977], 2006,

Worboys, M. *Spreading Germs*, Cambridge University Press, 2000

Secondary Sources: Articles & Papers

Alborn, T. Insurance against Germ Theory: Commerce and Conservatism in Late-Victorian Medicine*, Bulletin of the History of Medicine*, 75, 2001, pp.406-445

Atkins, P. J. Mothers' Milk and Infant Death in Britain circa 1900-1940, *Anthropology of Food*, 2nd September, 2003, 26.07.08. http://aof.revues.org/document310.html

Atkinson, B. Politics, *Kent in the Twentieth Century*, ed. N. Yates, Woodbridge: Boydell & Brewer, 2001, pp.153-199

Austin, K. H.G. Wells, *Bygone Kent*, volume 26, no.12, December, 2005

Bashford, A. Cultures of Confinement, in *Isolation: Places and Practices of Exclusion*, eds. Caroline Strange & A. Bashford, London, Routledge, 2003, pp.133-150

Berridge, V. *Health and Medicine*, in *The Cambridge Social History of*

Britain: Social Agencies and Institutions, ed. Francis M.L. Thompson, Cambridge University Press, 1993, pp.171-243

Brand, J. The Parish Doctor: England's Poor Law Medical Officers and Medical Reform, 1870-1900, *Bulletin of the History of Medicine*, 35, 1961, pp.97-122

Brown, J. Charles Booth and Labour Colonies 1889-1905, *Economic History Review,* volume 21, no.2, 1968, pp.349-360

Bryder, L. The First World War: Healthy or Hungry?, *History Workshop*, 24, 1987, pp.141-157

—. Comments on 'The Historical Decline of Tuberculosis' by Leonard Wilson *Journal of the History of Medicine*, 46:3, 1991, pp.358-362

—. 'Wonderlands of buttercup, clover and daisies': Tuberculosis and the open-air school movement in Britain, 1907-39, in *In the Name of the Child: Health and Welfare 1880-1940,* ed. Roger Cooter, Routledge, 1992, pp.72-95

—. A Health Resort for Consumptives: Tuberculosis and Immigration to New Zealand, 1880-1914, *Medical History*, 40, 1996, pp.453-471

Bynum, W. F. Darwin and the Doctors: Evolution, Diathesis, and Germs in 19th Century Britain, *Gesnerus*, volume 40, pt.1-2, 1983, pp.43-53

—. The evolution of germs and the evolution of disease. Some British debates 1870-1900, *History and Philosophy of Life Sciences*, 24, 2002, pp.53-68

Byrne, D. & Keithley, J. Housing and the Health of the Community, *Unhealthy Housing: Research, Remedies and Reform,* eds. R. Burridge & D. Ormandy, London: Routledge, 1993, pp.41-66

Campbell, M. What tuberculosis did for Modernism: The influence of a Curative Environment on Modernist Design and Architecture, *Medical History*, 49, 2005, pp.463-488

Cantor, D. The Diseased Body, *Medicine in the Twentieth Century,* eds. R. Cooter & J. V. Pickstone, London: Harwood: Academic Publishers, 2000, pp.347-366

Carter, K. C. The Development of Pasteur's Concept of Disease Causation and the Emergence of Specific Causes in Nineteenth Century Medicine, *Bulletin of the History of Medicine*, 65, 1991, pp.528-548

Chalke, H. D. The Impact of Tuberculosis on History, Literature and Art, *Medical History*, 6, 1962, pp.301-318

Cockerell, T. D. A. Municipal Activity in Britain, *American Journal of Sociology*, volume 11, no.6, May, 1906, pp. 817-829

Coker, R. Civil Liberties and Public Good, *Medical History*, 45, 2001, pp.341-358

Comaroff, J. Medicine: Symbol and Ideology, in *The Problem of Medical*

Knowledge, eds. Peter Wright & Andrew Treacher, Edinburgh University Press, 1982, pp.49-69

Cominos, P. Late-Victorian sexual respectability and the social system, *International Review of Social History*, viii, 1963, pp.19-48

Condrau, F. "Who is the Captain of all these Men of Death?": The Social Structure of a Tuberculosis Sanatorium, *Journal of Interdisciplinary History*, volume 32, no.2, Autumn, 2001, pp.243-262

Craddock, S. Engendered/Endangered: Women, Tuberculosis and the Project of Citizenship, *Journal of Historical Geography*, 27, 3, 2001, pp.338-354

Craig, R. & Whyman, J. Kent and the Sea, *The Economy of Kent, 1640-1914,* ed. Alan Armstrong, Boydell Press, 1995, pp.161-205

Cronin, J. E. The British State and the Structure of Political Opportunity, *Journal of British Studies,* volume 27, no.3, 1988, pp.199-231

Crowther, M. A. Paupers or Patients? Obstacles to Professionalisation in the Poor Law Medical Service Before 1914, *Journal of the History of Medicine and Allied Sciences*, 39:1, January, 1984, pp.33-54

Diamond, J. M. 'AIDS: Infectious, Genetic, or both?', *Nature,* 328, July, 1987, pp.199-200

Dolin, P. J., Raviglione M. C. & Kochi, A. Global Tuberculosis Incidence and Mortality during 1990-2000, *Bulletin of the World Health Organisation*, 72, 2, 1994, pp.213-220

Dorling, D & Pritchard, J. The Geography of Poverty, Inequality and Wealth in the UK and Abroad: Because Enough is Never Enough, *Applied Spatial Analysis and Policy*, 3:81, 106, 2010, pp. 81-105

Dutton, D. J. The Unionist Party and Social Policy 1906-1914, *The Historical Journal*, volume 24, no.4, December, 1981, pp.1005-1048

Eyler, J. M. Poverty, Disease, Responsibility: Arthur Newsholme and the Public Health Dilemmas of British Liberalism, *The Millbank Quarterly*, volume 67, supplement, 1, 1989, pp.109-126

Fairchild, A. L. & Oppenheimer, G. M. Public Health Nihilism vs Pragmatism: History, Politics and the Control of Tuberculosis, *American Journal of Public Health*, 88, July, 1998, pp.1105-1117

Farrant, S. London By The Sea: Resort Development on the South Coast of England 1880-1939, *Journal of Contemporary History*, volume 22, no.1, 1987, pp.137-162

Fee, E. & Porter, D. Public Health, Preventive Medicine & Professionalisation, in *Medicine in Society: Historical Essays,* ed. A. Wear, Cambridge University Press, 1992, pp.249-277

Figlio, K. Chlorosis and chronic disease in nineteenth century Britain: the social constitution of somatic illness in a capitalist society, *Social*

History, 3, 1978, pp.167-197

Gandy, M. & Zumla, A. The Resurgence of Disease: Social and Historical Perspectives on the 'New' Tuberculosis, *Social Science and Medicine*, volume 55, issue 3, August, 2002, pp.385-396

Gilbert, B. B. Health and Politics: The British Physical Deterioration Report of 1904, *Bulletin of the History of Medicine*, 39, 1965, pp.143-153

—. David Lloyd George: Land, The Budget and Social Reform, *The American Historical Review*, volume 81, no.5, December, 1976, pp.1058-1066

Groos, A. TB sheets: Love and Disease in La Traviata, *Cambridge Opera Journal*, 7, 3, 1995, pp.233-260

Haroutunian, L. M. Albert Camus and the White Plague, *Modern Language Notes*, volume 79, no.3, May, 1964, pp.311-315

Hastings, P. & Yates, N. Health and Social Welfare, *Kent in the Twentieth Century,* ed. N. Yates, Woodbridge: Boydell & Brewer, 2001, pp.229-286

Jones, G. 'The Captain of all these Men of Death': The History of Tuberculosis in 19th and 20th Century Ireland, *Clio Medica*, 62, 2001, entire issue

Joyce, A. H. Early Sanatoriums in Kent, *Bygone Kent,* volume 8, no.6, 1987

Koerber, A. From Folklore to Fact: The Rhetorical History of Breastfeeding and Immunity, 1950–1997, *Journal of Medical Humanities*, 27, 2006, pp.151-166

Lawlor, C. & Suzuki, A. The Disease of the Self: Representing Consumption, 1700-1830, *Bulletin of the History of Medicine*, 74:3, 2000, pp. 458-494

Lawlor, C. Consuming Time: Narrative and Disease in Tristram Shandy, *Yearbook of English Studies*, volume 30, 2000, pp.46-59

Lawrence, C. Incommunicable Knowledge: Science, Technology and the Clinical Art in Britain 1850-1914, *Journal of Contemporary History*, volume 20, 1985, pp.503-520

Laybourn, K. The Guild of Help and the Changing Face of Edwardian Philanthropy, *Urban History*, 20, 1993, pp.43-60

Levene, A. Powell, M. & Stewart, J. Patterns of Municipal Health Expenditure in Inter-war England and Wales, *Bulletin of the History of Medicine*, 78, no.3, 2004, pp. 635-669

Lewis, J. Providers, 'Consumers', the State and Health-care Services in Britain, in *Medicine In Society*, ed. A. Wear, Cambridge University Press, 1992, pp.317-347

MacKinnon, M. Poor Law Policy, Unemployment and Pauperism, *Explorations in Economic History,* 23, 1986, pp.299-336

Marwick, A. The Labour Party and the Welfare State in Britain, 1900-1948*, American History Review*, volume 73, no.2, 1967, pp.380-403

Mazumdar, P. M. H. The Eugenists and the Residuum: the Problem of the Urban Poor, *Bulletin of the History of Medicine*, volume 54, 1980, pp.204-215

McCarthy, O. R. The Key to the Sanatoria, *Journal of the Royal Society of Medicine*, volume 94, August, 2001, pp.413-417

McFarlane, N. Hospitals, Housing and Tuberculosis in Glasgow, 1911-1951*, Social History of Medicine*, 2 (1), 1988, pp.59-85

McKeown, T. & Record, R. G. Reasons for the Decline of Mortality in England and Wales during the Nineteenth Century, *Population* Studies, 16, 1962, pp.94-122

Mendelsohn, J. A. Medicine and the making of Bodily Inequality in 20th Century Europe*,* in *Heredity and Infection*, eds. Jean-Paul Gaudillière, & Ilana Löwy, Routledge: London, 2003, pp.21-81

Mooney, G. Public Health versus Private Practice: The Contested Development of Compulsory Infectious Disease Notification in Late-Nineteenth Century Britain*, Bulletin of History of Medicine*, 73, 1999, pp.238-267

Moorman, L. J. Tuberculosis and Genius: Ralph Waldo Emerson, *Bulletin of the History of Medicine*, 18, 1945, pp.361-370

Morgan, K. O. Lloyd George and Germany*, The Historical Journal*, volume39, no.3, September, 1996, pp.755-766

Mortimer, P. P. Mr. N. The Milker, and Dr. Koch's Concept of the Healthy Carrier, *The Lancet,* 353, 1999, pp.1354-1356

Musto, D. F. Quarantine and the Problem of AIDS, in *AIDS – The Burdens of History*, eds., Elizabeth Fee & Daniel M. Fox, Berkeley, University of California Press, 1988, pp.67-86

Newsom, S.W.B. Stevens' Cure: A Secret Remedy, *Journal of the Royal Society of Medicine*, volume 95, 2002, p.463-467

Nye, R. A. Sociology: The Irony of Progress*, Degeneration*, eds. J. E Chamberlin & S. Gilman, Columbia University Press, New York, 1985, pp.49-71

Pelling, M. The Meaning of Contagion: Reproduction, Medicine & Metaphor, in *Contagion Historical & Cultural Studies*, eds. Alison Bashford & Claire Hooker, London: Routledge, 2001, pp.15-38

Pelling, M., Berridge, V., Harrison, M. & Weindling, P., Chapter Four, *Caring for Health: History and Diversity,* ed. Webster, C., Oxford University Press, 2001

Perkin, H. J. The 'Social Tone' of Victorian Seaside Resorts in the North-West, *Northern History* 11, 1976, 87-94

Pickstone, J. V. Establishment and Dissent in Nineteenth Century Medicine: An Exploration of Some Correspondence and Connections Between Medical and Religious Belief Systems in Early Industrial England, *Church and Healing,* ed. W. J. Shiels, Oxford, Blackwell, 1982

Porter, D. Enemies of the Race: Biologism, Environmentalism & Public Health, in Edwardian England in *Victorian Studies*, 34:2, 1991, pp.159-178

Porter, R. The Case of Consumption, *Understanding Catastrophe*, ed. Janine Bourrau, Cambridge University Press, 1992, pp.179-203

—. Consumption: Disease of the Consumer Society? *Consumption and the World of Goods,* eds. John Brewer & Roy Porter, London: Routledge, 1993, pp58-84

—. Diseases of Civilisation, *Companion Encyclopaedia of the History of Medicine,* volume 1, eds. W. F. Bynum & R. Porter, London: Routledge, 1993, pp.585-600

Richardson, T. Labour, *The Economy of Kent, 1640-1914,* ed. Alan Armstrong, Boydell Press, 1995, pp.235-2161

Riley, J. C. Ill Health During the Mortality Decline: The Friendly Societies' Experience, *Bulletin of the History of Medicine*, 1987, pp.563-588

Rose, N. Medicine, History and the Present, in *Reassessing Foucault: Power, Medicine and the Body,* eds. C. Jones & R. Porter, London: Routledge, 1994, pp.48-72

Soloway, R. Counting the Degenerates: The Statistics of Race Deterioration in Edwardian England, *Journal of Contemporary History*, volume 17, 1982, pp.137-164

Springett, V. H. Tuberculosis - Epidemiology in England and Wales, *BMJ*, 1, 12th February, 1972, pp.422-423

Sturdy, S. & Cooter, R. Science, Scientific Management, and the Transformation of Medicine in Britain c.1870-1950, *History of Science*, xxxvi, 1998, pp.1-47

Sturdy, S. Hippocrates and State Medicine: George Newman Outlines the Founding Policy of the Ministry of Health, in *Greater Than the Parts: Holism in Biomedicine 1920-1950*, eds. C. Lawrence & G. Weisz, Oxford University Press, 1998, pp.112-134

Sutherland, G. *Social Policy in the Inter-War Years, Historical Journal,* volume16, no.2, June, 1973, pp.425-426

Szreter, S. Healthy Government? Britain c.1850-1950, *Historical Journal,*

34, 2, 1991, pp.491-503

—. The Importance of Social Intervention in Mortality Decline, 1850-1914: A Reinterpretation of the Role of Public Health, *Social History of Medicine*, 1988, pp.1-37

Thomas, K. Health & Morality in Early Modern England, *Morality & Health,* eds. Allen M. Brandt & Paul Rozin, London, Routledge, 1997, pp.15-34

Tomes, N. The Private Side of Public Health: Sanitary Science, Domestic Hygiene and Germ Theory 1870-1900, *Bulletin of the History of Medicine*, volume 64, 1990, pp.509-539

Trostle, J. Early Work in Anthropology and Epidemiology: From Social Medicine to the Germ Theory, 1840-1920, *Anthropology & Epidemiology,* ed. Craig R. James, 1986, pp.25-57

van Helden, P. D. The Economic Divide and Tuberculosis, *EMBO Reports*, volume 4 (supplement), June, 2003, S24-28

Waddington, K. The Science of Cows: Tuberculosis, Research and the State in the U.K., 1890-1914, *History of Science*, xxxix, 2001, pp.29-48

Weindling, P. Health and Medicine in Inter-War Europe*, Medicine in the Twentieth Century,* eds. R. Cooter & J.V. Pickstone, London: Harwood Academic Publishers, 2000, pp.39-50

Williamson, P. The Conservative Party 1900-1939: From Crisis to Ascendancy *A Companion to Early Twentieth-century Britain,* ed. C. Wrigley, Oxford University Press, 2003, pp.3-22

Wilson, L. G. The Historical Decline of Tuberculosis in Europe and America: Its Causes and Significance, *Journal of the History of Medicine,* 45, 1990, pp.366-396

Winter, J. M. Public Health and the Political Economy of War, 1914-18, *History Workshop*, 26, 1988, pp.163-173

Woods, R. I., Watterson, P. A. & Woodward, J. H. The Causes of Rapid Infant Mortality Decline in England and Wales, 1861-1921, Part I, *Population Studies,* 42, 1988, pp.113-132; Part II, Population Studies, 43, 1988, pp.343-366

Worboys, M. Spreading Germs, *Medical Innovations in Historical Perspective*, ed. J.V. Pickstone, MacMillan, London, 1992

—. The Sanatorium Treatment for Consumption in Britain 1890-1914, in *Medical Innovations in Historical Perspective*, ed. J.V. Pickstone, MacMillan, London, 1992, pp.47-71

—. Was There a Bacteriological Revolution in Late Nineteenth Century Britain?, *Studies in History, Philosophy, Biology & Biomedicine and Science,* 38, 2007, pp.20-42

Yeo, S. Working Class Associations, Private Capital and the State in the late Nineteenth Century and Early Twentieth Centuries, in *Social Work, Welfare and the State,* eds. Noel Parry, Michael Rustin and Carole Satyamati, London: E. Arnold, 1979, pp.48-71

Internet

Armytage, W. H. G. The Stock Question, The Social Context of Eugenic Thought, *The Galton Institute Newsletter*, issue no. 15, December, 1994, http://www.galtoninstitute.org.uk/Newsletters/GINL9412/social_context.htm

Collins, C. *Cholera and Typhoid Fever in Kent,* Paper no.004 www.kentarchaeology.ac.

Friendly Societies Research Group, Newsletter, Issue 11, September, 2003 www.open.ac.uk/socialsciences/friendly-societies-research-group/newsletters.php

Gehrke, J. Georgist Thought and the Emergence of Municipal Socialism in Britain, 1870-1914, http://schalkenbach.org/on-line-library/scholars-forum/municipal-socialism-in-britain/

Moloney, C. T. *Inflaming Infirmity: Some Medical-Literary Interfaces of 19th Century Tuberculosis,* 2009 www.lmi.org.uk/medical_society/12/12Moloney.pdf

Mearns, Reverend A. *The Bitter Cry of Outcast London: An Inquiry into the Condition of the Abject Poor,* 1883 www.attackingthedevil.co.uk/related/outcast.php

Szreter, S. *A Central Role for Local Government? The Example of Late Victorian Britain*,16.10.08. www.historyandpolicy.org/papers/policy-paper-01

Tressell, R. *The Ragged Trousered Philanthropists,* 19.10.11. http://www.unionhistory.info/ragged/browse.php

Theses & Dissertations

Cheney, D. *The Hateful Ordeal at Seven Star Street – The Operation of the Contagious Diseases Acts in Dover 1870-1886,* MA dissertation, University of Kent, 1990

Cronje, G. *Pulmonary Tuberculosis in England and Wales 1851-1910*, University of London PhD thesis, 1989

Moloney, C. T. *George Eliot, Henry James and Consumption: A shadow on the lung of the Victorian Psyche*, unpublished PhD thesis, Birbeck College, University of London, 1999

Roberts, A. *Feeding and mortality in the early months of life; changes in medical opinion and popular feeding practice, 1850-1900*, unpublished Ph.D. thesis, University of Hull, 1973

Sharp, G. C. *The Aristocracy and the Development of Seaside Resorts: The Radnor Family and the History of Folkestone 1840-1914*, MA dissertation, University of Kent, 1989

Walton, J. K. *The English Seaside Resort, A Social History, 1750-1914,* D.Phil thesis, University of Kent, 1977

Watkins, D. *The English Revolution in Social Medicine 1899-1911*, PhD thesis, University of London, 1984

INDEX